HORSE HEALTH MANAGEMENT

HORSE HEALTH MANAGEMENT

Kang Yu
Joe Cooper
Alan Palmer

Kruger Brentt
Publishers

2023

Kruger Brentt Publishers UK. LTD.
Company Number 9728962

Regd. Office: 68 St Margarets Road, Edgware, Middlesex HA8 9UU

ISBN: 9781787150607

Disclaimer:

Every possible effort has been made to ensure that the information contained in this book is accurate at the time of going to press, and the publisher and author cannot accept responsibility for any errors or omissions, however caused. No responsibility for loss or damage occasioned to any person acting, or refraining from action, as a result of the material in this publication can be accepted by the editor, the publisher or the author. The Publisher is not associated with any product or vendor mentioned in the book. The contents of this work are intended to further general scientific research, understanding and discussion only. Readers should consult with a specialist where appropriate.

Every effort has been made to trace the owners of copyright material used in this book, if any. The author and the publisher will be grateful for any omission brought to their notice for acknowledgement in the future editions of the book.

For information on all our publications visit our website at http://krugerbrentt.com/

PREFACE

A horse is a swift and strong animal. It can easily run long distances. If you look at history, you will know the important part they played in it due to their loyalty. Moreover, they also helped and saved their masters. For instance, Chetak was a renowned horse. In addition, Arabian horses are popular worldwide. A horse is a vegetarian and domestic animal. It is very beneficial as well. A horse has four feet, two eyes, a nose, two ears and a tail. Their feet are quite slim but really strong. It allows them to run fast and for long.Moreover, one can find horses in different sizes, colours and shapes. All this depends on their breed and genes. In addition, the quality and quantity they eat daily also impact their health. Horses are in many colours. There are white, red, brown, black, grey horses and also sometimes they have a mixture of colours. Almost every country in the world has horses. The Arabian horse is popular for running very fast.Foals are young horses or baby horses. A mother horse gives birth to one foal at a time. About 5000 years ago, horses managed to domesticate humans. A horse lives up to 25 to 30 years. However, it does depend on their living condition.Horses like living in grassy areas or field where they can eat the grass, leaves and all other types of greenery available. Humans keep horses in a stable which is a building made of wood to keep horses.

The present book contains ten chapters covering all related disciplines. These chapters include *Introduction to horse health, Basic equine care and management, Hoof care, Horse health and vaccinations, Disorders such as colic, laminitis, and internal parasites, Infectious diseases in horses, Equine physical therapy and rehabilitation, Body condition scor-card of horses, Shelters, stalls and horse facilities, Caring for the geriatric horse.* This book shows style of horse keeping that will protect the health and well-being of your horses and also evaluates the latest diagnostic aids, including rapid developments in molecular biology, while emphasising that they are no substitute for clinical observation and skills.The book is also supported with a comprehensive glossary and index in the end. This text is designed for veterinary practitioners, scientists, students, technicians and nurses working with horses.

We are grateful to all those persons as well as various books, manuals, periodicals, magazines, journals etc. that helped in the preparation of this book. In spite of the best efforts, it is possible that some errors may have occurred into the compilation and editing of the book. Further queries, constructive suggestions and criticisms for the improvement of the book are always welcome and shall be thankfully acknowledged.

Kang Yu

Joe Cooper

Alan Palmer

CONTENTS

1

INTRODUCTION TO HORSE HEALTH

Horse, (*Equus caballus*), a hoofed herbivorous mammal of the family Equidae. It comprises a single species, *Equus caballus*, whose numerous varieties are called breeds. Before the advent of mechanized vehicles, the horse was widely used as a draft animal, and riding on horseback was one of the chief means of transportation.

GENERAL FEATURES

In prehistoric times the wild horse was probably first hunted for food. Research suggests that domestication had taken place by approximately 6,000 years ago. It is supposed that the horse was first used by a tribe of Indo-European origin that lived in the steppes north of the chain of mountains adjacent to the Black and Caspian seas. Influenced by climate, food, and humans, the horse rapidly acquired its present form.

The relationship of the horse to humans has been unique. The horse is a partner and friend. It has plowed fields and brought in the harvest, hauled goods and conveyed passengers, followed game and tracked cattle, and carried combatants into battle and adventurers to unknown lands. It has provided recreation in the form of jousts, tournaments, carousels, and the sport of riding. The influence of the horse is expressed in the English language in such terms as *chivalry* and *cavalier*, which connote honour, respect, good manners, and straightforwardness.

HORSE BODY

A horse's body resembles a table, and while sitting in the saddle - you are right in his most vulnerable spot. The longer the table, the more fragile the middle point. This is why training should focus on building the horse's back muscles that hold your body's weight while riding, bending into a concave arch. This is why it's so crucial for the horse's back legs to be as under the barrel as possible - this is how the "table" shortens and your body weight is less of a burden for the horse. If your horse's back muscles are strong, they will not be strained.

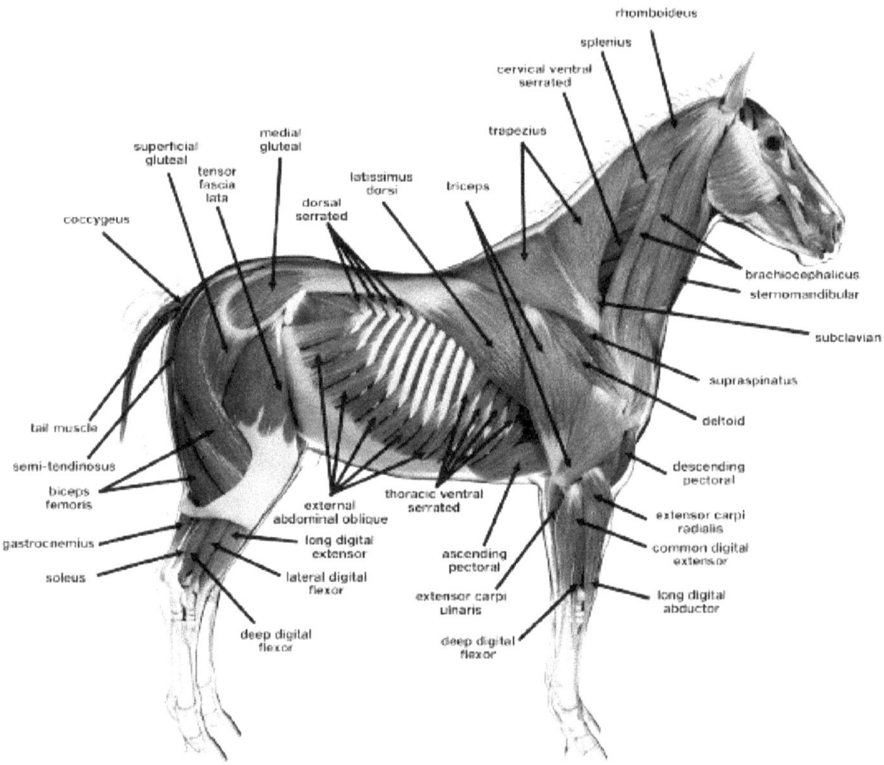

Fig. 1 Horse muscles anatomy

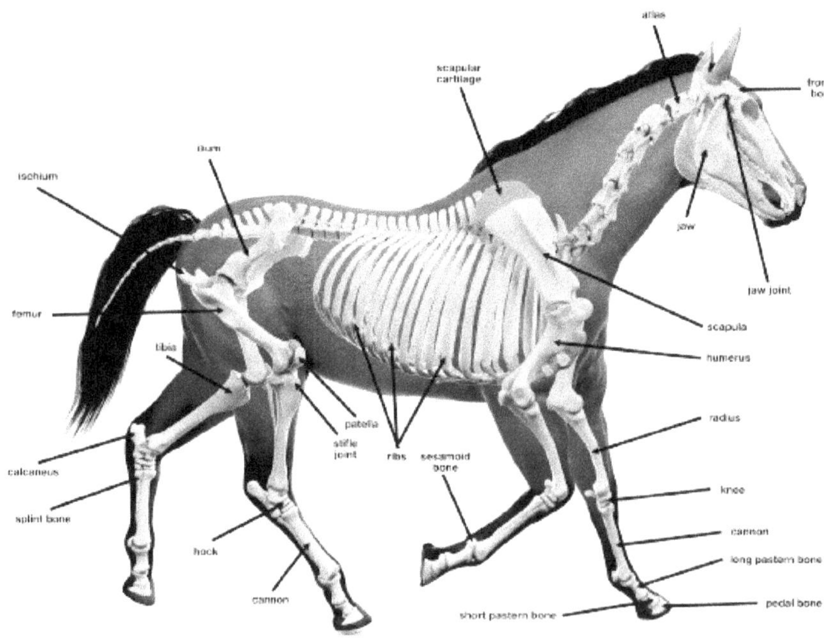

Fig. 2. Horse anatomy skeleton

Horse head

The horse's head is quite heavy – it can weigh approximately 16 kg if the horse is big. You should remember about this, especially when you allow the horse to "hang" on a bit and you "carry" his head's weight with your arms throughout the whole ride by holding the reins. After an hour of such exercise, you can really wear yourself out – which is why it is so important to train your horse to "carry" his own weight.

The horse's head – namely, its proportions in regards to the rest of the horse's body – differs depending on the animal's race and type. Cold-blooded horses have big heads, which allow them to additionally ballast the front of their bodies, which gives them exceptional pull strength. On the other side, saddle horses with small heads (in regards to the rest of their bodies), such as Arabs, are perfect for long or quick runs (rides, races). Relatively small heads lessen the burden on the front of their bodies. It is, however, good to keep in mind that a small head might mean that the horse has anatomical defects – overbreeding and a tiny skeleton.

Anatomy of horse head

The horse's head can be divided into two parts: top (neurocranium) and bottom (viscerocranium - the muzzle part).

The top part consists of:

- Occiput – is right behind the ears, exactly where the bridle comes (namely, the occiput strap of the bridle), it is a part that joins the horse's head with his neck.
- Crown – is between the ears and in front of them. It is a part, which lines are marked by the eye fovea, temples with the temporal fovea, forehead, eye sockets, and eyes.
- Forehead – is under the ears on the front of thc horse's head, usually covered with a forelock that grows out of the crown.

The bottom, muzzle, part consists of:

- Nose.
- Nostrils (along with the external part - nostril wings).
- Upper and lower lip (with chin).
- Cheeks with jaw below them (flat wide jawbones that stick out) and branches of the jaw (bottom edges of the jaw) and chin groove.
- Muzzle groove and edges.

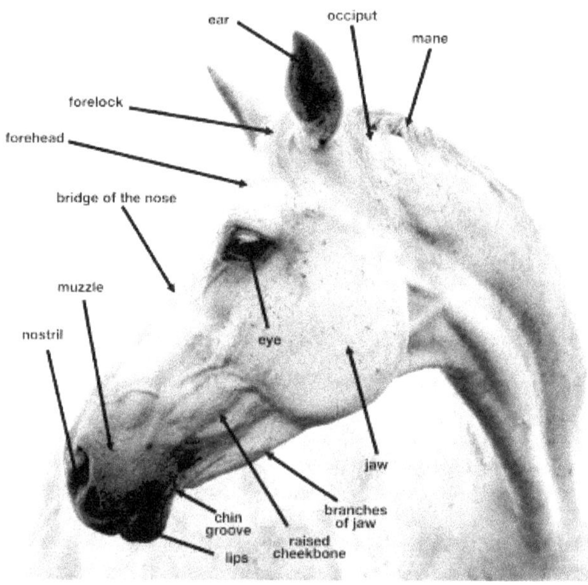

Fig. 3 Horse head diagram]

Types of horse head builds

The type of horse's head always depends on his race. We differentiate 4 basic types:

Noble head, straight profile:

It is the most perfectly balanced shape of the head, where the forehead-nose line remains straight. It is characteristic for breed and racing horses with a long top part of the head and short bottom part, with a broad forehead.

Dished (concave) face:

Characteristic for Arab and half-Arabs with a broad forehead, big eyes, and nostrils, but most of all – concave line of the nose, and small falcate ears.

Roman nose:

Characteristic for cold-blooded, and racehorses such as Lipizzaners, and Kladrubers; the head has a convex line of the nose, short top part (neurocranium) and elongated bottom part (viscerocranium), narrow forehead, small eyes, and nostrils in regards to the head's size, and long ears.

Types of horse ears

Horse ears differ depending on the type of the steed:

- cold-blooded horses have fleshy ears with "blunt" tips, namely, rounded ones, often covered with hairy fur, placed diagonally towards the horse's head,
- warm-blooded horses have lighter, thinner ears, placed vertically, with pointy tips.

The description above is for normal ears. Among anomalies, we can distinguish:

- hare ears - long and narrow,
- donkey ears - thick, long, and rather broad,
- lop ears - flopping to the sides,
- pig ears - flopping to the front,
- mouse ears - short and small with rounded tips.

The anomalies listed above – incorrect shapes of the horse's ears are only the so-called beauty faults, which do not translate into any health issues or physical abilities.

However, you should pay attention to the ears' "mobility" – if the horse moves his ears too much, it might speak for his temper (hyperactivity, nervousness), a complete lack of thereof might mean that the horse is deaf.

Horse eyes

While speaking of the horse's head, it would be a misunderstanding to omit the eyes - namely, their placing that allows the horse to see a particular perspective.

Horse teeth and his age

The saying goes "never look a gifted horse in the teeth." Why shouldn't we, though? You can learn the horse's age by his teeth.

While assessing the horse's age, you should mostly pay attention to his incisors, especially the sockets into the cutting surface of the teeth – the deeper they go, the older the horse. Additionally, while looking at the horse's jaw's intersection, you can see that his teeth go to the front as he grows older and start "leaning."

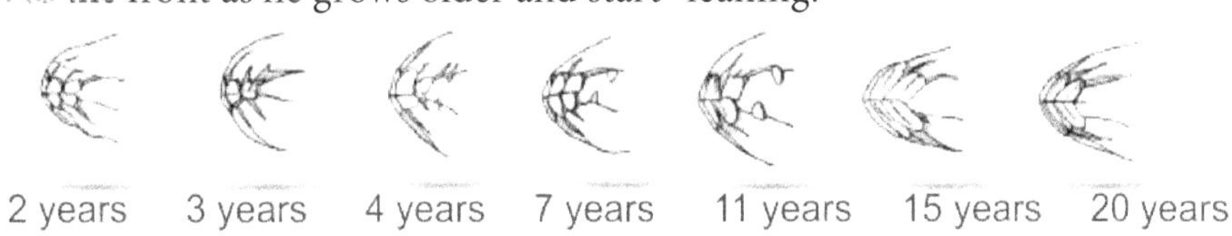

Fig. 4 Horse's teeth and his age

Horse neck

The horse's neck is his lever. Its muscles, length, and proportions in regards to the rest of the horse's body parts say volumes about his condition and sports predispositions but also about the quality of your training. For example, a neck that's too short may be a hindrance in jumping, where the proper basculing is crucial. Basculing is maintaining the proper position of the horse while jumping – stretching the horse's body over an obstacle with neck low and back bent in an arch, which allows for jumping over really high obstacles while keeping balance. At the same time, a neck that is too long might make it impossible for the horse to keep balance while performing difficult dressage figures.

Relaxing the horse that affects the health of his back starts from the neck. The neck is always crucial for maintaining balance – both while performing complicated dressage figures and while jumping. During training, you should go interchangeably for its stretching (relaxing), then gradual shortening (proper training), and final extension (stretching at the end of a ride).

Anatomy of horse neck

The horse's neck consists of the following parts:

- Left and right side,
- back of the neck/forelock,
- throat.

A horse that has been well trained should have well-developed muscles along the neck. A horse that is incorrectly ridden has usually very strong throat muscles because he has to keep his head and neck high, which results in a lack of relaxation.

Types of horse necks

We differentiate three types of horse's neck:

- Ideal (straight) neck – correct and most desired because it means that the horse has a straight trachea, which allows him to take in more air in a shorter period of time, which is crucial during intense effort.
- Swan neck – both the upper and bottom edge of the neck create an arch, which is often observed in Arab horses.
- Close-coupled neck – the bottom part of the neck remains convex but the upper part is concave, which causes the horse to carry his head high and, as a result, trip often. The convex bottom part blocks the airflow through the trachea, which makes it difficult for the horse to breathe – this is why this type of horse neck is considered the least desired and most flawed one.

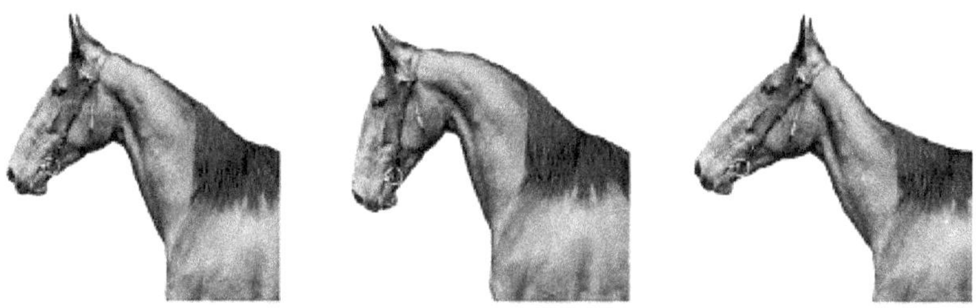

Ideal neck Swan neck Close-coupled neck

Fig. 5 Types and settings of horse neck

Fortunately, swan and close-coupled necks happen rather rarely - most horses have straight profiles of the neck. However, they differ in setting:

- Highly set neck – it is not an imperfection in dressage or combined driving.
- Properly set neck.
- Low set neck – it is not seen as a flaw in Welsh ponies and horses used for long and difficult routes, as well as carriage horses, as it helps them overcome the resistance while pulling.

Horse barrel, or the trunk

The horse's torso along with the back is the part of the horse's body that protects all his most important organs.

Horse withers - the highest point

The point where the neck ends and the torso begins is called the withers. The withers is a place of origin for crucial muscles, so it is very important for the horse to have it properly shaped – it should be visible, properly high, and broad, stretching to the back. An indefinite, flat, or too pointy withers might be caused by faulty training, malnutrition, adiposis, or simply flawed anatomy.

Withers that's sticking out too much will be susceptible to abrasions by the saddle and other injuries. Withers too flat will cause the saddle to shift to the sides.

The withers is a spot that defines the horse's height – we always measure the horse from the ground to the top of the withers.

How should the proper horse chest look

The chest must be broad, long, and deep enough to store all crucial organs: heart and lungs. Horses with broad chests will be heavier and slower. Those with narrow chests might not be fit for riding as it is more difficult for them to move with the rider on their backs, having less space for heart and lungs (smaller organs and worse exertional abilities).

Types of horse chests:

- Correct – averagely broad breast, nicely arched ribs.
- Narrow – too narrow breast, too little space for organs – heart, lungs.
- Broad – broader breast, inclinations for swaying gaits.

Horse flank – a sensitive point

A filled, not much concave flank (the space between the horse's trunk and croup on both sides) says a lot about his nutrition and condition. The flank is a very sensitive point of the horse's body, below it you can find his kidneys. You should omit this place while bathing your horse (especially on cold days) with cold water and treat it much more delicately while cleaning.

Horse spine – or horse back

The horse's back is a kind of "linking" between the rear and the front of the horse. It should be properly shaped and muscled to shift the rider's weight to his back and front limbs.

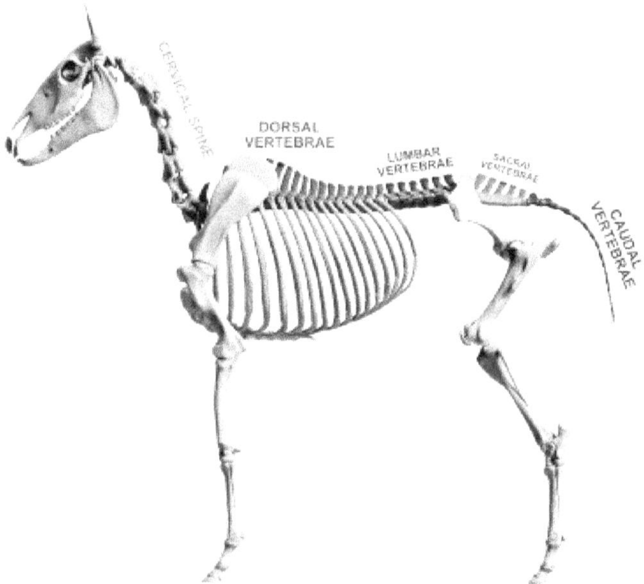

Fig. 6 Horse's spine divided into sections

Types of horse back

- Correct back.
- Roached-back (convex) – a short and arched upwards back, strong but also stiff and hard – the horse would tend to walk uncomfortably, roughly.

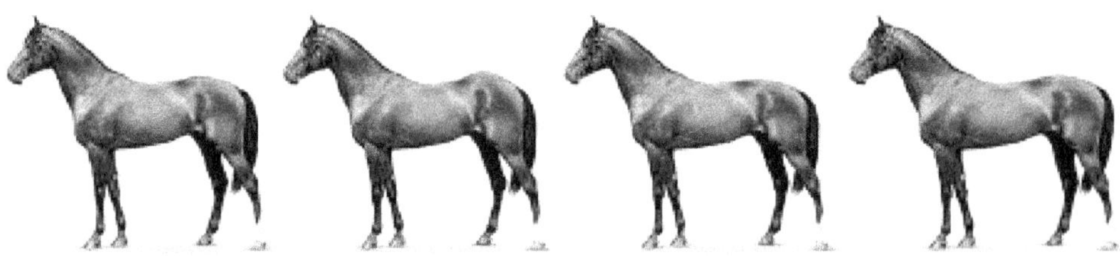

Correct back Swayback Roached-back Long backed

Fig. 7 Types of horse backs

- Swayback (concave) – is caused by insufficient cohesiveness of the vertebrae, which makes the spine weak – you can often observe that type of back in cold-blooded horses, and old steeds, and mares that have given birth to several foals – it then might be an acquired characteristic, not an innate one.
- Long backed – improperly muscled.

Front and back limbs

Horse's limbs – tendons, joints, and hooves are most prone to injuries and ailments, which is why we will try to say the most about them. What is important, is that a lot of anomalies stem from the owner's negligence or wrong use (e.g. too much load when the horse is too young – bone splits, wrong diet – unfit for the horse's needs, too much protein leads to laminitis, etc).

You should really pay attention to the state of the horse's limbs – their condition often says whether it's possible to use the horse. The build of the horse's legs depends on the race – their muscles, proportions, length, flexibility, strength.

Hot-blooded horses have dry, compact limbs, while cold-blooded horses have rather thick but weak limbs. The joints should have clear edges – if they are oval, it can suggest issues with the horse's lymph.

A slightly bad posture of the limbs is pretty common. If they impact the horse's riding value, you can often say only while actually riding on his back. The case is very different when it comes to serious faults, which can lead to premature exhaustion of the joints and tendons of the limbs.

Front limbs – function and build

Their basic function is to keep up the horse's body and buffer shocks during movement. They are closer to the horse's center of gravity than the back legs – which is why they are more ballasted (e.g. during landing from a jump). This is why they more often get injured.

Types of build of the front limbs - as seen from the front:

- Correct.

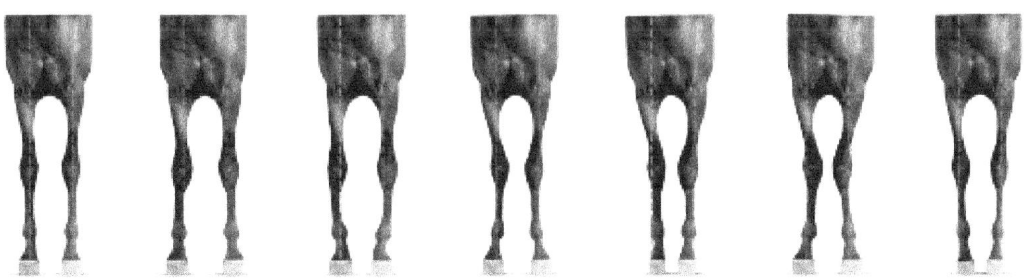

Correct Base wide Bowlegged Toes-out Base narrow Knock- kneed Pigeon-toe

Fig. 8 Front horse legs anatomy

- **Base narrow** – when the limbs are not parallel but come closer together at the bottom, this often causes strickling in horses (stepping on the back legs with the front ones).
- **Base wide** – the limbs from knees down go to the outside, which causes stiffness of gaits.
- **Pigeon-toed** – the fetlock-hoof axes go inwards, which causes the horse to make outward arches while walking.

- **Toes-out** - the fetlock-hoof axes go outwards and the limb goes on an inward arch, which causes strickling.
- **Bowlegged** – the front limbs resemble the walls of a barrel in shape. This puts too much load on the inner side of the horse's limbs and outside tendons.
- **Knock-kneed** – the axes of the limbs are broken in the knee joint to the inside, which makes the horse's legs look like a big X. This does not guarantee good support and balance, causing the horse to walk in inwards arches and strickle.

Back limbs posture - as seen from the side:

- Correct.
- Camped-under – shifted too far under the belly.
- Camped-out – shifted too much in front of the chest, it causes exhaustion of tendons and joints, this type of posture should not be mistaken with laminitis!
- Knee sprung – the leg's axis is broken to the front in the knee joint. This type of birth defect does not have to be an issue if it doesn't cause stumbling and problems with balance or affects the swiftness of gaits.
- Calf-kneed – with carpus shifted to the back.

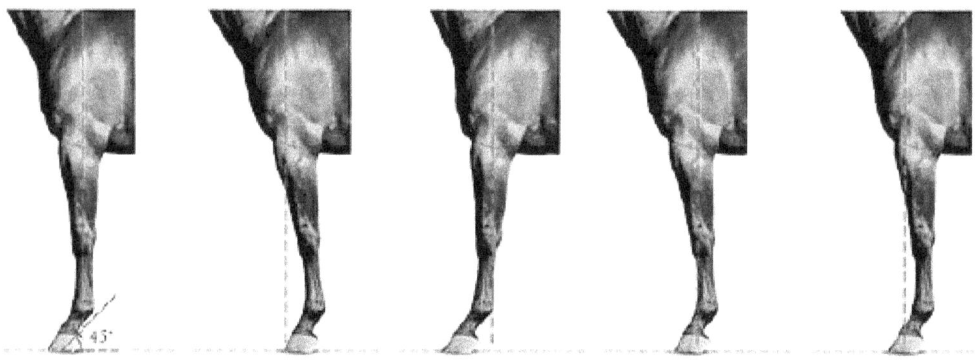

Correct Camped-under Camped-out Knee sprung Calf-kneed

Fig. 9 Horse's front limbs posture

The horse's shoulder blades are the top part of the front limbs, which decide the horse's physical capabilities. They should be long enough, diagonally positioned, which provides the horse freedom of movement.

Long, wide, and diagonal shoulder blades allow a sport horse to reach higher speed. In a carriage horse, you would want a more steep shoulder blade – which increases the horse's strength.

Back limbs – function and build

In the back limbs, there are the gaskin and hock. The other parts are pretty much the same as in the front limbs. The function of the back legs is to carry the horse's croup, power the gaits, increase dynamics and strength while jumping, they also help break the resistance of a pulled weight on a race track.

The hock should be thoroughly looked at while buying a horse as if it is burdened with faults, they can disqualify the horse from being used when they get worse.

Among the most common issues with the hock, you can find:

- **Spavin** – or bone spavin, the most serious and incurable fault – it is a bone growth, which often deforms the joint and causes knitting of small bones, which makes the horse unable to move. Spavin is induced by injuries caused by excessive effort. At first, it manifests itself through inflammation and lameness, which continues after the inflammation is cured – during more intense movement.
- **Bursitis** – an egg-shaped swelling of the top part of the bulb of the heel. Acquired bursitis – a skin protrusion. True bursitis – an inflammation of the heel bursa that does not cause lameness, being a so-called beauty defect.
- Popped splint – a bone growth caused by growth of the capitulum of a splint bone. In most cases, it does not cause lameness but when it's placed on a short and narrow joint, it might spread to neighboring tendons, irritating or even damaging them.
- **Bog spavin** – a convex protrusion that may be caused by overgrowth of the fascia that is responsible for keeping tendons around the hock, inflammation of said tendons, or position of the heel bone. Bog spavin might be birth or acquired defect. It does not have to cause lameness.
- **Windgalls** – they can happen both around the fetlock and the hock joints – it is a soft swelling, often as big as a (hen) egg. It is caused by a growing joint pouch full of synovia and exudative fluid – it might be the effect of inflammation after excessive training effort or wrong diet (too much protein). Articular windgalls – while pressing against a joint, the windgalls move onto its other side – this is the worst kind of windgalls.
- The hock may also be too short and too narrow, which will cause it to get damaged more quickly and more often.

Types of horses' back legs - as seen from the back:

- Correct.
- **Narrow** – limbs are placed too close to each other.
- **Knock-kneed** – analogous to the front legs posture.
- **Stands close** – analogous to base narrow in the front legs.
- **Stands wide** – analogous to bow-legged in the front limbs but the legs go to the outside, it's pretty rare (when happens, it is with starved horses, raised in a very harsh environment).

- **Bow-legged** – back legs resemble a barrel's walls in shape. The hocks are far away from each other, the legs go inwards, during movement, the horse makes arches with his legs and turns his hooves while taking steps, which becomes a serious functional defect.
- **Cow-hocked** – when the limbs' axes are broken in hocks to the inside (as in cows), with an advanced fault of posture, this causes excessive overload of the back limbs (tendons and ligaments).

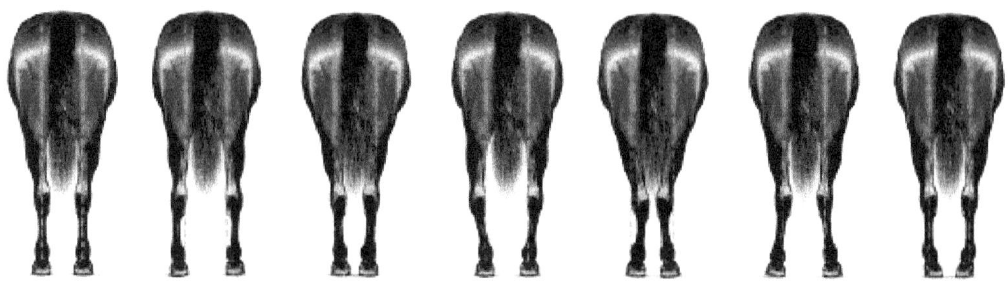

Correct Stands wide Narrow Bow-legged Cow-hocked Knock-kneed Stands close

Fig. 10 Types of build of horse's back legs

Posture of back legs - as seen from the side:

- Correct.
- **Camped under** – causes excessive use of tendons and ligaments, straining of periosteum, shortening of the gait, and furthers stepping or hitting of the back legs against the heels of the front ones.
- **Camped out** – with the limb far to the back, which shifts the body weight strongly onto the back (spine), which can, in turn, become roached-back. It causes slower, less effective gaits.
- **Sickle hocked** – when the cannon bone's bottom end is shifted to the front, which causes the hock to be placed at too wide of an angle. This can cause an overload of the joint (tendons and ligaments).
- **Leg too straight** – when the whole back leg is almost perfectly straight, which decreases the amortization in gallop and while jumping over obstacles.
- With weak hock (short and narrow one).
- Tied cannon bone.
- With bursitis.
- With bog spavin.

Horse pastern – faults, anomalies, ailments

Another important part of a horse's leg is the cannon bone. Its faults cause weakening of the limb.

Forms of faults in the pastern of a horse:

- Pastern is too straight.
- Calf-kneed (short, straight pastern).
- Buck-kneed.
- Pastern with thin hock.
- Coon-footed – when the outer edges of the pastern are not parallel and they come closer together at the top of the carpus.
- Pastern too long – disproportionate to the length of the cannon bone.
- Tied-in – too narrow and thin.

Defects of the pastern may cause various types of anomalies and ailments:

- The pastern might have a bony growth at 1/3 of the bone's length on the inner side. This is caused by inflammation resulting from excessive physical effort or mechanical injury.
- You may observe oblong convex protrusions that are a result of periosteum inflammation. This usually occurs in young horses that were used too harshly (in racing). While these changes form, they are painful and cause lameness.
- Windgalls – mentioned above.
- Tendon strain.

Faults of the fetlock in horses

- Normal, correct fetlock.
- Badly angled, too long fetlock.
- Steep fetlock – causes the horse's gaits to be unpleasant, harsh.
- Coon-footed – causes the joints and tendons to wear out quickly.
- Fetlock with ringbone.

Horse hooves - types and build

You could say that there's no horse without hooves and you would be 100% right. Thus, you should also pay attention to uneven detrition of the hooves' walls and any damages. Also, to oversensitivity while cleaning the hooves – apart from the characteristic smell, sensitivity is the first symptom of a rotting hoof.

Among the most common hooves' issues, we can find:

- Hoof too small or too big.
- Narrow hoof – causing vanishing of the frog.

- Flat hoof – which often leads to mechanical damage of the hoof when moving on hard or rocky ground.
- Diagonal hoof – one of the walls is either perpendicular or concave as a result of a faulty posture.
- Valgus hoof – caused by birth or acquired shortening of the flexor tendons – the back wall of the hoof does not touch the ground, the horse leans mostly on the front part of the hoof.
- Hoof with sharp edges – occurs in camped-under and camped-out posture of the front or back legs as a result of wrong cleaning and shoeing.
- Hoof with blunt edges – occurs in camped-under posture of the front legs or camped-out posture of the back ones.
- Steep – the front wall of the hoof is very steep, while the side walls are almost vertical. This is either a birth defect or a result of ailments and contracture of the tendons.
- Crooked – one of the hoof's walls is convex while the other one is concave – caused by an uneven distribution of the horse's weight, which is usually a result of a faulty posture of the limbs.
- Post-laminitis – with deformed hoof walls with transverse rings, caused by acute inflammation of the hoof material.

Croup and tail

The croup is evaluated based on its length, width, muscles, and angulation. Lack of proper proportions of the croup e.g. a croup that is too short might not allow you to use him with a saddle.

We differentiate three types of croups as seen from the side:

- Normal croup – the pelvis' slope is at 15-25 degrees to the ground.
- Flat croup (horizontal, straight) – the pelvis' slope is at less than 15 degrees, usually in noble horses, especially Arabs, which allows for an elongated, quicker gait. However, a horse with such a gait loses the strength of movements, which is not great for jumping, carrying weight, or quick starts (racing), but is perfect for combined driving, and dressage.
- Sloping croup (truncated) – at 30-40 degrees slope, which gives the horse more strength, making this type of croup good for carriage. A slightly sloping croup would also be good for jumping (great strength of takeoff), however, such a croup would not allow the horse to reach high speed.

And three types of croups as seen from the back:

- Normal croup – well-muscled and wide enough, of rounded oval shape.
- Lines of the quarter as seen from the back shape sort of a "roof," which top is at the end of the spine – sacrum. With proper muscles, this type of a croup can be only a beauty defect.
- Typical for cold-blooded horses croup that has top of the hips almost at the same level as sacrum. You can clearly see an indentation into the sacrum.

While speaking of the horse's croup, we should also mention the horse's tail, which:

- Protects the horse from insects.
- Helps him keep balance and steer while moving.

The horse's tail can be positioned normally, high (often in Arab horses) or low (in cold-blooded horses). The hairs of the mane and tail differ depending on the type of the horse – cold-blooded ones have thick, coarse hair, while hot-blooded horses have the opposite hair – silky and thin.

Horse skin and its products

The horse's skin is covered with hairs, which color depends on the horse's skin color. Gray horses have pink skin, while other colored horses have either dark gray or black skin.

The most important product of the horse's skin is the hoof with the bulb of the heels in the back part.

Other products contain:

- **Chestnuts** – elliptic in shape, placed on the inner side of the legs – above knees on the front legs, and above hocks on the back legs. They often grow, sticking out of the horse's silhouette more and more, to fall out with time, leaving a flat, callused skin lesion.
- **Ergots** – tumor masses that appear on the backside of fetlock joints, which are surrounded by long hairs.

Both chestnuts and ergots are believed to be atavistic – a remaining part of the primogenitor, from the no longer existing horse's toes that evolved into hooves.

ORIGIN OF HORSE DOMESTICATION

Archaeological evidence indicates that the domestication of horses had taken place by approximately 6,000 years ago in the steppelands north of the Black Sea from Ukraine to Kazakhstan. Despite intensive study over a long period of time, many questions remain about the early development of the species as it underwent domestication. One crucial question involves whether domestication was limited to a single location or occurred in multiple areas. Tied to this question of origins is whether domesticated horses spread throughout Eurasia or whether the practice of horse domestication spread to new areas, with local breeders capturing their own wild horses and introducing them to the domestic horse gene pool. Modern genetic techniques have been used to answer these questions, but different regions of the horse genome (that is, the complete nucleic acid sequence of a horse's genetic code) have yielded different answers.

Results of studies of mitochondrial DNA (mtDNA), which is inherited only from the mother, showed a great deal of diversity among individuals and strongly supported the idea that wild horses from many different geographic areas contributed to the domestic horse. The mtDNA data clearly indicated that there were multiple sites of domestication, with a large number of mares in the first populations, and that genetic input from local wild horses had been introduced into the domestic gene pool as domesticated horses spread. The mtDNA data also showed that the modern horse is a mixture of ancient lineages, all of which can be traced back to an "Ancestral Mare," which lived 130,000 to 160,000 years ago; thus, there is no clear mtDNA signature for modern horse breeds.

In contrast, studies have revealed that the domestic horse is dominated by a single, paternally inherited Y chromosome lineage, in which there is almost no variation. An exception was a study of horses in southwestern China that found that some southern Chinese populations of male horses possessed a Y chromosome variant that was not present in any other breeds that had been tested. This variant may represent a different paternal lineage that survived in the region, or it may represent a recent mutation. The lack of variation on the Y chromosome would seem to indicate a very narrow origin for the domestic horse.

However, the differences in variation between maternal and paternal lineages may reflect the differences in how breeders treated mares and stallions. It is possible that throughout history far more mares contributed to the founding of the domestic horse than stallions, because stallions can be difficult to handle. In addition, most selection is directed toward the males, because at the level of the individual they can produce such a large number of offspring compared with females. (In other words, it is likely that a small number of relatively cooperative stallions may have been used to impregnate large numbers of mares.)

Studies examining other regions of DNA have revealed a high genetic diversity in horses, which is consistent with mtDNA results; however, pinpointing where domestication events have taken place remains elusive. For example, research at the turn of the 21st century indicated that there appeared to have been an independent domestication event in the Iberian Peninsula (the region containing Spain and Portugal), which served as a refuge for many species, including horses, during the Pleistocene and Holocene glaciations.

Some two decades later, genetic studies cast doubt on whether such an event took place in Iberia, since those horse lineages became extinct before leaving significant genetic traces in the genomes of modern horses. In addition, genetic studies of other proposed centres of horse domestication, such as Anatolia and the Caucasus (which have long histories of horse utilization), have not turned up proof of single independent domestication events.

Most evidence indicates that humans spread domestic horses from western Eurasia and that domestic populations were supplemented with wild individuals which increased the genetic diversity of domestic horses. Based on modern genetic analyses, the answers to the questions surrounding horse domestication are that the horse has a diverse ancestry, that there was more than one domestication event, and that domestic horses have been widely interbred throughout the history of their domestication.

FORM AND FUNCTION

A mature male horse is called a stallion, the female a mare. A stallion used for breeding is known as a stud. A castrated stallion is commonly called a gelding. Formerly, stallions were employed as riding horses, while mares were kept for breeding purposes only. Geldings were used for work and as ladies' riding horses. Recently, however, geldings generally have replaced stallions as riding horses. Young horses are known as foals; male foals are called colts and females fillies.

SENSES

The extremely large eyes placed far back on the elongated head admirably suit the horse for its chief mode of defense: flight. Its long neck and high-set eyes, which register a much wider range than do the eyes of a human being, enable the horse to discern a possible threat even while eating low grasses. Like human vision, the horse's vision is binocular, but only in the narrow area directly forward. Evidence suggests that a horse's vision is limited in its ability to register colour; horses can detect yellow and blue but not red and green. While visual acuity is high, the eyes do not have variable focus, and objects at different distances register only on different areas of the retina, which requires tilting movements of the head. The senses of smell and hearing seem to be keener than in human beings.

COLOUR AND PATTERN

From the dun of the primitive horse has sprung a variety of colours and patterns, some highly variable and difficult to distinguish. Among the most important colours are black, bay, chestnut (and sorrel), palomino, cream, and white.

The black colour is a true black, although a white face marking (blaze) and white ankles (stockings) may occur. The brown horse is almost black but has lighter areas around the muzzle, eyes, and legs. Bay refers to several shades of brown, from red-brown and tan to sandy. Bay horses have a black mane, tail, and (usually) stockings. There is a dilution (or lightening) gene—called silver or silver dapple—that mainly influences the dark colours of the coat. Chestnut is similar to bay but with none of the bay's black overtones. Lighter shades of chestnut are called sorrel. The palomino horse runs from cream to bronze, with a flaxen or silvery mane and tail. The cream is a diluted sorrel, or very pale yellow, nearly white. White in horses is variable, ranging from aging grays to albinos with blue eyes and pink skin and to pseudoalbinos with a buff mane or with brown eyes.

The chief patterns of the white horse are gray, roan, pinto, sabino, and appaloosa. Gray horses are born dark brown or black and develop white hairs as they age, becoming almost all white in advanced years. Roan refers to white mixed with other colours at birth: blue roan is white mixed with black; red roan is mixed white and bay; and strawberry roan is white and chestnut. The pinto is almost any spotted pattern of white and another colour; other names, such as paint, calico, piebald, skewbald, overo, and tobiano, refer to subtle distinctions in type of colour or pattern. Appaloosa (leopard complex) is another extremely variable pattern, but the term generally refers to a large white patch over the hips and loin, with scattered irregular dark spots. Studies of five coat-colour genes in DNA samples from ancient, predomesticated horses have shown that these horses predominantly carried the genes for black or bay. Scientists believe that it is very likely that these horses also carried the dun dilution gene. The leopard (Appaloosa) mutation was also discovered, which was found to be consistent with some cave paintings dating to 25,000 years ago that depict spotted horses. Mutations for chestnut, tobiano, and sabino were also observed and were dated to 3,000 years ago, whereas the buckskin variant had emerged by about 1,000 years ago. Most of the variation in coat colour appeared after domestication occurred and was likely the result of artificial selection by humans.

REPRODUCTION AND DEVELOPMENT

The onset of adult sex characteristics generally begins at the age of 16 to 18 months. The horse is considered mature, depending on the breed, at approximately three years and adult at five. Fecundity varies according to the breed and may last beyond age 20 with Thoroughbreds and to 12 or 15 with other horses. The gestation period is 11 months; 280 days is the minimum in which the foal can be born with expectation to live. As a rule, a mare produces one foal per mating, twins occasionally, and triplets rarely. The foal is weaned at six months.

The useful life of a horse varies according to the amount of work it is required to do and the maintenance furnished by its owner. A horse that is trained carefully and slowly and is given the necessary time for development may be expected to serve to an older age than a horse that is rushed in its training. Racehorses that enter into races at the age of two rarely remain on the turf beyond eight. Well-kept riding horses, on the contrary, may be used more than 20 years.

The life span of a horse is calculated at six to seven times the time necessary for its physical and mental development—that is, 30 to 35 years at the utmost, the rule being about 20 to 25 years.

Ponies generally live longer than larger horses. There are a number of examples of horses that have passed the usual limit of age. The veterinary university of Vienna conserves the skeleton of a Thoroughbred mare of 44 years of age. There have been reports made of horses living to their early 60s in age.

To keep your horse healthy, it is important to vaccinate it against certain diseases, deworm it regularly, and properly care for the teeth and feet. Horses are also susceptible to conditions such as colic and laminitis, which can greatly diminish the horse's usefulness, or even end in death. The purpose of this paper is to give you an overview of health issues facing horse owners. The best advice is to establish a regular health care program with a local veterinarian who has interest and expertise with horses. Let the veterinarian help you make health care decisions. It is also important to find a farrier who you are comfortable working with and who can help you make decisions regarding the care and maintenance of your horse's hooves.

FEEDING YOUR HORSE

Horses must have access to an adequate amount of good quality feed in the form of roughage (pasture, hay or chaff) to keep them in good body condition. A guide to the amount to feed is generally 1–2 kg per 100kg of body weight each day or:

- Pony (measuring up to 13.5 hands, 200–350kg)
- feed 3–7kg each day
- Galloway (measuring 13.5–15 hands, 350–500kg)
- feed 7–10kg each day
- Horse (measuring 15–16.5 hands, 500–650kg)
- feed 10–13kg each day
- Heavy Horse (measuring 16.5+ hands, 650+kg)
- feed 13+ kg each day

You may need to supplementary feed if:

- a horse is being worked regularly
- there is not enough pasture
- the horse is losing body condition.

Provide a salt lick or mineral block in paddock. Check with your veterinarian about suitable supplementary feeds – grass clippings and many food scraps are not suitable feed as they can cause a horse to become ill.

Water for horse

Clean water must always be available for horse. A dam or self-filling trough is best and should be checked frequently. Bath tubs can be used but must be checked daily and re-filled if needed.

Buckets are not suitable as a permanent water supply (they can be tipped over).

If your water supply is not self-filling it must be checked daily.

As a guide, a horse may drink 25-45 litres per day in hot weather.

Shelter for horse

Horses need shelter from sun, wind and rain. Suitable horse shelters include:

- trees
- a walk-in shed
- a stable.

A waterproof rug can protect the horse from cold weather but check it daily to ensure it is not rubbing, slipping or leaking.

EXERCISE AND SPACE FOR HORSE

Horses must have enough space to walk and run around, unless they are exercised daily. Stabled horses must have enough space to walk forward, turn around, lie down and roll. Sick horses may need to be confined under the directions of a veterinarian.

Horses must not be tethered long-term. It is only acceptable for short periods of time. Where tethered the following requirements must be met:

- access to water at all times
- exercise off tether daily
- ability to lie down and stand without restriction
- tether must be attached by a swivel to a collar or halter
- twice daily inspection
- access to shelter at all times, for horses this may be shelter from a tree as well as a physical shelter
- be able to graze freely

Paddocks for your horse

To prevent injury and escape of horses:

- keep fences in good repair
- prevent threats such as loose wires
- be aware of attractions such as a neighbouring horse
- remove rubbish and weeds regularly

HORSE GENERAL HEALTH CARE AND MAINTENANCE

Feet care

Horse's hooves need to be trimmed every 6-8 weeks by a farrier. This prevents them chipping or becoming too long and uncomfortable for your horse. Shoes are needed if the horse is to be ridden on hard or rocky ground.

Teeth care

Horse's teeth need to be checked by a trained and competent equine dentist at least once a year for a horse kept in a paddock. Unchecked teeth can become sharp, causing pain and mouth injuries.

Horses under the age of 5, as well as grain fed horses, need a dental check at least once every 3 to 6 months.

Worming your horse

Worm your horse regularly to prevent build up of worms in the stomach and intestines. Many worming pastes require use every 6-8 weeks. Follow the directions on the product as dosage frequency and amounts vary.

Reducing the build-up of manure in your horse's paddock is a simple way to reduce worm contamination of pastures.

HORSE VACCINATIONS

Your veterinarian will advise what your horse should be vaccinated for and how often. They may recommend vaccination for diseases such as tetanus, viral respiratory disease and strangles.

Monitor your horse's body condition

Do not let your horse get too fat or too thin:

- a horse is too thin if its ribs are showing (you should be able to feel, but not see, a horse's ribs)
- a horse is too fat if it has a round rump, big belly and crested neck

A horse's body condition must not be allowed to become less than body condition score 2.

Laminitis

Some horses may develop laminitis, a very painful hoof condition. In some cases severe damage may develop that is untreatable and require the horse to be "put down".

Common causes of laminitis are obesity or too much green pasture or grain and ponies are particularly susceptible.

Always consult a vet if your horse appears lame, uncomfortable or stands in water for long periods. Further information about Laminitis.

Colic in horses

Colic refers to a range of digestive tract (gut) problems. Colic can be very painful and can have very serious consequences, including death.

If you suspect your horse has colic seek urgent veterinary attention. Symptoms in your horse include:

- lying down or rolling frequently
- teeth grinding
- restlessness
- repeatedly kicking
- looking at their flanks or sides.

Notifiable diseases in horses

Horses can suffer from a variety of diseases, some of which are notifiable in Victoria.

Company of other horses

Horses are herd animals and need the company of other horses. This can be in the same paddock or a neighbouring paddock. Keeping a horse on its own may lead to behaviour problems in the paddock or when out riding.

SUPERVISION AND MONITORING OF YOUR HORSE

Check your horse at least daily, ensuring it is not injured or ill and has adequate feed and water.

Consult a vet if the horse is injured or ill. Horses that are handled frequently are usually easier to manage for farrier, vet or dentist visits.

Stallions

Stallions are difficult to manage and are not suitable as companions. All colts and stallions should be desexed (gelded), by a veterinary practitioner, unless they are to be used for breeding. Geldings and mares are much more controllable companions than stallions.

Disposal of your horse

If you can no longer care for the horse, you must arrange for it to be cared for by someone else, sell it or have it euthanised. It is much kinder to have the horse humanely destroyed than let it suffer from neglect.

Selling a horse can be done privately such as through a friend or in the paper, or the horse can be taken to a saleyard for public auction.

Riding your horse

If you have little or no experience riding a horse you should:

- seek professional training or lessons from a riding instructor
- join a pony or adult horse club or a riding establishment.

This will help you to learn to ride properly and enjoy your time with the horse.

It is essential to use properly fitting riding equipment. This will ensure your safety and prevent injury to your horse. Consult your local saddlery or riding instructor for advice on appropriate equipment.

BREEDING HORSES

Breeding horses should not be done indiscriminately and should only be done by experienced people (or with advice from experienced people), it is:

- expensive
- time consuming and
- requires special facilities and knowledge.

Things to consider before buying a horse

Buying a horse is a big investment of time and money, you need to consider the following before purchasing a horse:

- Can you provide all basic health and welfare requirements to keep your horse happy and healthy?
- How much time do you have to spare? Keeping a horse requires a substantial time commitment.
- Keeping a horse is expensive, do you have enough money to care for your horse?
- Do you have a suitable property to keep the horse on?
- Is your property appropriately fenced and suitable for catching and working the horse?
- Is it close to home so you can visit your horse daily?
- Do you have enough pasture or other feed for your horse?
- Do you have enough money to feed the horse if the pasture becomes inadequate?

Can you afford to purchase gear and other items, including:

- a saddle
- saddle blanket
- bridle

- grooming gear
- feed and water containers
- riding clothes (including a suitable hard hat and riding boots)
- costs to access to a pony club or riding lessons.

PASTURE FOR HORSES

Horses should have ample time on good quality pasture. The opportunity to graze and exercise improves condition, prevents boredom-related behaviors (eg, cribbing and weaving), and reduces the risk of large-intestinal impactions. Grazing on grass also helps reduce the incidence of gastric ulcers. Reducing the time spent in poorly ventilated barns reduces exposure to many inhalant allergens incriminated in development of recurrent airway obstruction. Access to good forage provides a natural source of vitamins and fiber. If horses are fed in groups, sufficient space should be allowed to minimize competition and to ensure that even the most submissive horse has access to an adequate diet. Feeding hay and grain in elevated feeders off the ground reduces ingestion of sand, infective parasite eggs, and animal excreta.

Safe, durable fencing should be used for pastures and paddocks to reduce the risk of self-trauma. Double fencing between paddocks minimizes transmission of contagious disease between horses. Overcrowding should be avoided. Overgrazed pastures, which result from overstocking, lead to extremes in ground conditions (eg, dust or mud), contribute to increased parasite burdens, and favor overgrowth of potentially toxic plants.

Excessive dust increases the risk of respiratory infections among young horses by inhalation of soil saprophytes, such as *Rhodococcus equi*. The risk of this potentially fatal bacterial pneumonia on farms where the disease is enzootic can be reduced by minimizing exposure of young (<4 mo old), susceptible foals to aerosolized *R equi* using environmental control strategies such as decreasing dust formation on pastures and paddocks, housing foals in well-ventilated areas, rotating pastures, reducing the size of mare-foal bands, irrigating and planting dirt areas with grass, and removing feces frequently from stalls, paddocks, indoor arenas, and pastures.

Breeding mares earlier in the season to ensure foaling during colder weather may reduce the number of susceptible foals exposed to dry, dusty summer conditions. On farms where *R equi* is endemic and foal morbidity and mortality rates are high despite attempts at pasture management, the incidence of disease can be reduced with preventive administration of 1 L of hyperimmune plasma containing high concentrations of antibodies against *R equi* to newborn foals within the first week of life, followed by a second dose 25 days later.

Overstocking in barns and pastures favors outbreaks of other contagious respiratory infections caused by viral and bacterial pathogens spread between horses via aerosolization of respiratory tract secretions. Enteric infections with *Clostridium difficile* and *C perfringens* can become endemic on some farms. An increased incidence of *Clostridium* diarrhea in newborn foals has been associated with foaling on dirt, gravel, or sand surfaces, and with stall confinement or limited turnout on dry lots during the first 3 days of life.

Whenever possible, horses should not be pastured on sandy soils, because sand ingestion during grazing predisposes to colonic and rectal sand impaction, chronic diarrhea, and weight loss. If sandy pastures are unavoidable, the risk of sand colic can be reduced by feeding psyllium at regular intervals and by providing trace mineralized salt with equal parts of bone meal.

In addition to properly feeding and exercising your horse, other aspects of general care are needed to keep your horse healthy throughout his or her life. These include routine veterinary care for vaccinations, parasite control, and dental care; grooming and hoof care; and protection from the elements.

Importance of Veterinary Care

Adult horses should have a complete veterinary examination at least once a year. Geriatric horses (older than 20 years old) should see their veterinarian twice a year or more frequently because illness is more common in older animals and it can be identified sooner. Your veterinarian may recommend a wellness program for your horse, including routine blood tests.

Signs of Illness

You should monitor your horse regularly for signs of illness, such as during daily feeding and grooming times. General signs of illness include a lack of appetite, diarrhea, coughing and sneezing, or a discharge from the eyes or nose. Illness can also show up as a loss of hair or itchy areas on the skin. Problems with the musculoskeletal system are often seen as lameness (such as not putting weight on a particular leg), reluctance to move, or head bobbing. If your horse shows any of these signs for more than a day or two, a visit with your veterinarian is a good idea.

Giving Medication

Generally, administering medication to a horse is not difficult if you use common sense and follow good handling principles for keeping both you and your horse safe. Maintain physical contact with the horse by keeping your shoulder pressed against the horse's shoulder or flank (depending on where and what you are treating) and make sure to use a sturdy halter and lead rope (hooked to the left halter ring). *Never* let a loop of any rope that is attached to your horse get wrapped around any part of your body.

If you need to apply medication to the horse's feet or lower front legs, lift the hoof to be treated and cradle it between your knees. If you need to treat the rear legs, in addition to lifting the hoof, you will also need to bend the hock. If your horse "dances" around, have another person lift the other leg *on the same side* as the leg that you need to treat.

Oral medication is usually in the form of "horse pills" (called boluses), pastes, or drenches. When administering oral medication, identify the toothless gap directly behind your horse's incisors and in front of the molars. Insert your thumb into this gap while holding the horse's head down with your hand. Firmly pull the horse's tongue out through the gap and, and gently hold it outside the mouth. You can now administer a bolus by placing it behind the "top" of the tongue with a balling gun.

Always lubricate the bolus with something like petroleum jelly or vegetable oil to keep it from getting caught in your horse's throat. Drenching guns and paste syringes can be placed far back in the mouth for administration of the fluid or paste. Hold your horse's head level or tilting slightly upward until he or she swallows the medicine.

Some medications can be administered only by injection, which is usually given in the neck area or thigh. Ask your veterinarian for a demonstration and guidance to make sure you know how to give the injection properly.

Regardless of type of medication or how it is to be given, it is important to read and follow all label instructions regarding use and storage.

VACCINATIONS

Vaccination is a key component of preventive medicine in horses. Vaccinations are given to stimulate the immune system against infection before exposure to disease. Several vaccines are routinely given to horses as the core defense against serious infectious illness. Several others are important in certain regions and situations. Your veterinarian can advise which vaccines are necessary in your local area and circumstances (see Table: Vaccines Required or Recommended for Horses).

Foals born to a vaccinated mare are usually protected against most infectious diseases for up to 6 months, so long as the foal consumed the antibody-rich mother's milk known as colostrum within 6 hours of birth. In this case, vaccinations should be delayed until maternal immunity has waned. Otherwise, the vaccination will be ineffective.

Vaccinations should be administered by your veterinarian or other properly trained individual. If you administer vaccines yourself, learn how to do it properly. Use only vaccines from a reliable source who can verify that they have been kept clean and refrigerated. Poor-quality vaccines increase the risk of adverse reactions, which can range from inflammation at the site of the injection, fever, and malaise, to serious allergic reactions that affect the entire body (for example, anaphylaxis).

Parasite Control

Animals that graze on grasses, including horses, ingest parasite eggs that are found throughout the environment. The actual parasite burden for any individual horse depends on its age, the number of horses on the same pasture, and the pasture's size and quality. Internal parasites of horses can cause many intestinal problems, including gastrointestinal upset, diarrhea, and potentially colic.

The primary intestinal parasites of horses include roundworms (both large and small strongyles), tapeworms, pinworms, and stomach bots. These worms can cause damage to the digestive tract and blood loss, and interfere with absorption of essential nutrients.

The greatest damage is caused by strongyles (also called redworms or bloodworms), and most parasite control programs are designed around strongyle control. Young horses typically are infested with more parasites and have more signs than older horses.

Most intestinal parasites are ingested while horses are grazing, from eggs and larvae deposited on the grass and upper layers of the soil. The tapeworm lifecycle involves small mites (specifically, orbatid mites) that feed on tapeworm eggs and thus contain tapeworm larvae. These mites live on grasses and are ingested while grazing. Stomach bots are larvae of flies. The adult fly deposits eggs on the muzzle, legs, and chest of horses during the spring. When the eggs are licked by the horse, they hatch and are ingested by the horse. The larvae attach to the wall of the stomach and remain for a period of time (usually until the following spring). The bot pupae then pass into the feces, where they hatch as adult flies.

All horses should be on a deworming program that consists of either a periodic deworming treatment (usually by administering a paste) every 4 to 8 weeks or a daily dewormer in the feed. Pasture management and good grooming practices are also very important aspects of parasite control. You may want to periodically submit samples of your horse's feces to your veterinarian to check for the type and number of intestinal parasites.

External Parasites

As outdoor animals, horses are also bothered by flies and ticks. These can cause sores and subsequent infection on the head, neck, ears, face, abdomen, and legs. Irritation from external parasites can also cause general upset, failure to grow and thrive, and decreased appetite (for example, fly "worry"). Horses should be checked regularly for ticks or signs of fly damage. Fly control includes proper manure management and stall cleanliness. Many different insecticidal salves, lotions, sprays, and rubs are available that can be used to remove ticks and decrease insect irritation and annoyance. Consult your veterinarian or extension service about an appropriate control program for your area and circumstances.

Grooming

Grooming is an important part of daily maintenance for horses. Daily brushing and currying helps remove dirt and debris that can allow bacteria a place to multiply. During grooming, you can also check the overall condition of your horse's skin and find sores, infections, bumps, or welts when they first arise. Vigorous currying is required to remove dirt, and horses generally enjoy it. Hair that is bound up (tail bags and mane braids) should be taken down every 10 to 14 days for brushing and cleaning. Horses can be bathed with equine shampoo, but baths should be kept to a minimum to avoid drying out the skin and coat. Horses should not be bathed when winter temperatures are below freezing, because horses need to be dry to resist the cold.

Hoof Care

Hoof care is an important part of the daily grooming routine. The hooves should be "picked" daily to remove manure, dirt, and stones, and checked for signs of bruising, odor, discoloration, or discharge. The shoes should also be checked for wear and tightness of the nails. Hoof dressings may be needed, but care should be taken to apply them appropriately. For example, water-repellent dressings can be important to keep hooves dry and healthy during wet weather. However, excessive use of emollient dressings can soften the hooves and lead to problems. Antifungal solutions should be applied every 1 to 2 weeks during winter and wet weather to prevent thrush. Your veterinarian and farrier can provide information on when and how frequently to treat your horse's feet.

Horses' hooves grow constantly and require trimming about every 6 weeks. Horses need to be trained to stand properly so that their hooves can be trimmed correctly and damage to the foot can be avoided. Foot trimming is best left to your farrier or veterinarian if you do not have experience with this procedure.

Shoes

Horse shoes provide traction on some surfaces and help prevent wear and tear of the hooves. The need for horse shoes depends on several factors, including foot conformation and health as well as the types of surfaces the horse will travel on. Horses with tender or bruised feet require shoes for protection, as do horses working on hard or rough surfaces.

Various kinds of corrective shoes are available for particular hoof or lameness problems. For example, horses with cracked hooves or splayed feet may need a barred shoe for support, while horses with other specific lameness problems may need a shoe that slows down or stabilizes the gait. Veterinarians, farriers, and trainers can provide more information on the shoes needed for any particular problem.

NUTRITION OF HORSES

During the last 20–30 yr, there has been an increased awareness of equine nutrition and its importance to the health of the horse. In every stage of life, nutrition is the foundation for equine health and longevity. The dietary needs of a horse change as it goes through each life stage. The great varieties of commercial feeds on the market attest to the recognition of different diets for different life stages. Horses must be provided with an adequate supply of energy, protein, vitamins, and minerals and have access to fresh, clean water.

Adequate fresh water intake is essential for every horse. Storage tanks, troughs, or pails should be placed so the horse can reach in comfortably. Because most horses are reluctant to put their head in a trough or pail below eye level, the water level should be kept high. If water levels get too low, many horses will refuse to drink. The optimal temperature for drinking water is 68°–78°F (20°–26°C). Horses will reduce water intake if the water temperature is too cold or too warm. When daytime temperatures exceed 100°F (38°C), water in exposed pipes or hoses will be dangerously hot and should not be used for drinking or bathing.

The nutrient energy requirement of the horse depends on its level of activity, the energy content of the diet, and the capacity of the animal's digestive system. The size and weight of the newborn foal is influenced by the nutrition of the pregnant mare. Horses fed for rapid body and skeletal growth may develop bone abnormalities or be more prone to lameness conditions. A balanced diet should be fed according to the desired rate of gain within the sound parameters of good health. The best measure of growth in a young horse is weight, and the best description of size of a horse is a combination of height and weight. A high correlation between the measure of the heart girth and body weight in the horse has been reported. In young, growing horses, monthly measurements are helpful to monitor growth changes.

There are several reasons to know the weight of horses. Many feeding requirements are based on percentages of the horse's weight. Most feed recommendations are stated in the amount of feed (in pounds or kilograms) the horse should receive based on body weight. In young horses, "developmental orthopedic disease," although a multifactorial condition, can be related to rapid growth or imbalances in energy, protein, and minerals. The proper balance of protein, calcium, phosphorus, zinc, and copper is important in supporting healthy endochondral ossification and in stabilizing bone collagen and elastin synthesis. The amount of nutrients required in the diet for normal bone development are dictated by rate of growth. Excessive energy intake contributes to osteochondrosis by decreasing bone density and cortical thickness.

Deficiency of protein must be severe to interfere with endochondral ossification. Rapidly increasing protein intake may produce faster bone growth; however, if the diet lacks adequate minerals to support this increased growth, altered endochondral ossification can be seen. Calcium and phosphorus balance affect bone density, rate of growth, and cartilage thickness. Inadequate amounts of copper and zinc have been associated with an increased incidence of osteochondrosis and osteodysgenesis.

Some of the most common mistakes made when feeding young horses include feeding excessive grain and leafy legumes (eg, alfalfa, which results in too high an energy intake), feeding a diet with too little zinc or copper to support rate of growth, and feeding a diet with an improper calcium:phosphorus ratio. Cereal grains and grass forages are low in calcium, phosphorus, protein, and lysine. Excess energy from cereal grains may be more detrimental than excess energy from grass forages; one reason may be that energy from grain is derived from starch, whereas energy from grass forage comes from microbial production of volatile fatty acids. Starch, but not volatile fatty acids, stimulates insulin secretion, which has been implicated in stimulating hormone changes that contribute to osteochondrosis.

Older horses often have dental problems that compromise feed intake and mastication. Extruded or soft pelleted feeds are ideal. Hay should be good quality, leafy, and easy to chew. The most variable dietary requirement for any horse is energy. A certain amount of energy is required for maintenance and daily activity. Metabolic demands are increased for such activities as growing, performance activity, or lactation. In some activities, such as racing, jumping, or polo, the energy requirement may be increased by as much as 100%.

Diet manipulation can help treat, control, and prevent other disease conditions. Horses with recurrent airway obstruction should be fed as dust-free a feed as possible. Adding water or oil to grains decreases dust. Hay should be thoroughly soaked and fed close to the ground. If complete pelleted feeds are fed, hay can be removed completely from the diet. On sandy soils, hay should be fed off the ground to reduce sand ingestion. Dietary management can be used to reduce the risk of gastric ulcers. Alfalfa hay, with its high calcium and protein concentration, acts as a buffering antacid and has a protective effect on the nonglandular squamous mucosa. Small hay meals fed frequently or access to pasture also reduces the risk of gastric ulceration.

Nutritional management for Quarter horses with hyperkalemic periodic paralysis is focused on decreasing dietary intake of potassium and increasing renal potassium losses. Dietary manipulation includes avoiding high-potassium feeds such as alfalfa hay, brome grass, canola oil, soybean meal or oil, and sugar or beet molasses and replacing them with timothy or bermuda grass, beet pulp, and grains such as oats, corn, wheat, or barley. Affected horses should be exercised regularly and have access to pasture.

Heavily muscled breeds of horses, including Quarter horses, draft horses, and Warmbloods, are prone to myopathies associated with increased muscle glycogen stores and polysaccharide storage inclusions in type II muscle fibers. Successful management of this condition, known as polysaccharide storage myopathy, focuses on increasing the fat content of the diet and eliminating or reducing grain intake.

Management practices to reduce the risk of impaction include ad lib access to fresh water, adequate exercise, good quality feed, and good dental care. If impaction has been a problem, poorly digestible feeds (eg, mature forages) should be replaced with low-fiber, highly digestible forages (eg, growing grass or legume hays). A complete pelleted or extruded feed helps maintain soft feces.

Grazing lush pastures or consuming large amounts of legume hay and the development of laminitis have long been associated. Anecdotal observations indicate that pasture-associated laminitis occurs at times of rapid grass growth (eg, spring and early summer and in the fall after rainfall) that favor accumulation of certain carbohydrates such as fructans, starches, and sugars. Some horses and ponies may be more susceptible to pasture-associated laminitis because of genetic predisposition and other metabolic factors, including obesity, peripheral insulin resistance, and hyperinsulinemia. Strategies to reduce the risk of laminitis focus on limiting the intake of nonstructural carbohydrates such as fructans from pasture and other feedstuffs.

Horses and ponies with a history of recurrent laminitis should have limited pasture access during periods of rapid grass growth, such as spring and early summer. Nonstructural carbohydrate content also tends to increase during the morning, reaches maximal values in the afternoon, and then declines overnight. Therefore, a popular recommendation is to turn "susceptible" individuals out on pasture overnight or during the early morning and to remove them from pasture by mid-morning. Stemmy, mature pastures should be avoided, because mature grasses may contain more fructans. Turning susceptible individuals onto pasture that has been exposed to low temperatures in conjunction with bright sunlight (eg, as in the fall after a flush of growth followed by cool sunny days) should be avoided, because colder temperatures reduce grass growth and result in concentration of the fructan.

If feeding forage, lush legume hays should be avoided, because they tend to have higher nonstructural carbohydrate content. Soaking hay before feeding may help reduce the amount of fructans being fed. Grain and sweet feeds should be avoided.

The terms mature, senior, and geriatric refer to horses that have completed their growth cycle. However, because aging is a continuous process, there is no discrete age range for each category. Improved methods of overall care, management, and diet have enabled horses to live into their 20s or 30s. This increased longevity means they are used in a variety of leisure or competitive activities well into their teens or 20s.

Good management of still-active older horses means recognition and evaluation of conditions that occur with age (eg, arthritis, hyperadrenocorticism, gastric ulcers, laminitis, navicular disease, kidney or liver dysfunction), followed by therapeutic management and special dietary considerations. Horses with arthritis require a balanced diet with adequate minerals. In horses prone to hyperadrenocorticism, the use of fat-supplemented feeds with highly digestible fiber and reduced starch and sugar intake is important. Horses with liver or kidney conditions should not be fed legume hays and fat-supplemented feeds. Horses confined to stalls most of the time are more prone to intestinal problems and development of undesirable behaviors.

METABOLIC DISORDERS OF HORSES

Metabolism refers to all processes in the body that break down and convert ingested substances into the energy and nutrients needed to sustain life. Foods, liquids, and drugs all undergo metabolic processes within the body. Many foods are complex materials that need to be broken down into simpler substances, which in turn become "building blocks" for the body to use as needed. For example, protein is broken down into amino acids, which are used to build new proteins and regulate key metabolic reactions. Enzymes, are proteins that stimulate biochemical reactions for many metabolic processes. Whenever the function of an enzyme is altered, a metabolic disorder can develop. Metabolic disorders are important because they can affect energy production or damage tissues critical for survival. They may be inherited or acquired. Acquired metabolic disorders are more common and significant. Metabolic disorders may result in a substance rising to toxic levels (a storage disorder), or a necessary substance may not be produced, causing a deficiency.

Metabolic Storage Disorders

Metabolic storage disorders are characterized by the accumulation of a substance within cells due to the body's inability to break it down (metabolize it) because of a partial or complete lack of a certain enzyme. The missing enzyme may result in a substance building up to a toxic level. Although storage diseases are often widespread throughout the body, most signs are due to the effects on the central nervous system. Metabolic storage disorders can be either genetic or acquired.

Genetic (inherited) storage diseases are named according to the specific metabolic byproduct that builds up in the body. These diseases are progressive and usually fatal because specific treatments do not exist. Genetic storage diseases have not been reported in horses.

Acquired storage diseases can be caused by eating plants that contain inhibitors of specific enzymes. Eating locoweed plants (Astragalus or Oxytropis species) for a long time can result in an acquired neurologic storage disease. Several toxic components of these plants interfere with the activity of a specific enzyme. Horses are highly susceptible to locoweed intoxication.

Production-related Metabolic Disorders

Some metabolic disorders are caused by an increased demand for a specific element or nutrient that has become deficient. For example, in hypoglycemia, the animal's metabolic reserves are unable to sustain sugar (glucose) in the blood at a level needed for normal function. Likewise, in hypocalcemia, the level of calcium in the blood is too low. In some cases, dietary intake of a nutrient, such as calcium, is rapidly used up for an ongoing, high metabolic need, such as nursing a foal. Another production-related disorder of horses is exertional rhabdomyolysis, which is also called "tying-up." This condition is a syndrome of muscle fatigue, pain, or cramping associated with exercise. There are multiple underlying causes that result in similar signs. The syndrome may be sporadic, with single or infrequent episodes, or chronic, recurring often after mild exertion. Severe episodes require intensive supportive therapy to avoid kidney damage.

The difference between production-related metabolic diseases and nutritional deficiencies is often subtle. Typically, nutritional deficiencies are longterm conditions that develop gradually and can be corrected through dietary supplementation. Acquired metabolic diseases usually begin suddenly and respond dramatically to administration of the deficient nutrient (although affected animals may need dietary supplements to avoid recurrence). Because production-related metabolic disorders are serious and can develop suddenly, accurate and rapid diagnosis is essential. Ideally, diagnostic tests can be used to predict the chance of disease occurring so that it can be prevented or preparations can be made for rapid treatment.

METABOLIC STORAGE DISORDERS AND INBORN ERRORS OF METABOLISM

Genetic Storage Disease in Animals

Genetic storage diseases are named according to the specific metabolic byproduct that accumulates in the lysosomes. Animals are typically apparently normal at birth, then manifest clinical signs within the first weeks to months of life. These diseases are progressive and usually fatal, given that specific treatments do not exist.

In small animals, the gangliosidoses (GM_1 gangliosidosis and GM_2 gangliosidosis) occur in Siamese, Korat, and domestic cats and in Beagle crosses, German Shorthaired Pointers, Japanese Spaniels, Portuguese Water Dogs, English Springer Spaniels, Alaskan Huskies, and Shiba Inus. Sphingomyelinosis occurs in German Shepherd Dogs and Poodles and in Siamese and domestic shorthair cats. Glucocerebrosidosis occurs in Australian Silky Terriers and Dalmatians. Ceroid lipofuscinosis occurs in English Setters, Cocker Spaniels, Dachshunds, Chihuahuas, Salukis, Border Collies, and domestic cats. Mannosidosis occurs in Persian and domestic cats. Glycogenosis occurs in Silky Terriers and in domestic shorthaired and Norwegian forest cats. Globoid cell leukodystrophy (Krabbe disease) occurs in Cairn Terriers, West Highland White Terriers, Beagles, Bluetick Hounds, Poodles, and domestic shorthair cats. Mucopolysaccharidosis type I occurs in Siamese, Korat, and domestic shorthair cats, whereas type IV occurs in Siamese cats.

In dogs, mucopolysaccharidosis occurs in Miniature Pinschers, Plott Hounds, Rottweilers, Labrador Retrievers, Wirehaired Dachshunds, New Zealand Huntaways, Schipperkes, Welsh Corgis, Miniature Schnauzers, Chesapeake Bay Retrievers, German Shepherd Dogs, Rat Terriers, and mixed-breed dogs and is associated with lameness. Diseases associated with decreased RBC survival and anemia include pyruvate kinase deficiency in Basenjis, Beagles, and West Highland White and Cairn Terriers; phosphofructokinase deficiency in English Springer and American Cocker Spaniels; and porphyria in Siamese and domestic shorthair cats.

In large animals, alpha-mannosidosis occurs in Angus, Murray Grey, Simmental, Galloway, and Holstein cattle. Beta-mannosidosis occurs in Saler cattle and Nubian and Nubian-cross goats. Generalized glycogenosis (GM_1) occurs in Holstein cattle and Suffolk sheep. Generalized glycogenosis (GM_2) occurs in Shorthorn and Brahman cattle, and in pigs. Globoid cell leukodystrophy occurs in polled Dorset sheep.

Other identified diseases that are associated with neurologic signs and appear to be inherited include neuronal lipodystrophy in Angus and Beefmaster cattle, shaker calf syndrome of horned Hereford cattle, maple syrup urine disease of Hereford and polled Shorthorn cattle, and hereditary neuraxial edema of polled and horned Hereford and Hereford-Friesian cross cattle. There have been no reports of lysosomal storage diseases in horses; however, inherited diseases manifested by neurologic signs include inherited myoclonus of Peruvian Paso foals and congenital encephalomyelopathy in Quarter Horses.

Other inherited diseases that involve basic errors of metabolism in various tissues include goiter of sheep and goats, inherited parakeratosis (edema disease) of cattle, osteogenesis imperfecta of sheep and cattle, and possibly cardiomyopathy of cattle, the hypotrichoses, baldy calves, photosensitization of sheep, dermatosis vegetans of pigs and porcine stress syndrome, dermatosparaxia and Ehlers-Danlos syndrome of cattle, hemochromatosis of cattle, and Marfan syndrome in cattle. Many other inherited defects, especially those based on abnormal growth of collagen, cartilage, and bone, also are likely to have basic errors of metabolism of structural tissues. Many disorders of metabolism have been described involving dysfunctions of the immune system.

Acquired Storage Disease in Animals

Acquired storage diseases are due to ingestion of plants that contain inhibitors of specific lysosomal catabolic enzymes. Chronic ingestion of locoweed plants (*Astragalus* or *Oxytropis* spp) results in an acquired neurologic storage disease. Several toxic components, including locoine, swainsonine n-oxide, and indolizidine alkaloids, interfere with alpha-mannosidase activity. Horses are most susceptible to intoxication; however, cattle, sheep, and goats can also be affected.

2

BASIC EQUINE CARE AND MANAGEMENT

The horse world undoubtedly includes a wide variety of associations, disciplines, breeds, and types of horse owners. In the Sierra Foothills, horse ownership is just as diverse. You will find everything ranging from competition, breeding and pleasure horses, to the simple family pet, each of which encompasses a wide-range of breeds. Regardless of what type of horse owner you are, there is certainly never a shortage of opinions or advice related to how to best care for your horse. At the end of the day, the most important action is to evaluate what is best for each individual horse and to take responsibility as a horse owner.

The Sierra Foothill Research and Extension Center does not currently deal in equine health and research, although there are horses housed on-site to assist in the day to day cattle ranching activities. Our goal is to simply provide helpful information relative to the surrounding community. The series listed and portrayed below focuses on the most basic needs of every horse - regardless of breed, discipline, or region. If you have any questions about these basic needs or any other compelling questions related to your specific horse, please call your local equine veterinarian.

CARING FOR NEW ARRIVALS

Every horse entering a rescue/retirement facility should receive a complete physical examination upon its arrival. Permanent identification (e.g., microchipping, lip tattoo, freeze branding) of each horse is an economical, humane and unalterable tracking mechanism for a horse, and is included as part of the admissions procedures for many facilities. A health record must be established for each horse, clearly identifying the horse by name and/or number, age, gender and description. Medication and treatments should be given only under the direction of a veterinarian and recorded in the horse's health record.

Horses may be susceptible to transportation stress and disease following transport to a rescue/retirement facility. On arrival, new horses should be isolated from resident horses to prevent the possible spread of disease, preferably for 2-3 weeks. Handlers should carefully monitor recently transported horses for several days after long-distance transport. The temperature of these horses should be recorded daily for several days, and if not normal, the temperature should be recorded at least twice daily, i.e. morning and evening. If a horse's temperature exceeds the normal range, a veterinarian should be consulted.

MONITORING OF HORSES

Frequent observation of the horses in a rescue/retirement facility is paramount to ensure that they remain healthy. Horses should be observed routinely, at least once every 24 hours, paying particular attention during highrisk periods (e.g., inclement weather, foaling, introduction of new animals). The table below provides vital signs for an adult 1,200-pound (545 kg) horse at rest at 60°F. These criteria will vary according to age, physical fitness and environmental conditions. Younger horses tend to be at the higher end of the range.

PREVENTIVE HEALTH CARE IS A NECESSITY

Rescue/retirement facilities should consult with a veterinarian to develop a sound, integrated health care program appropriate to the facility and environment. Previous health records, if available, can assist a veterinarian in making recommendations that are most appropriate for the horse's needs, and should be requested.

PARASITE CONTROL

A parasite control program, one of the most important management matters to be considered, must be established in consultation with a veterinarian.1 An effective program will include the administration of chemical deworming agents, as well as manure and pasture management. Indiscriminate use of deworming agents is not advisable, as it adds to the growing problem of parasite resistance to such agents. With veterinary guidance, utilizing such tools as fecal egg counts to optimize use of dewormers, an effective and economical parasite control program, can be designed while minimizing parasite resistance.

VACCINATION

Administering the appropriate vaccinations is another tool which assists in controlling common infectious diseases of the horse. The specific immunizations needed by a particular group of horses depends upon several factors, including environment, age, breed, sex, use, exposure risk, geographic location and general management. Consult your veterinarian to determine the most effective vaccination program for your facility's horses.

NUTRITION

Formulating a diet for a horse should take into account the horse's state of health, geographic location, medical history, exercise/use, and individual metabolism. Special recommendations for feeding a starved horse are found at the end of this chapter. A veterinarian, perhaps assisted by an equine nutritionist, should be consulted to ensure current feeding programs are meeting each animal's needs.

GENERAL FEED REQUIREMENTS

A horse's daily diet should be adequate to maintain health and normal body functions, and should be fed on a regular daily schedule. In its natural state, the horse eats a variety of forages (mainly grasses) to meet its nutritional needs. Due to the small size of its stomach, the horse will normally consume its daily intake over 16 to 20 hours. When confined, horses should be fed at least twice daily; however, there appears to be no nutritional benefit when horses are fed more than three times daily.

Horses should be fed a forage-based diet (hay or pasture). For most mature horses that are not competing or exercising, a forage-based diet is usually adequate to meet caloric needs. Grain supplementation should be rarely needed. Fresh forage (pasture) can seasonally provide most of the horse's needs, but should be supplemented with dry forage (hay) to provide adequate dietary fiber.

Pasture provides additional health benefits to horses, allowing them to move and exercise as they normally do, and regular pasture turnout should be part of a horse's daily routine, unless otherwise directed by a veterinarian. In certain areas, minerals and trace minerals may be lacking (e.g., selenium in parts of the northern United States), and supplementation may be required, ideally as directed by a veterinarian.

There is rarely a need for horses in rescue and retirement facilities to be fed high-grain (high-energy) diets. If such diets are selected, attention should be paid to avoid nutritionrelated health problems, such as grain overload, laminitis, founder or obesity. To avoid problems such as colic, abrupt changes in diet should be avoided. To avoid major health problems, any changes in the type and quantity of feed should be introduced gradually over a period of several days. Feeds used in the horse's diet should be fresh, free of spoilage, toxic insects or contaminants, dust and molds. Horses should also have access to free-choice salt and appropriate minerals, as necessary.

When horses are fed in groups, some horses may "bully" others, and prevent other horses from eating. This may lead to some horses' overeating and becoming obese, while others may become thin and malnourished, even if adequate feed is being supplied.

To prevent such problems, adequate manger space or separate feeding areas should be available to minimize competition for feed. All horses should have simultaneous access to feeders so that all can eat at one time. Horses that "bully" others should be separated from less dominant horses to ensure that the less dominant horses receive adequate feed.

All feeds and supplements should be properly labeled and stored appropriately to avoid misuse. Owners and operators of retirement facilities would be well-advised to consult with their veterinarians prior to implementing nutritional supplements; such supplements may significantly increase the cost of care for the horses, but may not provide significant nutritional benefit. Feeds designed for other species, particularly medicated feeds and those containing urea, are unsuitable for horses. Feed troughs and buckets should be cleaned regularly.

FEED

Horses are known as "trickle feeders," meaning they constantly take in food throughout the day. If it were up to your horses, they would spend roughly 17-20 hours every day grazing on forage. Due to the scarcity of land with quality pasture, few domesticated horses have that luxury, so as owners we must compensate for their nutritional needs to the best of our abilities. Forage is the basis of an equine diet. This can include pasture, grass hay, legumes (ex. alfalfa), and/or beet pulp. These forages provide the essential proteins, carbohydrates, and fats every horse needs. Horses should consume 1.5%-3% of their body weight per day - with at least half of that being forage. That is 15-20 pounds of forage per day for an average-sized horse. Grain is not usually a necessary part of a horse's diet, but can be used as a supplement if needed or for horses expelling a lot of energy who may need an elevated calorie intake.

Equine dietary requirements can vary by region, age, breed, and level of activity. Talk to your equine veterinarian or equine nutritionist to make sure your horse is getting the nutrients he needs.

Determining Feed Requirements for Each Horse

The amount of feed required by a horse is made up of two factors:

- Maintenance needs, that is, the amount of feed that is required to keep the horse in good health.
- Activity needs (which include rate of work, growth, lactation and pregnancy)

Both requirements must be satisfied in order to maintain ideal body condition and weight.

SUPPLEMENTARY FEEDS

Cereal grains such as oats, corn and barley should be rarely needed for most horses at rescue and retirement facilities. Grains should only be added to the horse's diet to meet extra energy needs, such as those associated with exercise, late pregnancy, lactation, growth, and occasionally to help maintain proper weight, or during convalescence or recovery from surgery.

Cereal grains should always be measured by weight rather than volume when feeding (e.g., 1 pound, rather than 1 "coffee can"), as there are marked differences in densities, not only among types of grains, but also within different consignments of the same grain.

Oats tend to be safer to feed than other grains due to high fiber content. Most of the digestibility studies that have been conducted comparing crimped and whole oats indicate that there is, at most, a 6% increase in the digestibility of crimped oats, when compared to whole oats. Thus, in most cases, there is no real benefit to using crimped oats over whole oats. Prolonged storage of crimped oats reduces their nutritional value and should be avoided.

Corn and barley have a higher energy value than oats, and provide more calories on a per weight basis than do oats, and thus may be easier to overfeed. Barley's energy value lies between that of corn and oats. Its hard husk needs to crushed or cracked to aid digestion.

Young and growing horses have increased protein requirements compared to older horses. There are many ways to increase protein in a horse's ration, including feeding alfalfa hay. Meals such as soybean meal are often included in rations for young and growing horses also increase the protein content of the ration. They should be fed in small amounts and introduced gradually. Linseed meal is not an appropriate protein supplement for growing horses because it is low in the amino acid lysine, which is essential for normal development.

Many brands of blended horse feeds are on the market. Following the manufacturer's feeding guidelines provides a simple method of dietary supplementation recommendations (this information should be printed on the label, along with an analysis of ingredients).

In operations where small numbers of horses have similar supplementary feeding needs, premixed balanced feeds can save the facility work and ensure continuity of diet. When feeding commercially blended feeds, care should be taken to ensure the horse has access to its minimum daily forage (fiber) requirement of 0.5 to 1 pound dry matter/100 pounds bodyweight.

When horses are working and sweating, salt (sodium chloride) and possibly other electrolytes may need to be supplemented. Hand-fed horses should have salt supplemented daily, or have free choice access to a trace mineral/salt block. Advice on mineral deficiencies peculiar to any grazing area should be sought from a veterinarian or local extension nutritionist, and addressed accordingly.

CALCULATING HORSE BODYWEIGHT

Before accurate feed calculations can be made, the bodyweight of the horse should be estimated. Bodyweight assessment is also required when medicines, including dewormers, are administered.

The most accurate method of determining bodyweight is the use of electronic scales. To get the most accurate weight for a horse when using scales, weigh the animal just before feeding and watering.

This will help avoid variations caused by different gut-fill levels, and will allow subsequent weight measurements to be more standardized, and thus more meaningful. Weight tapes also can be useful in estimating a horse's body weight. While they may not give an accurate absolute measurement, they can be very effectively used to see if a horse is gaining or losing weight.

For those without scales, the Henneke Body Scoring System can help the average horseman, with practice, to establish and track changes in a horse's body condition. The "ideal" body condition is said to be when the horse's ribs can be easily felt, but not seen.

Expected Total Ration Comsumption By Horses

Class	Total consumption
	% bodyweight
Maintenance	1.5 - 2.0
Late Gestation	1.5 - 2.0
Lactation	2.0 - 3.0
Working	1.5 - 3.0
Weanling	2.0 - 3.0
Yearling	2.0 - 3.0
Two-year-old	1.8 - 2.5

WATER

Water is essential to your horse's overall health and well-being. A singular horse requires 5-15 gallons of water per day, so every horse should have access to clean, fresh water at all times. Your horse's water consumption can vary depending upon environmental temperature, diet, or level of exercise. It is important to pay special attention to your horse's drinking habits and note any changes. If your horse is a poor drinker or a heavy sweater, access to fresh, clean water alone may not be enough. Adding an over-the-counter, daily electrolyte supplement is a smart way to replace salt and the other minerals lost in sweat, and to help encourage your horse to drink. If your horse still isn't drinking enough water, contact your equine veterinarian for recommendations or other advice.

Every horse should have access to a sufficient amount of fresh, clean water to meet its individual maintenance and activity needs. A horse's daily water requirements may range from 5 to 20 gallons (20 to 70 liters), depending on air temperature, humidity, body weight, level of activity and health and physiological status (e.g., pregnant, lactating or growing).

As a general guide, horses need ½ to 1 gallon (2 to 4 liters) of water per 2 pounds of dry matter intake. This requirement increases with increasing air temperature; for example, an increase in ambient temperature from 55°F to 77°F (13°C to 25°C) increases water required by 15 to 20%.

As a practical matter, a horse should always have unlimited access to fresh water. Water troughs and containers should be regularly cleaned to prevent algae buildup. They should be located where they are protected from electrical problems, fouling, and freezing. In cold climates, horses preferentially consume warm water; if warmer water cannot be provided in cold climates, watering systems should be examined regularly to ensure that the water is not frozen. Automatic watering systems should be checked daily to ensure they are dispensing water properly.

In some disease conditions, such as severe diarrhea, rapid loss of water and essential body salts (electrolytes) can result. Fluid replacement necessary to overcome fluid loss should be administered by a veterinarian.

NUTRITION OF THE PREGNANT MARE

It is not common for rescue and retirement facilities to receive pregnant mares. However, if such mares are received, the non-working, non-lactating pregnant mare does not require an increase in feed above maintenance during the first eight months of pregnancy. During the last three months of pregnancy, the extra energy requirement, because of fetal growth and an increase in the mare's weight, is about 0.5% of bodyweight, as dry matter, so the total dry matter feed requirement becomes approximately 2.2% of bodyweight.

It has been estimated that a normal mare will produce milk equivalent to 3% of bodyweight in early lactation and 2% in late lactation. The milk production of pony mares is estimated at 4% in early lactation and 3% in late lactation. For example, this means an 1,100-pound mare (500kg) should produce 4 gallons (15 liters) of milk per day in the first three months and 2 ½ gallons (10 liters) per day in the last three months prior to weaning. Producing milk requires extra calories, and as a result, in dry matter intake, the lactating mare's nutritional needs are between 1 and 1.5% bodyweight above that which is required for maintenance.

Pregnant mares may also have additional health needs, such as vaccination against equine herpesvirus-1. Rescue and retirement facilities are encouraged to contact their veterinarians for advice on caring for pregnant, postpartum, and lactating mares.

NUTRITION OF GROWING HORSES

Growing horses need feeding above that which would be required to simply maintain their body weight because they need additional "building blocks" for growth. The feed required will vary with factors such as the expected mature weight, growth rate, age, and exercise. Young horses have a higher protein requirement than do mature horses. Their feed should contain 13 to 15% protein as weanlings. Yearlings may require 12 - 13% dietary protein, and two-year-olds require about 11% dietary protein. Young horses need approximately 3% of their bodyweight as dry matter intake, depending on dietary ingredients.

OVERFEEDING, OBESITY AND LAMINITIS (FOUNDER)

Excessive energy intake, both acute and chronic, is one of the causes of a common and crippling disease: laminitis. Laminitis affects the feet of horses and disrupts the sensitive and insensitive laminae, which secure the coffin bone to the hoof wall. "Founder" is a commonly used name for this condition. It is important to note, however, that there are many causal agents of laminitis, including stress, as well as various disease conditions.

In order to avoid laminitis, horses should not be permitted to become overly fat. Some equines, particularly ponies and donkeys, are able to utilize energy in feeds very efficiently; other obese horses may be affected with a condition known as insulin resistance/equine metabolic syndrome.5 Horses and ponies that tend towards obesity ("easy keepers") are considered to be more susceptible to laminitis, and should have restricted access to grains (if grains are fed at all), as well as spring and autumn pasture, which is low in fiber, and high in sugars. Low-energy forages such as grasstype hays should be fed in preference to higher energy legume hays (e.g., alfalfa).

Controlling the weight of horses using starvation diets is unacceptable. Such horses should first be examined by a veterinarian to rule out disease conditions that might affect weight, and then supplied with a balanced, reduced calorie diet, as well as free access to water.

REFEEDING THE STARVED HORSE

Unfortunately, some horses that arrive at rescue/retirement facilities have been subjected to long-term neglect and may suffer from starvation. Rehabilitating a starved horse presents many challenges for caregivers. In both horses and humans, the abrupt refeeding of a starved horse can cause dysfunction of the body's metabolic system, which can lead to failure of the heart and lungs and ultimately death. A veterinarian is vital to the recovery of these animals and should be consulted as soon as a starved horse arrives at the facility. Even under the best of care, horses subjected to prolonged malnutrition may die, even after having been placed with a responsible caregiver and having been provided an appropriate diet. Owners and operators of rescue and retirement facilities should realize that the financial costs of stabilizing malnourished horses may significantly exceed their market price, and that responsible management of chronically starved horses should include the option of euthanasia.

REFEEDING RECOMMENDATIONS

Days 1-3

Feed one pound (approximately 1/6 flake) of leafy alfalfa every four hours (total of six pounds per day in six feedings). Contact a veterinarian to evaluate the medical status of the horse.

Days 4-10

Slowly increase the amount of alfalfa and decrease the number of feedings so that by day six, you are feeding just over four pounds of hay every eight hours (total of 13 pounds per day in three feedings.)

Day 10 - Several Months

Feed as much alfalfa as the horse will eat and decrease feeding to twice a day. Provide access to a salt block. Do not feed grain or supplemental feed until the horse is well along in its recovery; early feeding of grain and supplemental feed complicates the return of normal metabolic function and can result in death.

- Provide clean, fresh water at all times.
- Deworming and correction of dental problems are very beneficial to the horse's recovery.

HEALTH MANAGEMENT FOR PERFORMANCE

When a horse begins showing signs of poor performance there are three major body systems to be considered: respiratory, cardiovascular and musculoskeletal.

Respiratory

Upper airway obstructions are caused by malfunctioning structures that lead to airflow obstruction. One common condition of the upper airway is known as roaring, or laryngeal hemiplegia. It can cause difficulties in active horses and can manifest as noises - "roaring" - during exercise.

The lower respiratory tract is at risk for viral diseases and bacteria that can affect the lungs. Performance horses are especially vulnerable. Common viral diseases are rhinopneumonitis (equine herpesvirus) and equine influenza. Performance horses have increased risk of exposure to these diseases and should be vaccinated.

Several risk factors are associated with the spread of viral diseases:

- Horse shows where lots of animals mingle
- Many animals of different age or immune states
- Transportation often causes stress in horses
- Stress acts as an immunosuppressive, which may cause the horse to pick up a virus

Preventive measures include:

- Quarantine horses coming or returning to the farm
- Don't share tack between new arrivals and those already on the farm
- Prevent nose-to-nose contact

- During transport, horses should be able to lower their heads, which helps clear the airway of dust and other particles
- If a disease outbreak occurs, control animal and human traffic to minimize spread

There are no specific treatments for viruses, but Montgomery recommends a low-dust environment and time to heal. If the animal has a low fever, they may go off their feed.

"Really, the most important thing is rest. I can't stress that enough, because once the clinical signs go away, the lungs are not completely healed," she says.

Viral respiratory infections can lead to complications such as bacterial pneumonia or inflammatory airway disease. Researchers are also investigating the connection between viral respiratory disease and recurrent airway obstruction (RAO or heaves) - a chronic, asthma-like condition.

Horses that perform at maximum lung capacity - such as racehorses -are also at risk for developing a condition called exercise-induced pulmonary haemorrhage. It's thought that damage to veins within the lungs results in pulmonary bleeding.

Cardiovascular (Heart)

High-performance horses often develop specific arrhythmias because of their low resting heart rates. Arrhythmias may appear during a regular physical examination or during a mandatory veterinary check:

- Atrioventricular block or dropped beat. The horse's heart beats at a normal rhythm with a pause every three or four beats at a regular interval. This is common in fit horses - as well as very fit human athletes - and should go away with exercise.
- Atrial fibrillation. This arrhythmia can occur without an underlying heart disease. The atria will start to fibrillate, or contract irregularly. In high performing horses, this can present as poor performance or exercise intolerance. This condition can be caused by low potassium. If an endurance horse is sweating a lot or on a diuretic, they may be at risk.

Murmurs result from turbulent blood flow through the heart, often caused by leakage in the heart valves. Small leaks can be clinically insignificant but still show up during an exam. Age can cause changes in the aortic valve, but unless there are performance concerns, it doesn't usually require further investigation.

Murmurs can also appear as a symptom of other problems such as dehydration or a low red blood cell count. These "functional murmurs" usually go away when the underlying problem is addressed.

Muscoloskeletal System

Over time the horses' body has evolved to run more effectively. Montgomery compares the body of a horse to a suspension bridge - the front limbs are attached only through muscles and function like a sling as the body is propelled forward.

The horse carries about 60 per cent of its body weight on the front limbs and uses the hind legs for power. The force of this impact can affect its legs and feet. Because the horse is evolved to run, its legs are made up of tendons and ligaments instead of muscle.

The horses' hind legs directly connect to the back muscles, which means problems with the hind limbs sometimes present as back pain. Because the horse will often shift its weight around to compensate for pain, this can create other problems and it can be difficult to isolate the source.

Certain issues also correlate to specific equine sports. Horses required to collect or shorten, their gait - such as barrel racers or dressage horses - often suffer from sore hocks. Similarly, horses involved in driving and show jumping where a high head carriage is normal are prone to developing back pain.

In racehorses, speed and fatigue can result in limb injuries. Back problems can also arise from several other sources: an improperly seated rider, a poorly fitted saddle or prolonged exercise on one lead. In racehorses, surface texture can also lead to musculoskeletal injuries. With a hard surface, the force of impact on landing increases. Soft surface can result in an increased strain of soft tissue structures.

Tying-up syndrome is another common disease in horses that can be related to exercise or an underlying disease. Signs include stiffness, firm and painful muscles, sweating, an elevated heart rate and dark brown urine. These signs should be considered an emergency situation, as the horse is in a lot of pain and the breakdown of the muscle - muscle necrosis - can affect the health of the kidneys.

3

HOOF CARE

The old saying 'no foot, no horse' still holds true today and whilst as an owner you can't do much mechanically to the hooves, daily care and observation are vital to avoid problems. For the sake of the organization, discussion here applies specifically to horses in rescue/ retirement facilities and should not be confused with any breed predilection or discipline.

HOOF GROWTH

As a general rule, adult horse hoof growth is approximately 3/8 of an inch (9 millimeters) per month, while hoof growth in a foal is approximately 5/8 of an inch (15 millimeters) per month. With that in mind, as a general guideline, an adult horse should be trimmed (or shod) in accordance with the needs of the horse. Foals should be trimmed every four weeks, or as needed.

KEEPING THE HOOVES BALANCED

Horses with balance hooves move better, and have less stress and strain on bones, tendons and ligaments. The ideal foot has:

- A straight hoof-pastern angle
  - A straight line from the pastern down through the front of the hoof wall.
  - This correctly lines up the bones between the pastern and coffin bone.
- Easy break over
  - The toe is not too long and is squared, rounded or rolled.
  - This allows easier movement with each step.
  - Too much break over can result in health problems.
- Adequate heel support
  - The shoe extends back to the end of the hoof wall and supports the back of the entire leg.

    - The back edge of the shoe is under a line drawn down the center of the cannon bone.
- Medial-lateral balance
    - The foot lands evenly from side to side as the horse walks.

START WITH A THOROUGH EXAMINATION

Upon entering a facility, a complete physical examination should be performed on every horse. As part of the examination, the feet should be evaluated carefully to identify any hoof wall cracks, bruises, lacerations or any other pathology that need the attention of the farrier or veterinarian. Any history of disease should be addressed at this time to help facilitate proper shoeing for the horse.

SPECIAL CONSIDERATIONS

Horses entering retirement/rescue facilities come in all shapes and sizes and often require the involvement of the veterinarian and the farrier to address hoof concerns specific for individual horses. For example, retired racehorses are shod in aluminum shoes with toe grabs; American Saddlebred horses may have been shod in stacks of pads.

For retired horses, it may be best to remove these shoes, balance the foot according to conformation, and shoe him, or trim him and leave him barefoot, according to his individual needs.

Some other items to consider are:

1. Hoof Wall Cracks/Quarter Cracks: A farrier should evaluate and address the crack for infection, necrotic tissue and, most importantly, stability. Stability of a hoof wall crack is necessary for the crack to heal, and for normal hoof growth to resume.
2. Navicular Disease: If history exists or a diagnosis is made, veterinarian and farrier involvement is necessary to facilitate the comfort and shoeing needs of the horse.
3. Laminitis: Accurate diagnosis, which may require radiographs, is necessary to determine the shoeing needs of the horse. Proper shoeing, good management and nutrition all play a vital role in foot care relative to laminitis.
4. Corrective Shoeing: May sometimes be necessary depending upon injury and conformation. Consultation with a veterinarian, working in conjunction with a farrier, is recommended.
5. Environment: Hoof care can be affected by the environment in which the horse lives. Moisture can soften hooves, and can lead to thrush and other problems. Cold weather slows hoof growth. Shoeing and trimming considerations must be addressed for each horse as an individual, in light of his environmental circumstances; for example, recommendations may be different for a frozen pasture versus a rocky pasture.

6. Management: Basic horse husbandry considerations such as good nutrition, shelter and dry bedding are all important in maintaining good, healthy feet. Some people advocate the use of feed additives for healthy hoof growth; these should be considered on the advice of a veterinarian.

STRUCTURE OF THE HORSES FOOT

Coronary band

This is located at the top of the hoof and is responsible for creating horn that makes up the hoof wall.

Periople

This is the outer layer of the hoof that forms a protective covering on the hoof wall. It is responsible for regulating moisture content in the horn, secreted from the perioplic ring above the coronet.

HOOF WALL

The hoof wall is the exterior of the hoof, made from a keratin-based substance.It provides a hard protective layer around the internal parts in the foot. It takes 9-12 months for the hoof to grow from the coronary band to the toe. In order for the horn to grow correctly and form a healthy foot, the horse must be provided with a good diet and be in good health. These factors must be checked if the horn starts to become brittle and weak or if the foot looks badly formed. A feed supplement of biotin may be helpful to promote good horn growth.

Sole

This is a tough structure that provides external protection to the sensitive sole underneath. It is slightly concave and is not weight bearing.

Frog

The frog has an extruding triangular structure which extends from the heel to halfway down the foot. Its function is to absorb concussion, provide grip and be a weight-bearing surface for the foot. It also ensures that a healthy blood supply reaches the foot. The grooves along each side of the frog allow for expansion when it makes contact with the ground.

INSIDE THE HORSES FOOT

Sensitive sole

This is found underneath the pedal bone, within the insensitive sole. It produces the new cells that replace lost layers of the insensitive sole.

Digital cushion

The digital cushion is found between the pedal bone and deep flexor tendon. It is an elastic, fibrous pad that absorbs concussion from ground impact. It also helps to push blood back up the leg.

Lateral cartilages

These are attached to the pedal bone and serve to protect the coffin joint. They also help absorb concussion.

Laminae

The insensitive laminae are supportive structures that attach to the hoof wall and interlock with the sensitive laminae. The sensitive laminae then attach and support the pedal bone. The divide between sensitive and insensitive laminae can been seen as a white line on the sole of the foot.

Conformation

This is extremely important, as the feet are obviously essential to the horse. They should be even and round in shape and in proportion with the rest of the horse. The fronts should be of equal size and shape and so should the hinds.

The front feet should slope forwards and be at a 45 degree angle to the ground, and on through the fetlock and pastern. The hind feet should be at an angle of 50-55 degrees to the ground. The hoof wall should be smooth and free from cracks. Any lines could indicate poor nutrition or past cases of laminitis.

Poor conformation in the feet can result in strains to tendons and ligaments, tripping and bruising. Many foot conformational faults can be improved by a good farrier and over a period of time.

COMMON AILMENTS IN HORSES FEET

In most cases of lameness, the cause is usually found in the foot.

Bruised soles

These are caused by an injury to the sole of the foot, usually by standing on a hard object or concussion from hard ground. They can also be due to poor trimming or shoeing.

Symptoms are acute lameness that gets progressively worse, red or bruised areas seen on the sole, and reaction to pressure on the sole due to pain.

The treatment is to restrict movement and keep on a soft surface – a deep bed in a stable, sand school or woodchip area until sound. If in severe pain, call the vet who may prescribe anti-inflammatory drugs and check for any infection.

Thrush

This is caused by continuous exposure to a damp environment without sufficient care and attention to the feet, such as poor stable management, wet or damp bedding, and wet, muddy fields. It is a bacterial infection and if left untreated, it can move to the sensitive, internal structures in the foot. Symptoms are a black, smelly discharge around the frog, and possibly lameness if severe.

The treatment is to scrub out the foot and apply eucalyptus oil (available from most chemists) repeatedly along the grooves of the frog until it clears. The farrier should trim the sides of the frog to remove any damaged tissue. If there is infection and lameness call the vet and follow the advice – it may need poulticing.

To prevent thrush, keep the feet clean, scrub them out and apply eucalyptus oil at least once a week during the winter, and when necessary in the summer. Make sure that there is a dry area in the field, for example hard standing, if the horse is out all the time. Make sure bedding is kept clean and dry.

Seedy toe

This is the separation at the white line. It usually starts at the toe and gradually progresses up the hoof wall. The hole becomes filled with white, dead material.

It normally occurs when the toes are allowed to become too long, but it can be a result of laminitis or of concussion on hard ground.

This condition needs to be managed by regular, correct trimming by a farrier – the hole will then grow out. Some of the tissue may need to be cut away and packed with putty. There may be an infection so, if the horse is lame, call the vet, as antibiotics may be needed. The foot may then need to be tubbed with water and Epsom salts and poulticed.

Laminitis

This is caused by several factors, but the main reason is an overload of soluble carbohydrates in the digestive system, see our Laminitis advice

Symptoms are a reluctance to move, increased digital sesamoid pulse, walking heel to toe, and leaning back onto the hind feet.

Call the vet immediately and follow the treatment plan given. Remove the horse from grass and take him into a deep bed of shavings, cardboard or sand until sound.

To prevent laminitis, a properly formulated high fibre diet is necessary with strict weight control, and regular farrier attention.

Infections in the foot (pus in the foot)

This is caused by puncture wounds, seedy toe, or bruising. It is the most common reason for lameness.

Symptoms are an extreme lameness due to the inflammation in the foot, increasing pressure against the hoof wall, causing pain. There is an increased digital sesamoid pulse in the affected hoof, and reaction to pressure on the infected site due to pain.

Call the vet, as the infection (pus) should be released from the foot by digging out the infected area. This can also be done by a farrier. The horse will be sound or at least almost sound after this procedure.

The foot will then need to be tubbed and poulticed to draw out the rest of the infection. If not treated, the leg can begin to swell and the infection can spread through the foot and burst out of the coronary band. In extreme cases the vet may prescribe antibiotics alongside practical procedures. Also, ensure that the horse is covered for tetanus, as puncture wounds are an ideal way for tetanus to enter the body.

A vet should see all puncture wounds to the foot because if they are deep enough, they can infect the pedal or navicular bone. This is a serious condition and needs surgical attention. It can cause damage to sensitive, internal structures including tendons and could cause permanent lameness.

NAIL BIND/PRICK

This is caused by the farrier putting a nail too close to the sensitive part of the foot (nail bind) or actually piercing the sensitive part of the foot (nail prick).

Symptoms are lameness after shoeing, either immediately or up to a couple of days later.

To treat it, the farrier needs to remove the nail and the foot should be tubbed and poulticed as with a foot infection. Call the vet if lameness continues, or if the farrier recommends it. Check tetanus vaccinations are up to date.

SAND/GRASS CRACKS

A sand crack starts at the coronet band and works down, whereas a grass crack runs from the ground towards the coronet band. Both are caused by poor foot conformation or condition, poor or irregular farrier attention, or an injury.

Call the farrier for treatment. The cracks can be stopped from spreading by marking a groove in the hoof wall above or below the crack, or by putting clips around the start of a grass crack. With regular, correct farriery, the cracks should grow out.

Below is a list of actions you should perform regularly to ensure optimal hoof care.

KEEP BEDDING CLEAN AND DRY

Dirty, wet bedding provides the ideal environment for bacteria to build up within the feet. This can lead to conditions such as thrush. Thrush is a bacterial infection, often caused by Fusobacterium necrophorum, which occurs in the clefts of the frog. The bacterium that is commonly involved is anaerobic, meaning it does not like oxygen. It produces a black, foul smelling discharge within the affected cleft of the frog, often making the frog soft and sore. Treatment involves moving the horse on to clean dry bedding and paring back affected tissues. Topical solutions should be applied to the area, as recommended by your vet.

PICK OUT HOOVES AT LEAST ONCE DAY

Picking out the hooves is important in many ways and provides a vital opportunity to closely inspect all of the hoof structures.

The frog should be regularly inspected for damage, cuts and conditions such as thrush. The sole should be examined for puncture wounds and stones wedged beside the frog. The wall needs to be inspected for excessive growth or wear and the white line should be checked to ensure it is free from trapped grit which may cause opportunity for an infection if left.

If your horse has been out in damp muddy conditions and then brought in to a stable, it is important to pick out the feet, not only to carry out the checks previously described but also to remove the wet mud trapped in the underside of the hoof. Should this mud be allowed to remain in place it will leave the sole and frog damp for an extended period of time, which will result in the horn structures becoming soft and not as resilient as they should be.

Furthermore, picking out your horses feet regularly allows oxygen to penetrate the underside of the hoof, reducing the risk of conditions such as thrush developing.

CHECK THE CONDITION OF THE SHOES

If shoes are fitted, assess their wear after two to three weeks (depending on the workload). If they are worn significantly, the next re-shoeing appointment should occur sooner or the workload on abrasive surfaces should be reduced. This will help to avoid shoes becoming loose or moving on the foot before the farrier's regular visit.

Shoes should also be checked daily for any movement on the foot, as when horses move freely it is possible for them to catch their shoes. Typically, horses will often catch the front shoes with their hind shoes and either lose them completely or bend one heel up. This is a problem as it is possible for the nails in the shoe to be trodden back again which may puncture the sole.

If the shoe has moved dramatically and a punctured sole is suspected, professional advice should be sought immediately as any puncture wound can be problematic. Additionally, a deep puncture within the middle area of the hoof can be potentially fatal, if not dealt with correctly.

CHECK THE HORSE'S DIGITAL PULSE

Feeling your horse's digital pulse is a very useful way of assessing conditions that may be occurring within the hooves.

This is only helpful if you know what the digital pulse feels like when all is well. Once you know what is normal for your horse you will be able to tell your veterinary surgeon or farrier when it is abnormal for your horse.

One of the best places to find the digital pulse is over the outside of the fetlock joint, slightly towards the back. Use your thumb and forefinger and apply gentle pressure. A horse's pulse is slow at rest and often the fingers are moved away too quickly so make sure you wait patiently to feel the pulse.

FARRIER

Great care must be taken when selecting a farrier, so ask your vet for recommendations. Correct trimming and shoeing is vital to the horse's welfare, and any mistakes can lead to serious, lasting damage.

The horse's feet should be correctly balanced whether shod or unshod. Balance is important as inaccuracy can lead to lameness and aggravate navicular syndrome and laminitis. It can affect the whole movement and development of the horse and cause ongoing problems.

Shoes are not always needed. It depends on the amount and type of work the horse is doing. Sometimes only front shoes may be needed. The farrier will be able to advise on the best option for the individual horse.

Checklist

- Always check the horse's feet after the farrier has visited
- The horse should be sound. If he is even slightly lame or lame a few days later, the farrier must be recalled immediately to address the problem.
- Check the balance of the feet. The angle should be around 45-50 degrees from the ground at the front and 50-55 degrees from the ground at the back.
- The angle through the pastern, fetlock and hoof should be 45 degrees. When viewed from the heel, with the foot raised, the sides of the foot should be level. With the foot on the ground both sides of the hoof should be of equal length.
- If shod, the shoe should fit the foot with no gaps between the shoe and the foot. The clenches should be about one third of the way up the hoof wall from the floor. They should be in a straight line and be flush with the hoof. The toe clips should also be flush with the hoof wall.
- The sole of the foot should not be touching the ground in unshod horses.

The sides of the frog should be trimmed. The frog should be level or slightly below the edge of the hoof wall.

If any deviations from the checklist are found, speak to your farrier. There may be a reason for this, such as correction of conformational defects, but the feet may need to be re-checked.

COMMON HOOF PROBLEMS

Poor shoeing or trimming

- Long toes and collapsed heels
  - Strains flexor tendons and the navicular bone
- Short toes and long heels
  - Cause trauma to the coffin bone and joint
- Imbalanced hooves
  - Causes stress on supporting ligaments and joints

HOOF CRACKS

Causes

- Dry weather, or frequent changes from wet to dry
- Drawn-out trimming intervals and long toes
- Poor hoof quality, some horses may be born with it

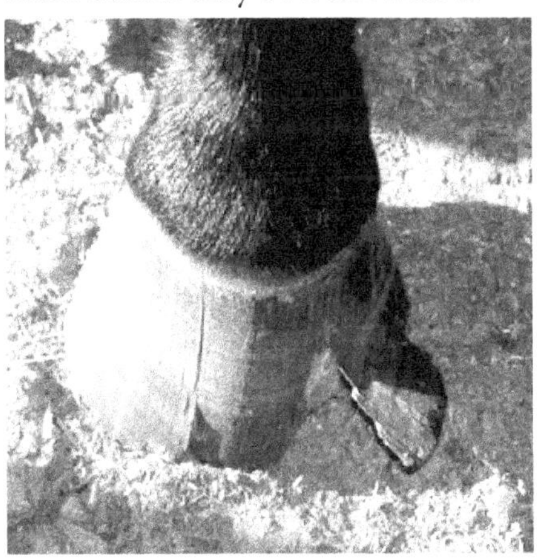

Fig. 1 Horse hoof blowout crack caused by long trimming interval.

Treatment tips

- Apply hoof moisturizers to the hoof wall and sole during:
  - Dry weather
  - Periods of brittle or cracking hooves

- Provide good nutrition and commercially available hoof supplements to improve hoof quality
- Regularly trim your horse's hooves

Types of hoof cracks

Horizontal cracks and blowouts

Horizontal cracks and blowouts occur following injury to the coronary band or blow to the hoof wall. This hoof problem generally doesn't cause lameness.

Grass cracks

Grass cracks commonly occur in horses with long, unshod hooves Trimming and shoeing can correct these cracks.

Sand cracks

Sand cracks result from injury to the coronary band or white line disease that breaks out at the coronary band. Sand crack may result in lameness.

Treatments can include:

- Determining the cause of the cracks and removing it
- Floating the hoof wall (not letting it bear weight)
- Patching the crack

It usually takes nine to 12 months for a horse's hoof to grow out.

THRUSH

Thrush is a foul-smelling black oozy liquid around the frog. Thrush occurs in wet, soiled conditions. Thrush invades the sensitive tissues of the hoof and causes lameness. You can treat by keeping your stalls or barn clean and dry.

Solar abscess

A solar abscess is an infection in the sole of the hoof. Solar abscesses lead to sudden or severe lameness. Causes of solar abscess include trauma, bruising, or a foreign body.

Treatments include:

- Removing the foreign body (if possible)
  - Keeping the hoof bandaged, clean, and dry
  - Keeping the hoof bandaged, clean, and dry

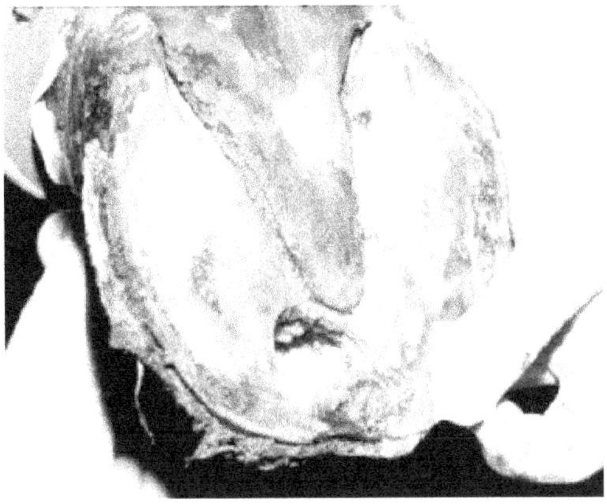

Fig. 2 Horse hoof with solar abscess.Soaking the hoof in warm water and Epsom salt

HOT NAIL

A hot nail is a horseshoe nail within a sensitive area of the horse's hoof. Hot nails will generally cause lameness.

Treatments include:

- Cleaning the nail hole with antiseptic, a wash that prevents germ growth
- Packing the hole or bandaging the foot
- Providing a Tetanus booster

STREET NAIL

A street nail is any foreign object that enters the horse's foot. Call your veterinarian immediately if your horse has a street nail. Treatment will depend on the location of the injury.

LAMINITIS AND FOUNDER

Laminitis is swelling of the sensitive laminae. The lamina is a connective tissue located inside the hoof. Swelling causes the coffin bone to rotate or sink downward within the hoof. There are several causes of laminitis.

Treatments include:

- Regular shoeing or trimming
- Keeping short toes
- Keeping frog and sole support

NAVICULAR

Navicular disease involves the navicular bone, bursa, ligamentous, and/or soft tissue structures. Horses affected by navicular will usually step toe-first because of heel pain.

Causes of navicular

- Inheritance (Quarter Horses and Thoroughbreds)
- Poor conformation
- Hoof imbalance
- Exercise on hard surfaces

Treatments

- Shoeing
- Keeping a short toe
- Elevating the heels
- Having a good break over
- Pads

NUTRITION

Nutrition can help some hoof problems

- Feed good quality hay.
- Correctly supplement vitamins and trace minerals.
- Provide constant access to fresh, clean water.
- Correct poor nutrition can lead to gradually improve hoof health.
- Cooperate with veterinarians and horse nutritionists to set up a good nutrition plan.

Research shows poor quality hooves can benefit from commercially available hoof care products that contain:

- Biotin (20 milligrams per day)
- Iodine (1 milligram per day)
- Methionine (2500 milligrams per day)
- Zinc (175 to 250 milligrams per day).

4

HORSE HEALTH AND VACCINATIONS

Horses are among the most important animals in human history; they have been used in wars, as a means of transport, and even facilitated work in mines. In the late 19th century, horses played a crucial part in developing the first antidote to cure diphtheria. Since then, the rate of contact between domesticated horses and humans steadily increased. Nowadays, for example, horses play an important role in animal-assisted therapy. Furthermore, the detection of infectious diseases that affect both humans and horses are crucial, especially in cases of highly transmissible diseases. Beside infectious diseases, non-communicable diseases (NCDs) such as skeletal and joint diseases or metabolic disorders are of concern to both. Several risk factors concerning the health of humans and horses exist. Therefore, this article will give an overview of OH with a focus on horses and their relation to the environment and humans, along with the influence of other factors such as climate change.

The goal of vaccination is to develop and maintain both individual and herd immunity against infectious diseases. Commercial vaccines are available for rabies, encephalomyelitis (Eastern, Western, and Venezuelan), tetanus, influenza, equine herpesviruses 1 and 4, botulism, equine ehrlichiosis (Potomac horse fever), equine viral arteritis, rotavirus, West Nile virus, and *Streptococcus equi* (strangles). Vaccination programs are formulated based on the animal's age, use, and level of exposure. Broodmare vaccination is important to provide active immunity for the mare and passive immunity for the foal via transfer of colostral antibodies. Vaccination guidelines for foals have been modified because of the interference of maternal antibodies with the initial vaccination response.

Routine vaccination is a critical component of developing a health maintenance program for horses. It is important to emphasize that there is no standard vaccination program that is suitable for every horse, and that individual programs should be developed with your veterinarian. Vaccinations help to prime the immune system to respond quickly when a horse is exposed to an infectious agent. Although vaccinations cannot guarantee disease prevention in all circumstances, they help minimize the risk of infection and aid in the prevention of certain diseases. Vaccination is not a substitute for other good management practices, and should be used in conjunction with proper nutrition, deworming, pasture management and minimizing stress and overcrowding for optimal results in each horse and herd. Ideally, all horses in a group should receive vaccinations and be on the same schedule when possible.

The vaccination program appropriate for an individual horse or herd needs to take into account things such as age, sex, geographic location, use of the horse, pregnancy status and risk for developing the disease. Currently, there are vaccines available for Tetanus, Encephalomyelitis, West Nile Virus, Rabies, Rhinopneumonitis (Equine Herpes Virus), Influenza, Strangles, Potomac Horse Fever, Botulism, Equine Viral Arteritis, Anthrax, and Rotavirus. The vaccines are administered by an intramuscular or intranasal route depending on the disease. Influenza and Strangles have both intramuscular and intranasal vaccines available. Adverse reactions to vaccination are not common but are a potential risk of vaccination. Signs of an adverse reaction may include muscle soreness, swelling, fever, anorexia, and lethargy. If the signs are severe or are not self-limiting, your veterinarian should be informed and may want to initiate additional therapy.

When considering a vaccination program for your horse, it is important to remember that each horse's immune system will respond a little differently to vaccination. Not every horse will be protected exactly the same or for the same amount of time following vaccination. A primary series of the vaccines with booster doses will be required for an appropriate immune response before exposure to the disease. It will take 1-2 weeks after a completed vaccine series for your horse to be protected against the disease. After the initial vaccine series, most horses will require annual or semi-annual booster vaccinations.

The following vaccination recommendations assume that foals are born to vaccinated mares and have absorbed adequate colostral antibodies with IgG levels >800 mg/dL.

Foals with failure of passive antibody transfer (ie, IgG levels <200 mg/dL) and/or foals born to unvaccinated mares can receive their initial vaccination for equine herpesvirus 1 and 4, tetanus, and Eastern and Western equine encephalomyelitis beginning at 3–4 mo of age, followed by a second dose 4–6 wk later and a third dose at 10–12 mo of age. These foals can receive their first dose of rabies vaccine at 3–4 mo of age, followed by a booster at 12 mo. Influenza vaccination can be started at 6 mo of age. Foals born to mares that have never been exposed to or vaccinated against West Nile virus can receive their first vaccination at 3–5 mo of age.

TETANUS

Clostridium tetani is present in all parts of the world. Tetanus occurs most commonly when wounds become contaminated with the organism from the soil. Vaccination is recommended for all horses and ponies on an annual basis. A horse with an unknown vaccination status that sustains an injury should receive a dose of tetanus antitoxin along with a dose of tetanus toxoid. A second dose of toxoid should be given 4 wk later. Foals from vaccinated mares should be given a three-dose series at 7 ,6, and 9 mo of age. Foals from unvaccinated mares should receive tetanus toxoid at 4 ,3, and 6 mo of age. Whenever a vaccinated horse experiences a serious wound, a tetanus booster may be indicated.

EQUINE HERPESVIRUS 1 AND 4 (RHINOPNEUMONITIS):

Two types of equine herpesviruses vaccine are available, EHV-1 and EHV-4. The EHV-1 virus is the primary cause of abortion and neurologic disease in horses. The EHV-4 virus is the primary cause of respiratory infections, especially in young horses. The control of rhinopneumonitis is by a combination of vaccination and good management practices. To prevent abortion, a killed EHV-1 vaccine should be administered to pregnant mares at 3, 5, 7, and 9 mo of gestation. Respiratory disease is best prevented using a combination vaccine of EHV-1 and EHV-4. There is no evidence that vaccination protects against the neurologic form of the disease. Vaccine recommendations for foals are three doses every 4 wk starting at 6 mo of age, and a booster at 1 yr of age. Pleasure and performance horses should be vaccinated every 3–6 mo, depending on the risk of exposure. Broodmares should have an EHV-4 vaccination 2–4 wk before foaling to ensure the availability of colostral immunity.

ENCEPHALITIS

Eastern equine encephalitis (EEE) virus has a wide distribution. This includes the eastern USA, Central and South America, and eastern Canada. In the USA, EEE is seen primarily in the southeastern states but has been reported in all states east of the Mississippi River. EEE in horses is nearly always fatal regardless of treatment. Infected horses usually become comatose, seizure, and die in 36–48 hr.

The virus of Western equine encephalitis (WEE) is primarily located in the western USA. In recent years, reports of WEE have not been common, probably as a result of adequate vaccination programs. The virus is not as pathogenic as EEE, and animals infected with WEE have a greater chance of survival. Mortality is usually 50%.

Venezuelan equine encephalitis (VEE) virus causes outbreaks of disease in horses in Mexico, Central and South America, and occasionally the southern USA. The VEE vaccine is a single vaccine or in combination with EEE and WEE. Its need is limited to those horses traveling to or located in endemic areas.

West Nile virus (WNV) disease is considered a zoonotic disease similar to the encephalitis viruses. The bird population allows for maintenance of the virus, which is then transmitted by mosquitoes to both people and horses. There is very little risk of disease from any infected horses. Vaccination protocols for broodmares, foals, and adult horses are the same as those for Eastern and Western encephalitis. Combination vaccines that include EEE, WEE, and WNV are available.

INFLUENZA

Influenza is one of the most frequent causes of viral respiratory disease in horses and is highly contagious among susceptible horses. Therefore, vaccination is recommended for all foals, broodmares, and horses at risk of exposure, usually as a result of showing, racing, or shipping. Young foals from vaccinated mares, because of maternal antibodies, should be vaccinated at 9, 10, and 12 mo of age. Foals from unvaccinated mares should be vaccinated earlier. The intranasal vaccine can be used every 6 mo in young, susceptible performance horses 2–4 yr old. A vaccination is recommended every 6 mo for horses exposed to other horses at equine events.

RABIES

Signs of rabies include the inability to eat or drink, disorientation, and incoordination. Rabies is fatal, and also poses a health risk to those who handle infected horses. Prevention in horses is primarily via vaccination. Broodmares should be vaccinated 4–6 wk before foaling. Foals from vaccinated mares should be vaccinated at 6 and 7 mo of age and again at 12 mo of age. Foals from unvaccinated mares should be vaccinated at 3, 4, and 12 mo of age. All adult horses should be vaccinated annually.

POTOMAC HORSE FEVER

Potomac horse fever (equine monocytic ehrlichiosis, equine ehrlichial colitis) is caused by *Neorickettsia risticii*. Vaccination is recommended in endemic areas, such as near freshwater streams, rivers, ponds, and heavily irrigated pastures. Annual boosters in the spring are recommended. Pregnant mares should receive a booster before foaling. Although the vaccine may lessen the impact of the disease, it appears not to prevent abortion in pregnant mares.

BOTULISM

Equine botulism is mostly seen in the Mid-Atlantic area of the United States, but the disease has also been reported worldwide. In the USA, the most common types are B and C botulism, although type A has been reported in the western USA. The spores of *Colostridium botulinum* are found in the soil and are resistant to light, drying, and heat. The Type B vaccine gives good protection in adult horses. Adult horses and broodmares in areas where botulism is a potential hazard should receive initially three doses at -30day intervals and then annual boosters. Foals from vaccinated mares in endemic areas should be vaccinated at 3 ,2, and 4 mo of age, because colostral immunity does not always occur. Foals from unvaccinated mares should be vaccinated at 4 ,2, and 8 wk of age. The use of Type B vaccine in areas where Type C occurs has uncertain results.

STREPTOCOCCUS EQUI INFECTION

Streptococcus equi infection (equine strangles, equine distemper) can be highly contagious. Use of the IM or intranasal vaccine is recommended only in those situations or on premises where the disease has been a problem. The IM vaccine involves three injections administered 2–4 wk apart, starting at 4 mo of age in foals, with a booster at 12 mo of age. If the intranasal vaccine is used, vaccination can begin at 6–9 mo of age, with a second dose given 3–4 wk later and a third dose administered at 12 mo of age. Adult horses, if in potential disease situations, should receive an annual vaccination. Broodmares on endemic farms should receive an annual booster using the IM vaccine 4–6 wk before foaling. Because of the increased risk of inducing immune-mediated purpura hemorrhagica, horses with titers to the SeM surface protein of S equi in excess of 1:1,600 may not need to be vaccinated.

ROTAVIRUS

Foal diarrhea as a result of rotavirus infection can be a severe problem on some breeding farms. Single cases or a farm outbreak can occur. Therefore, pregnant mares should be vaccinated IM at 8, 9, and 10 mo of gestation. This will increase the amount of colostral immunoglobulins. It is a vaccine for use in particular situations or areas of high endemicity.

EQUINE INFECTIOUS ANEMIA

In the acute state, equine infectious anemia (swamp fever) causes severe RBC destruction and anemia. Once infected, a horse can become a carrier for life and is a threat to other horses. The virus is transmitted by bloodsucking insects. Currently, the disease is uncommon, and most horse owners are aware of its dire consequences. A simple blood test, the Coggins test, is available to detect infected horses. A horse that tests positive cannot cross state lines and is required to be maintained in strict isolation for life. For horses participating in equine activities or being transported across state lines, proof of a negative Coggins test is required. Annual testing of every horse is recommended. No vaccine is available.

PERINATAL MARE AND FOAL CARE

Horse producers face many decisions that require them to understand the foaling process and the needs of newborn foals.

Parturition in the Mare Gestation Length

The normal gestation length of mares ranges from 320 to 380 days with an average of 338 to 345 days. Gestation length will be variable between mares and even the same mare from year to year. Gestation lengths shorter than 320 generally are considered premature and there is an expected need for veterinarian neonatal care procedures. Seasonal factors can impact gestational length. Mares foaling during long day lengths typically tend to have a shortened gestation, while mares foaling during shorter days have a longer gestation. All fetuses are not necessarily mature 320 days from the last breeding. As such, gestational length alone is not an adequate means of determining fetal readiness for birth.

Gestation lengths as long as 365 are not entirely uncommon; however, longer gestations may be a sign of impending foaling problems. For instance, extended gestation length is one of the problems associated with mares consuming endophyte-infected fescue hay or pasture.

Predicting Day of Foaling

The accuracy of breeding records leads to increased accuracy in predicted foaling dates. A predictor of 335 days (11 months) after the last breeding date is used frequently. The 335 days is actually shorter than the expected average, and as such, will allow for an increased watch before most mares will foal.

There are several conformational changes that indicate a mare is approaching the day of parturition (Table 1). These signs are variable between mares and will change with successive pregnancies. Mammary development and colostrum production in the mare are reliable indicators of fetal maturity and readiness for birth. The calcium concentration of mammary secretions in a majority of mares will increase significantly 1 or 2 days before foaling. Mares with mammary secretion of calcium concentrations greater than 200 ppm have a 54 percent probability of foaling within 24 hours, 84 percent probability of foaling within 48 hours and 97 percent probability of foaling within 72 hours. Most mares foal within a short period of time if the mammary secretion calcium increases to levels between 300 and 500 ppm. Mares with mammary secretion calcium levels lower than 200 ppm have a less than 1 percent chance of foaling within 24 hours of testing. This response can be quantified with testing kits developed specifically for mare's milk, which are available through veterinarians. Water hardness test strips have also been used.

Preparing the Mare for Foaling

Recommended procedures to prepare a mare to foal vary. Mares on rangeland will foal without any human intervention. Conversely, intensive monitoring and assistance are routine at neonatal clinics for newborn foals at major equine hospitals, and farms specializing in critical care of foals have foaling teams and special facilities. The vast majority of mares receive some type of preparation between these two extremes.

If not housed on the farm where she will foal, the mare should be moved to the location one month prior to the expected foaling date and isolated from resident mares. This will allow the mare to become accustomed to her new surroundings and develop location specific disease immunity before the stress of foaling. The foaling location should provide protection, natural or otherwise, from wet, cold weather and predators. Foaling mares are housed separately from other horses. Mares should be moved into foaling areas within several days to a week before the expected foaling day. If the mare does not foal within 2 to 3 days after being placed in a foaling stall, she should be walked daily to keep her muscles toned and prevent fluid buildup along the limbs and abdomen.

Mares pastured with access to fungus-infected fescue or fed fungus-infected fescue hay should have all fescue access removed 45 to 60 days prior to foaling. Mares with continued access will have a significant chance of prolonged gestation, low milk production and foaling problems. Drug therapies for prevention and treatment of fescue toxicosis are available from veterinarians.

Foaling paddocks, foaling sheds and foaling stalls have been used successfully. The covered areas in paddocks or stalls should provide a minimum of 200 square feet space for normally sized stock horses, although larger areas are preferred (16' X 16', 20' X 20'). Clean, large particle bedding such as green grass in paddocks or straw in stalls is desirable. Smaller particle bedding such as shavings may collect along the newborns nostrils. Cleanliness of the foaling area reduces mare and foal disease, so complete stripping of bedding material between foalings and use of disinfectants and cleaners approved by the attending veterinarian are essential. This is an increased need as compared to standard cleaning practices on-farm.

The general preparation of the mare, excluding vaccinations and standard health practices as recommended by the veterinarian, includes cleaning the mare's body, washing the perineal and mammary gland areas, and wrapping the upper half of the tail. If the mare has had a Caslicks procedure performed in the past, it must be opened before she foals, preferably approaching or at the time she enters the foaling stall.

Consult your veterinarian if a mare appears to be leaking an excessive amount of milk prior to birth, as it may be a sign of an impending abortion. Generally, this pre-foaling milk is not typically colostrum-rich. However, depending on your veterinarian's recommendation, the mare may be milked and the colostrum frozen to give to the foal shortly after birth. Without it, the foal is at an increased risk of infections. This early milk can be tested to determine whether or not it is rich in antibodies. Foals not receiving adequate transfer of antibodies from colostrum at birth may need veterinarian prescribed plasma transfers to boost their immunity. Therefore, it is important to locate a back-up supply for orphan foals or mares without an adequate supply of colostrum.

HEALTH PROGRAMS FOR THE FOALING MARE

Recommendations for which vaccines are needed and frequency of administration are influenced by factors such as geographical location and number of animals routinely arriving and departing from the farm. Owners must consult with their local veterinarian to develop vaccination schedules that will incorporate all the vaccines needed and administration times that will best maintain immunity for their specific operation. Recommended vaccinations typically include tetanus toxoid, encephalomyelitis, West Nile Virus, Influenza, Rhinopneumonitis, and possibly, Strangles and Rotavirus A. Several of these vaccines require multiple doses. The timing of vaccination is important as late gestation vaccinations will aid in the transfer of protection to the foal via the mare's milk. Schedules to administer vaccinations should be developed with your attending veterinarian's advice.

Recommendations on the types and administration of deworming drugs will also vary because of factors such as geographical location and stocking densities. Consult your veterinarian for the specific needs before starting a deworming program for pregnant mares. In general, deworming is recommendable every 2 to 3 months during pregnancy. Most anthelmintics are safe to use in pregnant mares, but be sure to read product labels! For example, organophosphates should not be used in late gestation and it may be prudent to avoid their use at all during pregnancy. Deworming the mare 1 to 2 days after foaling reduces the likelihood of transmission of Strongyloides westeri through the milk.

Foaling Process

Mare behavior will gradually change during the weeks preceding foaling. They usually show signs that they will soon go into labor. The timetable though is far from being absolute. Some mares may show all the signs, while others may show just a few and will be in labor before you expect it.

Labor is divided into three stages

Stage one begins with the onset of contractions and generally lasts 1 to 2 hours. During this time the mare becomes anxious and restless. She may appear to be colicky. She may kick at her belly, pace, lie down and get up, look or bite at her flanks, and sweat. She may frequently raise her tail and urinate. Generally, this is the first stage of labor. However, be aware that colic remains a possibility. Contact your veterinarian if such behavior is prolonged for more than an hour or two without progress towards foaling.

Mares may exhibit some of these signs periodically for several days before they actually progress into the foaling process. Most mares will foal at night and prefer, if not require, a quiet, dark place to foal without disruptions. Even though it is advised by most veterinarians to keep a frequent watch on mares approaching the foaling time, disruptions can delay the onset of this stage of labor. Watch systems that emphasize a quiet, dark, uninterrupted environment will help the mare.

During this phase of labor, contractions move the foal through the cervix and into position in the birth canal. The fetal membranes, Chorioallantois, may become visible at the mare's vulva. Stage one ends when the amniotic sac breaks, which is signaled by a rush of fluid.

Stage two is the actual expulsion of the foal. This phase moves relatively quickly and usually occurs within 15 to 20 minutes after the mare's 'water breaks.' Taking more than 30 minutes to deliver may indicate a need for intervention from qualified attendants. If labor seems to be progressing, wait and watch. Even in a normal delivery, the mare may stand up, lie down and roll several times in an effort to properly position the foal for delivery.

Normal presentation of the foal resembles a diving position, the front feet first, one slightly ahead of the other, hooves down, followed closely by the nose, head, neck, shoulders and hindquarters. If you notice hoof soles up, the foal may be backwards or upside down and you should call your veterinarian immediately. It is important that the presentation of the foal is correct, and that qualified assistance be provided if delivery presentation is abnormal. The mare will remain lying down for several minutes following foaling.

Stage three labor begins after delivery and is the phase during which the afterbirth, placenta, is expelled. Most placentas are passed within 1 to 3 hours after the foal is delivered. Call your veterinarian if the placenta has not passed within 3 hours. A retained placenta can cause serious problems, including massive infection and laminitis. A knowledgeable person should inspect the placenta to insure it was completely expelled and to check for other abnormalities that indicate a potential problem with the foal.

THE FOAL

The Newborn

The mare and foal will remain lying down for several minutes following foaling. The umbilical cord is usually still intact and blood continues to flow from the mare to the foal. The foal will move its head and body within minutes after birth. The umbilical cord should break as a result of this movement. If the umbilical cord is not broken within a few minutes after birth and has stopped pulsing, it may need to be broken by hand. The cord should break at a site approximately one inch from the foal's abdomen, where the cord's diameter is slightly narrower than the remainder of the cord. If it is necessary to manually separate the cord, it should be held firmly on either side of the intended break site, then twisted and pulled to separate. Never cut the cord, as twisting and pulling of the cord stimulate closure of the umbilical vessels and reduce the likelihood of bleeding from the cord stump. If bleeding persists following cord separation, pressure can be applied to the stump for several minutes by squeezing with a thumb and finger.

Foals should make attempts to rise within 30 minutes after birth. Nursing should occur soon after standing, usually within half an hour to an hour and a half. Nursing is important, as the first milk contains antibodies that develop the foal's immune system. If the foal has not nursed within 3 hours, the foal may be weak and in need of assistance or medical attention. Delayed nursing past 8 to 12 hours after birth impairs the transfer of antibodies from the mare to the foal, which puts the foal at risk of not being able to ward off infections. The foal's serum can be tested at 12 to 24 hours of age to evaluate IgG antibody levels. Treatments for low antibody levels include administration of colostrum, plasma immune products and plasma transfers.

The meconium or 'first feces' should be passed within the first 8 to 12 hours after birth. Most foals will also urinate within the first several hours of birth. The foal will lie down frequently the first several hours after birth and will sleep for short periods of time.

Recommendations for assisting the newborn foal varies; however, most veterinarians suggest avoiding help unless necessary for the health of the mare or foal. The decision to assist should be guided from an experienced individual, and a qualified person should conduct the assistance. Too much or unnecessary assistance may increase stress in the mare or foal, may be counterproductive to the health of the mare or foal, and as mares are naturally protective, can be dangerous. Several checks are routine to assist decisions on intervention.

After birth, the foal's nostrils may be covered with part of the placenta or bedding. These materials need removing if they constrict respiration. If the foal appears to not be breathing, respiratory assistance will be needed to inflate the lungs. The umbilical stump is treated with disinfectant, such as tame 2 percent iodine solution or 0.5 percent chlorhexidine (Nolvasan) diluted 1 to 4 parts water, shortly after it is broken. The umbilical stump should be treated once or twice daily for the first couple of days.

The foal should have an examination within 12 to 24 hours after it is born. Procedures include an ophthalmic exam, respiratory exam and visual checks for conformational abnormalities. As mentioned above, the foal's antibody levels in the serum should be tested for IgG antibodies, which should be above 800 mg/dl.

Early life handling of foals has benefits of imprinting acceptable behaviors around people. There are several publications on the timing and routines of imprinting. These sessions begin immediately after birth.

Foals and mares should be allowed access to paddocks or pasture within a couple of days post foaling. If weather and facility constrain access to paddocks, mares should be hand walked with the foals by their sides. Mares and foals should be turned into pastures or paddocks with other lactating mares within several days to a week after foaling.

The Nursing Foal

Foals receive their nutrition from the mare's milk exclusively for the first several weeks to one month of age. If allowed access to their dam's grain or grain by creep feeding, foals will begin to eat small amounts of grain rations within the first month of their life. Creep feeding provides supplemental feed to foals by using feeders constructed to restrict access of mares.

Vaccination and deworming schedules should be under the supervision of your attending veterinarian. The time to begin vaccinations depends on the vaccination of the mare prior to foaling. Vaccinations given to mares the last 30 days of pregnancy will assist the protection of the foal during the first several months of life. In general, foals born to mares with current vaccinations should receive their first vaccinations at 6 to 9 months of age as vaccinations at an earlier age may interfere with the foal's immune response resulting from the antibodies received in the mare's milk. If mares are not vaccinated before foaling, foals should receive their vaccinations beginning at 3 to 4 months of age. Owners should consult with their veterinarian to refine timing of vaccinations.

Orphan Foals

Orphan foals will require milk replacement. There are several commercially developed milk replacers. Preplanning for the potential need by locating suppliers before foaling will help access a supply in an emergency. Foals can be taught to drink in buckets. Holding the bucket with milk replacer near the foal, with milk on the person's fingers can encourage the foal to begin drinking the milk. The majority of foals will drink readily from the bucket after two or three offerings. Bucket placement at the level of the foal's chest will help access. Buckets that are left for the foal to drink need to be securely attached to the stall wall. The first several feedings may require handlers to hold the bucket and/or foal. Foals drink small amounts frequently, so a small, continual supply of fresh replacer will be required. Buckets will require cleaning to remove any left over residue or milk. Most label directions suggest free choice supplies of replacement, as the foal will regulate needs. Milk 'replacer' pellets, also called 'foal pellets,' are also an option. Additionally, the use of a nurse mare may be an option if a suitably mannered mare in early lactation is available.

A soft, pelleted or extruded grain source should be offered to the orphan within several weeks following birth. Depending on consumption patterns of grain, foals may be weaned off milk replacer around 2 months of age. Housing around other horses will help reduce stress in orphans. Placement of a companion animal, such as a small goat, with an orphan has been used successively to further reduce stress in orphans.

Management of orphans should encourage moving foals into normal management and contact with other foals as quickly as possible. Contact with other foals increase the desire to consume feed and provides the orphan a companion to reduce stress. Once over 2 to 3 months of age, most orphans can be placed with other foals going through the weaning process.

Parasite Control

Establishing a deworming program for equine parasites has become a somewhat controversial topic of discussion. Due to the emergence of resistant parasites (worms that are not killed by traditional dewormers), some of the emphasis is shifting to prevention and control, rather than just routine rotational treatment with anthelmintics. The American Association of Equine Practitioners (AAEP) recommends establishing a program with your veterinarian that works best for your horse and/or herd, in conjunction with these suggestions for environmental management:

- Clean and dispose of manure in the pasture at least twice weekly.
- Mow and harrow pastures regularly to break up manure and expose parasite eggs to the sun.
- If possible, rotate pastures by allowing other livestock to graze them.
- Group horses in a pasture by age to reduce exposure to certain parasites, and maximize the deworming program geared to that group.

- Prevent overgrazing and reduce fecal contamination by keeping the number of horses per acre to a minimum.
- Feed horses in a feeder for hay and grain rather than on the ground.
- Remove bot eggs from the hair routinely to prevent ingestion

Individual horses can be monitored for parasites with a fecal examination and egg count. The peak worm season is fall, winter, and spring. Treatment should be focused around these times. The effectiveness of different dewormers can be measured using a fecal egg count reduction test, which involves performing a fecal egg count before and after deworming your horse. Although it is critical to target the large and small strongyles in adults, as well as roundworms in foals, rotation of dewormers should not be done as often as every 4-8 weeks, because this may promote resistant worms. Ideally, a dewormer can be used for several treatments prior to rotation to a new drug. It is important to remember that treatment with ivermectin is done at 2 month intervals, while moxidectin is done at 3 month intervals. Equine tapeworms are difficult to identify in fecal examinations, and deworming for tapeworms is recommended biannually or annually with a product containing praziquantel (Zimectrin Gold, Combocare, Equimax), or double dose pyrantel pamoate or tartrate. A blood test has been developed that identifies antibodies to tapeworms in horses. This test is only available at one lab in the United States at the University of Tennessee's College of Veterinary Medicine. However, there are likely horses with tapeworms that this test will not identify, and it is more practical to be sure horses are dewormed annually for tapeworms. Consult your veterinarian for a deworming strategy that works best for your horse and/or herd.

5

DISORDERS SUCH AS COLIC, LAMINITIS, AND INTERNAL PARASITES

COLIC IN HORSES

Colic is a term used to describe a symptom of abdominal (belly) pain, which in horses is usually caused by problems in the gastrointestinal tract.

There are over 70 different types of intestinal problems that cause colic symptoms, which range from mild to severe (life-threatening) in nature.

Colic is one of the most common causes of death in horses, although the prognosis today is far better than it once was. This is largely due to improvements in the way in which we diagnose and treat colic, better anaesthetic drugs and monitoring and improved surgical techniques.

Early diagnosis and surgical treatment of more serious cases of colic remains one of the most important factors in giving horses the best chance of survival following colic surgery.

Causes

Colic can be due to something as simple as a gut 'spasm' resulting from a change in diet or routine i.e., a digestive upset or as serious as twisting of a part of the intestine with consequent strangulation of its blood supply.

The more common causes include impaction (where the intestine becomes clogged with semi-digested food material), displacement of a segment of bowel from its normal position, torsion or twisting, strangulation through hernias or holes, strangulation by fatty tumors wrapping around them and other causes of obstruction.

Like humans, horses are relatively sensitive to anything causing pain within the intestine.

This might be due to intestinal spasms (cramp), the gut wall being stretched by gas or feed material, the blood supply being shut off to part of the gut or intestine becoming stuck (entrapped) somewhere abnormal.

Occasionally there are non-intestinal conditions, such as laminitis, bladder stones or ovarian problems, that may initially look like symptoms of colic. This is known as 'false colic', but may still be very serious.

Treatment

Horses with colic may or may not need surgery. Almost all horses will require some form of medical treatment, but only those with certain mechanical obstructions of the intestine need surgery. The type of treatment is determined by the cause of colic and the severity of the disease. If the horse appears to have only mild pain and the heart and circulatory system are functioning normally, the horse may be treated using medication or other nonsurgical methods and the response evaluated. Ultrasonography can be used to evaluate the effectiveness of nonsurgical treatment in some cases. If necessary, surgery can be used for diagnosis as well as treatment.

If evidence of intestinal obstruction with dry, digested food is found, the main goal of treatment is to rehydrate and remove the intestinal contents. If the horse has severe pain and has signs indicating loss of fluid from the bloodstream (high heart rate and discoloration of the mucous membranes), the initial aims of treatment are to relieve pain, restore tissue blood supply, and correct any abnormalities in the composition of the blood and body fluids (such as an abnormal pH or electrolyte level).

If damage to the intestinal wall is suspected, specific medications may be administered to prevent or counteract the ill effects of bacterial toxins (called endotoxins) that leave the intestine and enter the bloodstream. If there is evidence that the colic episode is caused by parasites, one of the first goals of treatment would be to eliminate the parasites.

Pain Relief

Pain is mild in most cases of colic, and pain medication is all that is needed. This is the usual treatment if the cause of colic is believed to be a spasm of intestinal muscle or excessive gas in a portion of the intestine. If the pain is due to a more serious condition, such as an intestinal twist or displacement, some of the stronger pain medications may mask the signs that would be useful in making a diagnosis. For these reasons, whenever possible a thorough physical examination is performed before any medications are given. However, because horses with severe colic or pain may hurt themselves and become dangerous to people nearby, pain medication often must be given first. In addition, many horses with less severe problems may need pain relief until the other treatments have time to be effective.

Your veterinarian will chose a pain reliever that is least likely to cause side effects or changes in the horse's attitude. Examples include anti-inflammatory drugs, sedatives that also reduce pain, and narcotics. Although pain relief usually is provided by medications, pain can be reduced in other ways. For example, the veterinarian's use of a stomach tube during diagnosis will also remove any fluid that has accumulated in the stomach because of an obstruction of the small intestine. The removal of this fluid not only relieves pain caused by distention of the stomach but also prevents rupture of the stomach.

Fluid Treatment

Many horses with colic benefit from fluid treatment to prevent dehydration and maintain blood supply to the kidneys and other vital organs. The fluids may be given either through a stomach tube or intravenous catheter, depending on the particular intestinal problem. Intravenous fluids may be needed for several days until intestinal function has returned, blood electrolyte (salt) concentrations are balanced, and the horse can maintain its fluid needs by drinking.

Protection against Bacterial Endotoxins

Endotoxins are a part of the outer coating of certain bacteria. Endotoxins are released when the bacteria die or multiply rapidly. Normally, endotoxins are contained within the intestines, but if the intestinal lining is damaged, they can escape into the abdominal cavity or bloodstream. Endotoxins then trigger an inflammatory response (commonly called endotoxemia) that can include fever, depression, reduced blood pressure, impaired blood circulation, blood clotting abnormalities, and eventually death. One treatment is administration of antibodies or medications designed to neutralize the endotoxin. The effectiveness of this treatment is still being studied, with some studies finding a benefit and others that do not. Other treatments include anti-inflammatory medications and certain antibiotics. In cases of colic, your veterinarian will be on the alert for damage to the intestinal lining and the possibility of complications due to endotoxins.

Intestinal Lubricants and Laxatives

A common cause of colic in horses is obstruction of the large intestine by dried digested food, sometimes mixed with sand. In most instances, lubricants or fecal-softening agents given through a stomach tube soften the impacted material, allowing it to be passed. Intravenous fluids are often given during this procedure. The horse will normally need to be muzzled to prevent further impaction of feed while the obstruction is softening. Medications include mineral oil, dioctyl sodium sulfosuccinate (a soap-like compound), and psyllium hydrophilic mucilloid (an ingredient also found in some fiber products used by humans). When mixed with water, psyllium forms a gelatin-like mass that carries ingested food along the digestive tract. Horses that live in a sandy environment or that persistently develop impactions may be given psyllium powder in their feed, as directed by a veterinarian, to help prevent impaction.

Strong laxatives that stimulate intestinal contractions are not commonly used to treat impactions and, in fact, may worsen the problem. If an impaction does not start to break down within 3 to 5 days, surgery may be necessary to remove the impacted material.

Deworming Treatments

The larvae of large bloodworms, especially *Strongylus vulgaris*, can cause colic by interfering with the flow of blood to the intestines. The routine use of deworming medications has reduced the occurrence of this once-common type of colic. Intestinal damage caused by the larvae of small strongyles may also cause colic, diarrhea, and loss of condition, especially in young horses. Infections with the intestinal tapeworm *Anoplocephala perfoliata* are also associated with intestinal impactions. Horses with parasite infections are treated with deworming medications. Complications, such as pain or intestinal obstruction, must also be treated appropriately.

However, intestinal impactions can occasionally occur after the administration of deworming medication, especially in young horses with an inadequate history of deworming. This occurs when deworming drugs that are highly effective against *Parascaris equorum* cause a mass of paralyzed worms to obstruct the small intestine. Some affected horses may respond to medical treatment (fluids and intestinal lubricants), whereas others may require surgery to relieve the impaction. Your veterinarian can recommend an appropriate deworming program to minimize the likelihood of this occurring in other horses on the same property.

Surgery

Usually, surgery is necessary if there is a mechanical obstruction that cannot be corrected medically or if the obstruction also interferes with the intestinal blood supply. The latter condition causes death of the horse unless surgery is performed quickly. Occasionally, surgery is needed to diagnose the problem in horses with longterm colic that have not responded to routine medical treatment.

Horses with severe pain that do not respond to pain medications usually require surgery. However, some horses with mild or moderate pain may also require surgery, a judgement your veterinarian will make based on the physical examination.

Some of the common indications for surgery in horses with colic include:

- uncontrollable pain
- more than 4 liters of fluid retrieved from the stomach tube
- no intestinal sounds heard with a stethoscope
- abnormalities within a fluid sample from the abdomen
- evidence of an intestinal obstruction or displacement identified on rectal examination

If surgery is indicated, it is critical to perform it promptly to ensure the best chance of success and survival. This usually requires referral to an equine surgeon at a properly equipped facility. Depending on the cause and the extent of the damage, care after the surgery may include intravenous fluids, antibiotics, antibodies against endotoxin, anti-inflammatory drugs, or other medications. Each horse is individually treated based on its response to surgery and the development of any complications.

Outcomes for Colic

The survival rate for horses that undergo surgery to treat colic ranges from 50% to more than 80%. Your veterinarian can provide insight into the possible outcome for your horse based on physical examination findings. In general, survival rates are highest for horses with mild abdominal pain and are lowest for horses with severe pain. Horses with distended intestines, lack of abdominal sounds, red mucous membrane color, or impaired cardiovascular function (such as low blood pressure) tend to do worse than those without these signs.

Specific Causes of Colic and their Treatment

Colic can be caused by several disorders of the stomach and intestines. The most common ones are discussed here.

Distention and Rupture of the Stomach

Excessive gas or intestinal obstruction can lead to distention of the stomach. This may also be caused by overeating fermentable feeds such as grains, lush grass, or beet pulp. If untreated, this can rapidly progress to a rupture of the stomach. Signs include severe abdominal pain, increased heart rate, and retching. Once the stomach ruptures, the horse may act relieved or depressed. The outlook for survival is often excellent if the condition is recognized and treated soon enough, but stomach rupture is fatal.

Obstruction of the Small or Large Intestine

Signs of colic may occur if the small or large intestine is obstructed. The outlook depends on the location and can worsen if treatment is delayed, so rapid diagnosis and treatment are critical.

The most common condition that causes obstruction of the small intestine is impaction (blockage of the intestine by food or other materials that have been eaten). It has been linked to eating Coastal Bermuda hay and infection by the tapeworm *Anoplocephala perfoliata*. Young horses may be affected by impaction of the small intestine with ascarid parasites following deworming. Intussusceptions (a telescoping of a section of the intestine within an adjacent section) can also cause small intestinal obstructions, especially in horses younger than 3 years old. In the large intestine, the underlying cause of obstruction is not always known but has also been linked to coarse feed, insufficient water intake, and diseased teeth. In some areas sand may be the cause of intestinal obstruction and colic. This is especially true if there is not enough pasture and the horse is fed on the ground. The sand may accumulate in the large intestine and eventually cause a blockage. Morgan, Arabian, and Appaloosa horses may have a higher risk of impaction of the cecum compared with other breeds. Impactions also may develop because of other intestinal diseases or occur after prolonged hospitalization. Impactions within the cecum tend to occur in horses older than 8 years.

Signs in horses with impaction of the small intestine include mild to severe abdominal pain, reduced intestinal sounds, stomach reflux, and increased heart rate. Because the horse's condition may remain stable and the pain may be mild at first, many horses with this condition are not immediately referred for surgery. The condition often requires surgery, although it may respond to treatment with fluids, pain-relieving drugs, and mineral oil if identified early. A lack of normal intestinal contractions may occur after surgery. Adhesions within the abdomen are another potential complication.

In contrast, horses with impaction of the large intestine may display more mild signs and do not usually require surgery. Almost all respond well to administration of laxatives, fluids, and pain medications. If the obstruction occurs in the descending colon, however, surgery is often necessary. The outlook for horses with impactions of the large colon is excellent, with more than 95% of horses surviving the condition. For horses with impactions of the cecum, the survival rate ranges from 60% to 80% depending on whether they are treated medically or surgically.

Adhesions

Adhesions are fibrous connections between organs within the abdomen. They generally affect the small intestine. Adhesions develop in response to abdominal injury such as surgery, longterm distention of the intestine, inflammation, or migration of larval parasites. They can squeeze or kink the intestines, leading to an obstruction. Signs range from mild, recurrent colic to severe, continual pain. Treatment involves surgery to remove the fibrous tissue and the affected portion of the intestine. Medications are also given to try to reduce the formation of new adhesions. However, adhesions often recur and the longterm outlook for horses with extensive adhesions is poor.

Inflammation of the Small Intestine

Inflammation of the first part of the small intestine is a poorly understood condition of horses. The condition has several names, including proximal enteritis–jejunitis, anterior enteritis, and duodenitis–jejunitis. It has been reported in the southeastern and northeastern US as well as in England and continental Europe. There may be fluid or bleeding within the intestinal wall, or tissue death in more severe cases. The condition was more common in the United States in the 1980s but occurs less frequently and less severely now.

Varying degrees of abdominal pain are the most common sign of the disorder. Treatment may be either medical (such as placing a stomach tube and administering fluids, pain medication, and other drugs) or surgical. About half of the cases are fatal. Laminitis, or inflammation of the hoof, is a common complication that occurs in approximately 25% of affected horses.

Lipomas

Colic caused by lipomas (benign fatty tumors) is sometimes seen in horses more than 10 years old. If the tumor is attached by a stalk to connective tissue in the abdomen, then it may wrap around a part of the intestine, shutting off its blood supply. Signs may include depression and severe abdominal pain, with rapid worsening of condition. Treatment requires removal of the tumor by surgery, along with any damaged sections of the intestine. If the problem is detected early, the outlook is good, but if surgery is not done before signs are advanced, the chances for recovery are fair to poor.

Twisting or Displacement of the Small or Large Intestine

Twisting of the intestines (**volvulus**, sometimes also called a **torsion**) occurs when the intestine rotates around its attachment to the abdominal wall. This reduces the blood supply to the intestine, leading to colic. Horses with this condition are painful and have an increased heart rate. Rapid dehydration is caused by movement of fluid into the stomach and intestine. The horse's condition may worsen rapidly.

Portions of the small intestine can become trapped within mesenteric rents (defects within the connective tissue that connects the intestine to the body wall) or the epiploic foramen (a natural opening between the liver and major abdominal blood vessels). Signs can be vague and can vary from mild to severe pain. These entrapments require surgery to correct. If surgery is performed quickly, the outlook is good. However, the vagueness of signs can delay surgery and worsen the outlook.

Displacement, without twisting, of the large intestine may occur and also leads to obstruction. A **left dorsal displacement** occurs when part or all of the left colon gets displaced over the renosplenic ligament (an anatomical attachment between the kidney and the spleen). A **right dorsal displacement** occurs when the left colon becomes trapped between the cecum and the body wall. A portion of the colon may also be twisted in some of these horses. Horses with displacements of the large intestine do not usually worsen as rapidly as those with twisting.

Displacements of the large intestine can often be treated with medical management. Depending on the colon's location, treatment may include withholding food, administering fluids and pain medications, jogging or rolling the horse, or other medications. Surgery may also be necessary to relocate the colon, especially if pain is severe or if twisting is present.

Twisting of the intestines requires surgery to correct the positioning of the intestine. Removal of part of the intestine may also be required if it has been compromised by a lack of blood supply for too long. The outlook for recovery is good if the condition is detected and treated soon after it occurs. Adhesions (see above) may be a complication, especially if the illness is prolonged. Volvulus of the large colon can recur in as many as 20% of cases, but performing a colopexy (a surgical procedure that attaches the colon to the abdominal wall) may reduce the recurrence.

Inguinal Hernia

Inguinal hernias (commonly referred to as scrotal hernias) occur when the intestine passes from the abdomen into the inguinal canal that connects the testes to the abdomen. They occur in male horses, generally after breeding, trauma, or a hard workout. If the inguinal opening is large enough, part of the intestine may become trapped, causing colic. Hernias appear to be most common in Tennessee Walking Horses, American Saddlebreds, and Standardbreds. If the condition has been present for more than a few hours, the horse's condition worsens rapidly. A veterinarian may be able to push the hernia back through the abdominal wall (called reducing the hernia) if it has occurred in the last few hours. Otherwise, surgery is the usual treatment and may require removal of the testicle on the affected side, along with a portion of the intestine if it has become too damaged. The chances for survival appear to be breed-dependent, with Standardbred horses having a good outlook and Tennessee Walking Horses a fair to poor outlook. Presumably, this is because Tennessee Walking Horse stallions with inguinal hernias show few signs of pain, which may delay recognition of the problem and treatment.

Enteroliths (Intestinal Stones)

Enteroliths are hard masses composed of magnesium ammonium phosphate crystals that form around a foreign object (such as a piece of wire, stone, or nail) in the large intestine of horses. Enteroliths may be seen singly or in groups and are commonly found in horses in certain parts of the United States, including California, the southwest, Indiana, and Florida. Most horses with enteroliths are about 10 years old; horses younger than 4 years old are rarely affected. Enteroliths are commonly seen in Arabian horses. A common factor associated with formation of enteroliths may be the consumption of alfalfa hay, which results in a higher pH and increased concentrations of calcium, magnesium, and sulfur in the large colon.

Many horses with this condition have a history of recurring colic, which may indicate that the enterolith(s) had caused partial or temporary blockage of the large intestine. Depending on the location of the enterolith, the horse may be in severe pain. Heart and respiratory rates increase, and the mucous membranes may be pale or pink. Generally, intestinal distention is evident to the veterinarian on rectal examination, but the mass cannot usually be felt. In areas where the problem is common, x-rays may be used to identify the enteroliths.

Treatment involves surgery to decompress the intestine and remove the stone(s). The outlook is excellent. Veterinary practices in areas where this condition commonly occurs report survival rates of 95%.

LAMINITIS IN HORSES

Laminitis is a common, extremely painful and frequently recurrent condition in horses, ponies and donkeys.

It has significant welfare implications for owners. This condition affects the tissues (laminae) bonding the hoof wall to pedal bone in the hoof. This can result in the pedal bone sinking or rotating within the hoof under the weight of the horse. In extreme cases this can result in penetration the sole of the foot by the pedal bone. More than 7% of equine deaths are linked to the laminitis, with many animals having to be euthanased.

Etiology and Pathogenesis:

Three main disease states are thought to be associated with laminitis: 1) diseases associated with sepsis or endotoxemia, 2) endocrinopathic laminitis encompassing equine metabolic syndrome (including pasture-associated laminitis) and pituitary adenoma, and 3) supporting limb laminitis. The pathogenesis of laminitis remains controversial and most likely varies widely between these three primary causes. A fourth, less common cause is ingestion of shavings (sometimes inadvertently used for bedding) from black walnut heartwood; the pathophysiology of this type of laminitis appears similar to that of sepsis-related laminitis. The diseases causing systemic sepsis in sepsis-related laminitis are diseases commonly associated with gram-negative bacterial (or polymicrobial) sepsis and include ingestion of excess carbohydrate (grain overload), acute postparturient metritis (retained fetal membranes), colic (anterior enteritis, large colon volvulus), and enterocolitis. Laminitis secondary to equine metabolic syndrome most commonly occurs in overweight horses and ponies and is commonly exacerbated when grazing lush pastures. It is possible that laminitis occurring from an acute intake of lush pasture may be a combination of sepsis-related laminitis (similar to grain overload) and metabolic syndrome.

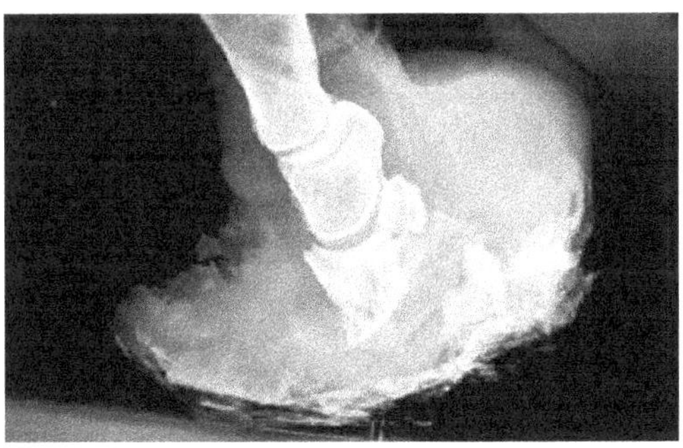

Fig. 1 X ray of severe equine laminitis case

Supporting limb laminitis can occur any time the horse places excessive weight on one limb for an extended period because of inability to use the other limb (eg, postoperative orthopedic procedures, radial nerve paralysis, or a septic joint or tendon sheath). The basic cause of laminar failure in laminitis is a failure of attachment of the laminar basal epithelial cells (LBECs) of the epidermal laminae to the underlying dermal laminae. Although this failure was thought to be primarily due to breakdown of the matrix molecules in the basement membrane and dermis (to which the LBECs attach) by matrix metalloproteases, studies have questioned the importance of matrix metalloproteases.

It appears that the LBECs may primarily be losing attachment to the underlying dermal laminae due to dysregulation of the hemidesmosomes (the adhesion complexes on the basal side of the LBECs that attach the cells to the underlying matrix molecules of the basement membrane) and possibly the associated cytoskeleton. Inflammatory mediators and enzymes (eg, proinflammatory cytokines, cyclooxygenase-2) are markedly increased in the laminae in the early stages of sepsis-related laminitis and may injure the LBECs or cause cellular dysregulation, leading to loss of attachment.

Hypoxia and ischemia due to aberrant vascular flow is also likely to play a role in LBEC dysfunction in sepsis-related laminitis but appears to occur later in the disease process. The pathophysiology behind laminitis associated with equine metabolic syndrome is not as well researched as sepsis-related laminitis, but work indicates that inflammatory signaling does not play a major role and that dysregulation of the LBECs is likely to result from insulin-related signaling, possibly through growth factor receptors such as IGF-1 receptor.

The pathogenesis of supporting limb laminitis is only now being intensively investigated. These studies indicate that the central pathophysiologic factor in supporting limb laminitis is decreased laminar blood flow due to a lack of movement of the supporting limb because of pain in the opposite limb. After loss of integrity of the laminar attachments, the distal phalanx can undergo three types of displacement depending on the forces placed on the foot and the pattern of laminar injury. Symmetrical distal displacement of the entire phalanx (usually termed "sinking") occurs when there is circumferential loss of laminar attachments, most commonly seen in severe cases of sepsis but also seen in equine metabolic syndrome.

Palmar rotation of the distal margin of the distal phalanx (usually termed "rotation") is the most common displacement seen, and most likely occurs due to a combination of loss of the dorsal laminar attachments (while maintaining some laminar integrity in the quarters and heels) and tension on the deep digital flexor tendon. Rarely, uniaxial/unilateral distal displacement of the distal phalanx occurs, most commonly to the medial side in the forelimb; this displacement can only be visualized on an anterior-posterior radiograph of the foot. In laminitis related to sepsis and equine metabolic syndrome, the forelimbs are most commonly affected, although the hindlimbs can also be affected in severe cases. In supporting limb laminitis, either a front or rear foot is affected depending on which opposite limb has the weight-bearing problem.

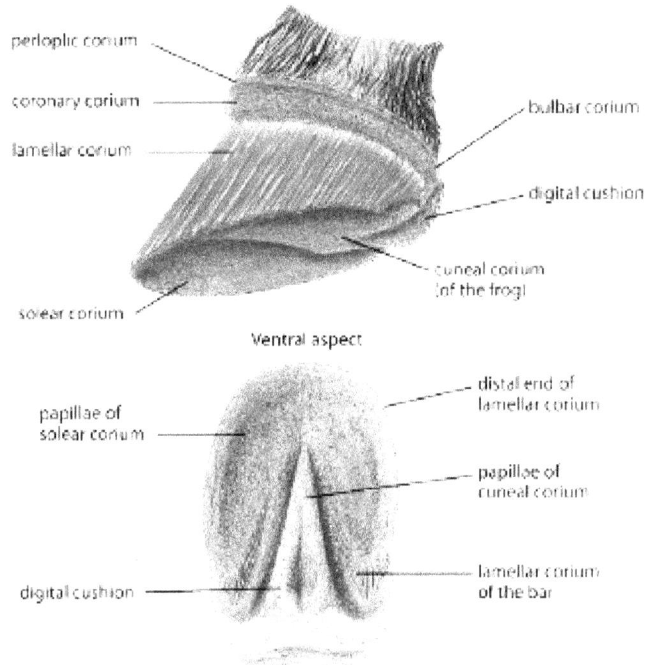

Fig. 2 Corium of the digit in the horse

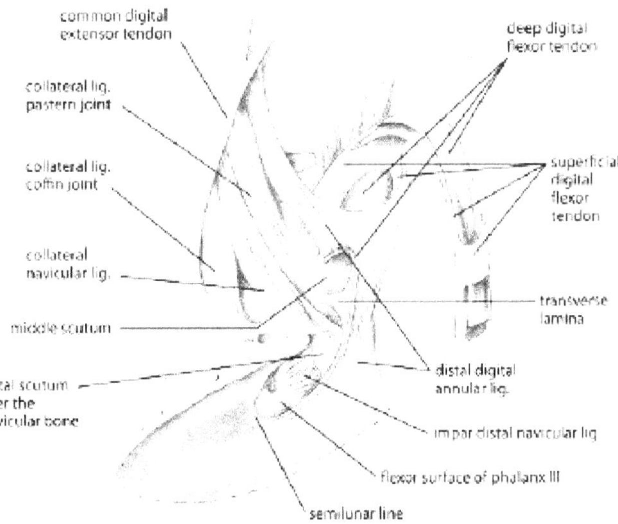

Fig. 3 Ligaments and tendons of the distal digit in the hors

Causes

While the exact mechanisms by which the feet are damaged remain a mystery, certain precipitating events can produce laminitis. Although laminitis occurs in the feet, the underlying cause is often a disturbance elsewhere in the horse's body. The causes vary and may include the following:

- Digestive upsets due to grain overload (such as excess grain, fruit or snacks) or abrupt changes in diet.
- Sudden access to excessive amounts of lush forage before the horse's system has had time to adapt; this type of laminitis is known as "grass founder."
- Toxins released within the horse's system.
- High fever or illness; any illness that causes high fever or serious metabolic disturbances has the potential to cause laminitis, e.g., Potomac Horse Fever.
- Severe colic.
- Retained placenta in the mare after foaling.
- Excessive concussion to the feet, often referred to as "road founder."
- Excessive weight-bearing on one leg due to injury of another leg or any other alteration of the normal gait.
- Various primary foot diseases.
- Bedding that contains black walnut shavings.
- Although controversial, prolonged use or high doses of corticosteroids may contribute to the development of laminitis in some horses.

Risk Factors

Factors that seem to increase a horse's susceptibility to laminitis or increase the severity of the condition when it does occur include the following:

- Heavy breeds, such as draft horses
- Overweight body
- High nutritional plane (feeding large amounts of carbohydrate-rich meals)
- Ponies, Morgans, miniature horses and donkeys
- Unrestricted grain binges, such as when a horse breaks into the feed room (if this happens, do not wait until symptoms develop to call your veterinarian— call immediately so corrective action can be taken before tissue damage progresses)
- Horses who have had previous episodes of laminitis
- Older horses with Cushing's disease

Signs

Signs of *acute laminitis* include the following:

- Lameness, especially when a horse is turning in circles; shifting lameness when standing.
- Heat in the feet.

- Increased digital pulse in the feet (most easily palpable over either sesamoid bone at the level of the fetlock).
- Pain in the toe region when pressure is applied with hoof testers.
- Reluctant or hesitant gait ("walking on eggshells").
- A "sawhorse stance," with the front feet stretched out in front to alleviate pressure on the toes and the hind feet positioned under them to support the weight that their front feet cannot.

Signs of *chronic laminitis* may include the following:

- Rings in hoof wall that become wider as they are followed from toe to heel.
- Bruised soles or "stone bruises."
- Widened white line, commonly called "seedy toe," with occurrence of seromas (blood pockets) and/or abscesses.
- Dropped soles or flat feet.
- Thick, "cresty" neck.
- Dished hooves, which are the result of unequal rates of hoof growth (the heels grow at a faster rate than the rest of the hoof, resulting in an "Aladdin-slipper" appearance).

Clinical Findings

Classically, laminitis is considered acute, subacute, or chronic. Acute laminitis is classically defined as the initial few days of clinical signs of laminitis (usually <3 days) in a horse in which the distal phalanx has not undergone displacement. Subacute laminitis is commonly used to define laminitis in which clinical signs have continued >3 days, but the horse still has no distal phalangeal displacement. Chronic laminitis is classically defined as the case in which distal phalanx displacement has occurred regardless of the duration of the disease. Early in laminitis, the horse is depressed and anorectic and stands reluctantly. Resistance to any exercise is marked, and the normal stance is altered in attempts to relieve the weight borne by the affected feet. If only the forelimbs are affected, the horse will stand with the forelimbs placed far forward (to decrease the weight on the front digits); the hindlimbs also are placed more forward to support more of the weight of the horse. If forced to walk, the horse shows a slow, crouching, short-striding gait. If all four limbs are affected, the animal will appear "camped out," with the forelimbs placed more forward than usual and the hindlimbs placed more caudally than usual. Each foot, once lifted, is set down as quickly as possible.

Clinical lesions

In the acute stage of laminitis, the entire hoof wall may be warm. An exaggerated and bounding pulse can be palpated and may be visible in the digital arteries. Pain can cause muscular trembling, and a fairly uniform tenderness can be detected when pressure is applied to the sole (most commonly in the toe region). The pulse rate (60–120/min) and respiratory rate (80–100/min) are commonly increased, primarily because of pain. Lameness is usually moderate to severe at this time. In exceptionally severe cases, for which the prognosis is unfavorable, a blood-stained exudate may seep from the coronary bands. These clinical signs do not always occur in endocrinopathic laminitis because of the insidious nature of the disease process, which can occur over months or years; the first clinical sign in many of these horses is toe bruising due to solar compression by the slowly displacing distal phalanx. Radiographic evidence of displacement of the distal phalanx can be present as early as the third day after the onset of disease in horses with sepsis/endotoxemia. However, an MRI study has shown that, in the acute case, the horse may have normal-appearing distal phalanx on radiographs, despite destruction of the entire dorsal laminar attachment that is visible on MRI.

Subacute cases may exhibit any or all of the above clinical signs but to a lesser degree. Often, there is only a mild change in stance, with reluctance to walk and some increased sensitivity to concussion on the soles of the affected feet. There may be no demonstrable heat in the coronary band or increase in digital pulse. The acute and subacute forms of laminitis tend to recur at varying intervals and may develop into the chronic form.

During and immediately after displacement of the distal phalanx (classically termed chronic laminitis once displacement occurs, regardless of the temporal aspect of the disease course), the horse is usually extremely lame and may spend a great deal of time recumbent. In severe cases, the foot may prolapse through the sole cranial to the frog, or the coronary band may separate; both occurrences gravely affect the prognosis. Longterm cases of chronic laminitis are characterized by changes in the shape of the hoof and usually follow one or more attacks of the acute form. Especially with cases of rotation of the distal phalanx, bands of irregular horn growth (laminitic rings) may be seen in the hoof, close at the toe and diverging at the heel (due to minimal hoof growth from the dorsal coronary band). The hoof itself becomes narrow and elongated, with "dishing" of the dorsal surface of the hoof wall with a steep angle to the hoof wall proximally and a much more horizontally oriented wall distally.

As the displacement of the distal phalanx progresses in longterm cases, the sole becomes flattened or somewhat convex in outline on the ground surface immediately cranial to the apex of the frog. The gait is similar to that already described, and when standing, the body weight is continually shifted from one foot to the other. Radiography commonly reveals rotation and some bony resorption of the dorsal solar margin of the distal phalanx in longer term cases.

Diagnosis

In acute laminitis, diagnosis is usually straightforward and is based on the history (eg, grain overload) and posture of the horse, increased temperature of the hooves, a hard pulse in the digital arteries, and reluctance to move. Abaxial sesamoid nerve blocks of the forelimb digits in the very lame horse allow assessment of possible involvement of the hindfeet (by walking the animal a few steps) and enable full assessment of the soles of both feet (for solar prolapse, etc). These nerve blocks also make it possible to obtain good quality lateral and anterior-posterior radiographs of the foot without severe duress to the horse. Lidocaine should be used for the nerve block, because it will last only a short time (ie, not long enough for the animal to move excessively and further damage the laminae); applying a temporary pad to the foot not being radiographed (to protect that foot) is also recommended. Gross observation and distinct measurements of the hoof wall and sole thicknesses from the radiographs allow determination of whether distal displacement, rotation, both distal displacement and rotation, or unilateral sinking has occurred. Depending on the radiographic diagnosis of the type of phalangeal displacement present, there is usually time while the nerve block is still effective to apply a temporary type of pad or shoe.

Treatment

Acute laminitis constitutes a medical emergency, because phalangeal displacement can occur rapidly. Despite prompt therapy, the prognosis is guarded until recovery is complete and it is evident that the hoof architecture is not altered. Most animals should be administered NSAIDs, with flunixin meglumine being the drug of choice if the horse is still systemically ill (ie, enterocolitis). Phenylbutazone is usually used in the early chronic stage when the horse is lame but does not have signs of systemic disease such as sepsis/endotoxemia. Close attention to the potential toxicities of NSAID therapy, particularly with phenylbutazone, is required. Because phenylbutazone accumulates in the tissue (unlike flunixin or most other NSAIDs), it is best to skip a day every 5–7 days to "clear the system" (flunixin can be administered that day). NSAIDs should be used according to label instructions and, if used in combination, the dosage of each drug should be reduced accordingly. Another option for treatment of chronic laminitis in horses at risk of renal or GI complications is the COX-2-selective NSAID firocoxib.

Other options for analgesia include detomidine, butorphanol, morphine, or a constant-rate infusion of a "cocktail" of sedatives and analgesics. For treatment of possible ongoing ischemia, acepromazine is the only drug found to effectively increase digital blood flow in some studies; however, this has been questioned again by a study using laminar microdialysis catheters in which urea clearance (an indicator of blood flow) was not changed in horses administered acepromazine. In a horse at risk of or in the early stages of sepsis-related laminitis, digital hypothermia (cooling of the foot by placing it directly in ice water) has been popularized again by several experimental studies consistently demonstrating efficacy in protection of the structural integrity of the lamellar tissue; in one clinical study of enterocolitis cases in two hospitals, risk of developing laminitis was decreased 10-fold in septic/endotoxemic horses in which continuous digital hypothermia was performed.

During the first 2–3 wk, it is important to remove standard shoes, because shoes place the majority of stress on the hoof wall and therefore the laminae. The feet should be padded with a soft, resilient substance such as a 1- to 2-in. thick piece of closed-cell foam cut to the diameter of the foot. Pads to provide sole support can also be made from different putties available to farriers. Decreasing padding (or beveling the pad) in the region dorsal to the apex of the frog decreases the stress on the dorsal laminae. Styrofoam insulation (2 in. thick) can be used in small equids but usually provides minimal support in larger animals. Other temporary shoes (eg, Redden Ultimate and wooden or EVA clog) that can be applied without severe concussion can provide different physical properties depending on the type of displacement (and veterinarian/farrier preference) in the first few weeks.

Shoeing laminitic horses with metal shoes is usually not a good option until ~3–4 wk after the onset of laminitis, when the laminar structure may be stabilizing. The type of shoeing depends on the type of displacement. In a horse with distal phalangeal rotation, an attempt is made to begin realigning the palmar surface of the distal phalanx to the sole, while not allowing excessive forces on the laminae.

The breakover of the shoe is moved as far caudally as possible, and some of the caudal hoof (from the frog apex caudally) is removed to allow realignment to the sole. This may have to be performed in combination with raising of the heel (with wedge pads, etc), which still allows alignment of the distal phalanx to the solar surface while avoiding excessive changes in relation to the ground surface, thus preventing excessive tension on the deep digital flexor tendon and therefore the dorsal laminae. It may be appropriate to place some type of resilient putty on the solar surface to provide support to the distal phalanx in horses in which some degree of laminar instability is still suspected. Multiple types of shoes can be used, including heart bar shoes, egg bar shoes, and natural balance shoes. Steward clogs are an important option for treating horses with distal displacement of the distal phalanx; these allow the horse to maximize comfort because of being beveled in multiple directions (and therefore minimizing laminar stress). Some farriers/clinicians also use clogs in cases of rotation of the distal phalanx.

Surgical options include deep digital flexor tenotomy, to neutralize the pull of the deep digital flexor tendon, and dorsal hoof wall resections. Deep digital flexor tenotomy is most commonly performed in cases of chronic rotation that do not respond to the above shoeing techniques; it should always be accompanied by aggressive derotation via rasping of the caudal foot. The farrier and veterinarian must address subluxation of the coffin joint subsequent to deep digital flexor tenotomy in most cases (usually by applying adequate heel wedging to neutralize the subluxation). Hoof wall resections are performed much less frequently than in the past. Generally, only a partial hoof wall resection is performed (usually on the distal hoof wall) because of the severe digital instability caused by removing the entire dorsal wall in an extensive hoof wall resection.

PARASITE CONTROL IN HORSES

Internal parasites represent a significant health threat to horses. Internal parasites (worms) are organisms that live a portion of their life cycle in a host animal. They live in internal organs, body cavities and tissues, and gain their nutritive source by feeding on the host animal and ingested nutrients. Part of their life cycle also occurs in the external environment, typically pastures. The horse is affected by many different species of parasites. The nature and extent of damage varies with the parasite. Parasites cost the horse owner in several ways:

- It is expensive to feed parasite burdened horses (they require more nutrients).
- Parasites rob the horse of intended nutrients.
- Parasites can cause anemia.
- Parasitized young horses grow slower.
- Parasites can reduce reproductive and athletic performance.
- Parasite burdens can suppress the horses' immune system, making them more susceptible to other infections.

Signs of Parasitism

The signs of parasitism are common among different parasites infecting the horse and include:

- Weight loss
- Dull, rough hair coat
- Potbelly
- Decreased stamina or lethargy
- Coughing
- Diarrhea
- Colic
- Tail rubbing

There are numerous internal parasites that can infect horses, but only a few commonly cause significant health problems. It is important to understand the life cycle of these parasites. Successful prevention and control programs are effective because they interrupt the life cycle of parasites. The primary class of internal parasites that cause health problems for horses are nematodes (such as large and small strongyles), roundworms and tapeworms. Other internal parasites of minor significance such as threadworms, pinworms and botfly larvae are often considered when designing a parasite control program.

Types of Internal Parasites

Large strongyles, small strongyles, ascarids, tapeworms, pinworms, bots, and threadworms are common internal parasites that infect horses. In adult horses, small strongyles and tapeworms are the largest concerns. Each type of parasite impacts the horse differently and has unique infective states (time in the parasite's life cycle when it can infect the horse). The age of a horse will also impact which species of parasites they are more susceptible to; for example, ascarids are more likely to be found in foals and weanlings than mature horses. A large concern with internal parasites is resistance to dewormers (known as **anthelmintic resistance**). Some parasite species have become very resilient, adapting to survive dewormer treatments. This is of particular concern with ascarids and small strongyles.

Large Strongyles

Three species of large strongyles affect horses: *Strongylus vulgaris, Strongylus edentates,* and *Strongylus equinus.* Large strongyle larvae are found on pastures and are ingested while the horse grazes – the larvae "swim" up blades of grass in water droplets to increase their chances of being eaten. Once ingested, *S. vulgaris* larvae migrate to the large intestine, and can then migrate to the blood vessels and burrow through the walls of arteries and disrupt blood flow. Because of this, *S. vulgaris* are commonly known as "bloodworms" and are considered the most pathogenic and damaging of the large strongyles. The other two species of large strongyles will migrate from the digestive tract into the liver and then back to the large intestines, but these are not as damaging since they do not affect the blood stream to the same extent. Currently, large strongyles are not a large concern for domestic horses, as treatment strategies from decades ago have substantially reduced their presence.

Small Strongyles

Similar to large strongyles, there are a number of different species of small strongyles found in the horse. Small strongyles (*Cyathostomes*) have a similar life cycle to large strongyles in that they are found on pasture grasses, ingested by the horse as larvae, and then move through the digestive system. However, once the small strongyle larvae reach the large intestines they do not migrate into other organs or tissues. Small strongyles are unique in that they often burrow into the walls of the large colon and cecum, becoming what we call "**encysted**." This makes management of small strongyles difficult, because while encysted, these parasites can remain in the body for up to two years and are not affected by most dewormer treatments. They will wait until conditions within the intestines are ideal for maturation, and then emerge from the intestinal wall to mature and produce eggs. Small strongyles are prolific and have become resistant to most dewormers currently available. Small strongyle resistance to deworming is one of the primary reasons recommended deworming protocols have changed within the past decade. It is assumed that all grazing adult horses are infected with small strongyles, but clinical symptoms are rare.

Ascarids

Ascarids (*Parascaris equorum*), or roundworms, typically affect younger foals and weanlings, as most horses develop immunity to them by the time they are yearlings. Foals ingest ascarids as eggs, consuming them from many different places in their environments. Unlike many other equine parasites, ascarids are not just found on pasture grass; they can be found on many surfaces such as buckets, troughs, and even the udder of the mare. Once ingested, ascarid eggs develop into larvae in the small intestine. Hatched larvae then migrate through a series of tissues; they move from the small intestine to the liver and then to the lungs. Once in the lungs, the parasites are coughed up, swallowed, and then migrate back to the small intestine for maturation. Similar to small strongyles, they are developing resistance to certain types of dewormers, which could lead to problems with dewormers remaining effective against ascarids in the future.

Tapeworms

There are three species of tapeworms found in horses, but the most common one is *Anoplocephala perfoliata*. Tapeworms (Fag. 5) are unique in that they have two hosts in their life cycle; the first is the oribatid mite, and the second is the horse. Mites consume tapeworm eggs, which then develop into larvae inside of the mite. Horses then ingest the mites while grazing, and the mite moves to the small intestine of the horse where it releases the tapeworms. Adult tapeworms then continue to move through the small intestine until they arrive at the ileocecal junction. This is the junction between the ilium (the last part of the small intestine) and the cecum. Here, the tapeworms attach to the gut wall and may cause inflammation of the intestinal tract. Colic has been reported to be caused by tapeworms. Additionally, obstruction, ulceration, or thickening of the intestines can occur because of heavy tapeworm loads.

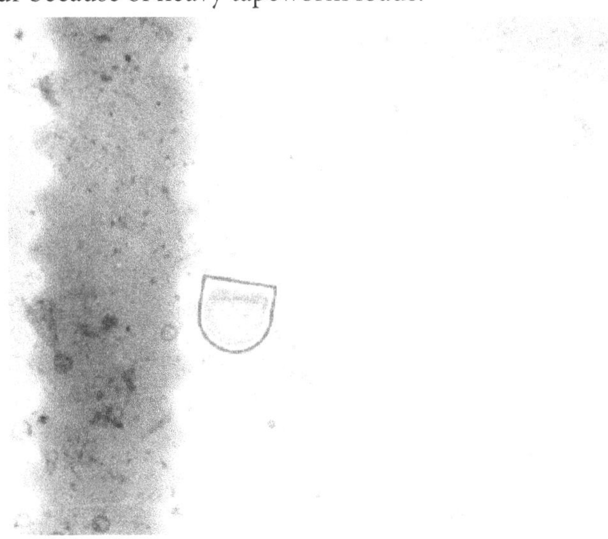

Fig. 5. Tapeworm egg at 100x magnification. Tapeworm eggs are an unusual sighting in a fecal sample

Pinworms

Pinworms (*Oxyruris equi*) are ingested by the horse as eggs and can be found in the horse's environment. Once ingested, pinworms mature in the horse's intestines. Adults then emerge out of the anus and lay eggs along the horse's skin there, which makes the horse itch and rub its tail. Unlike other parasites mentioned, pinworms do not cause much harm to the horse internally, but instead cause unattractive hair loss from the horse scratching its tail. They are not a large concern from a health perspective, but treatment for this species of parasite is still recommended to reduce irritation.

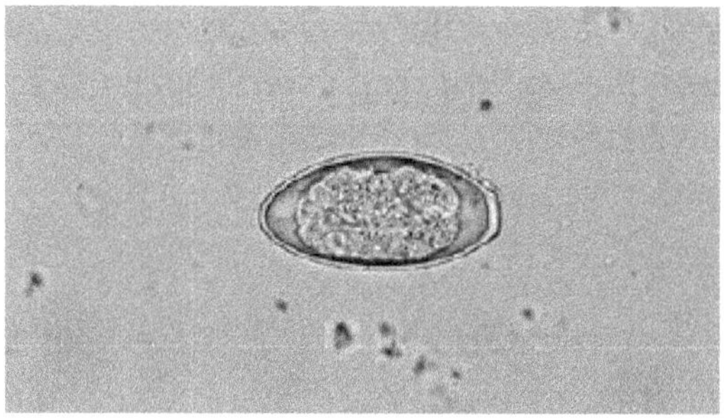

Fig. 6. Pinworm eggBots

Bots, often referred to as stomach bots, are unique because they are both internal and external parasites. The most common species of bot fly found in horses is *Gasterophilius intestinalis*. The adult bot fly, an external parasite, is a flying insect resembling a bee that lays yellow-oval shaped eggs on the horse's coat. Eggs are found primarily on the lower forelimbs (and to a lesser extent the neck and mane). The eggs will remain there until stimulated to hatch by the horse's saliva as it bites or licks the affected area. The newly hatched larvae burrow into the gums of the horse where they will stay for about four weeks. The parasites then move to the lining of the stomach where they stay for nine months before being passed in manure. Possible minor oral lesions and damage to the stomach lining can occur from stomach bots, but no serious health problems are generally caused by bots.

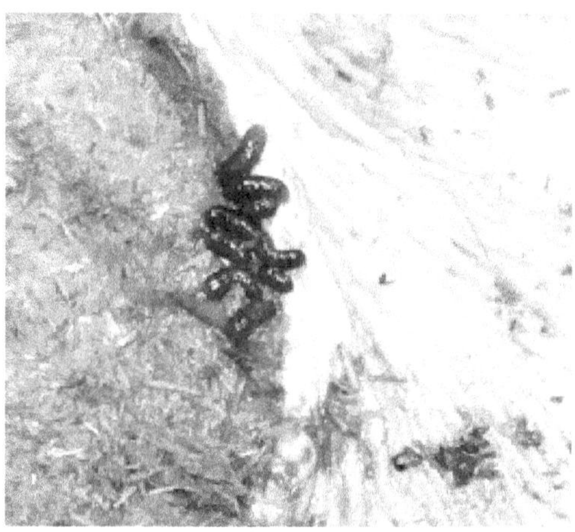

Fig. 7 Stomach bots

Threadworms

Threadworms (*Strongyloides westeri*) are internal parasites that primarily infect foals. Though they can be seen in older horses, they are rarely found in horses over 8-10 months due to developed immunity. Foals become infected in three different ways: by ingesting larvae through the mare's milk, from the larvae penetrating the foal's skin, or ingestion of the larvae from the environment. Larvae migrate to the lungs and end up in the small intestine. Diarrhea is often associated with threadworm infestation and can cause dehydration. Due to current dewormer treatments, threadworms today are quite rare.

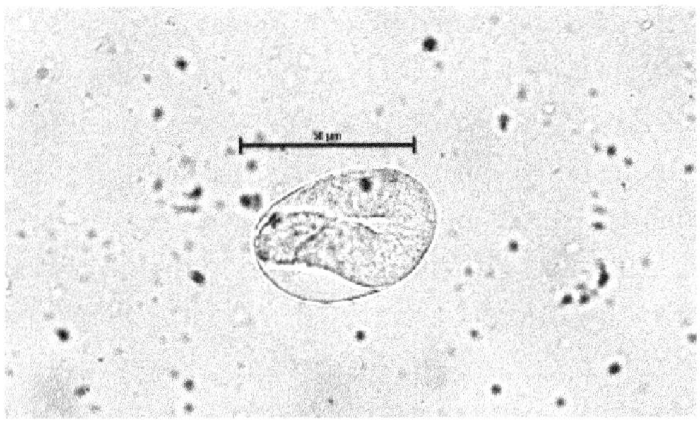

Fig. 8 Threadworm egg as seen under a microscope at high resolution

Control of internal parasites is a cornerstone of equine management and a continual endeavor. Control programs should be tailored to each farm situation and require a cooperative program between the horse owner and the veterinarian. The principal internal parasites of horses are nematodes. Unfortunately, many species of adult cyathostomes have developed resistance to standard doses of the benzimidazoles and the tetrahydropyrimidines. Among intensively managed horse populations, treatment with macrocyclic lactones (eg, ivermectin, moxidectin) does not suppress strongyle egg counts for as long as previously expected. Among foals, weanlings, and even yearlings, there are increasing reports of ascarids becoming resistant to ivermectin and moxidectin.

A program of anthelmintic resistance involves multiple parasites and multiple drug classes, and must consider horses of all ages. No single parasite control program is ideal for all horses. Age of the horse, population density, region of the country, climate, method of confinement (eg, stall or pasture), and pasture size and quality can affect the choice of parasite control programs. As horses age, they develop resistance to reinfection with certain parasites, such as *Strongyloides westeri* and *Parascaris equorum*. Resistance to most strongyles is incomplete. Although anthelmintics are the primary method of parasite control, other factors such as pasture management and stable environment are also important. The parasites of greatest concern in horses are large strongyles, small strongyles, roundworms, pinworms, stomach bots, and tapeworms.

GI parasites can cause acute medical problems as well as chronic debilitation. They may be responsible for diarrhea, intestinal impactions or irritation (colic), and poor performance. The result can be slow growth in young horses, poor performance, acute bouts of colic, and death in severe instances. The migrating ascarids (*Parascaris equorum*) are the primary cause of pulmonary inflammation and intestinal rupture in foals and weanlings. The control of large strongyles with improved anthelmintics has allowed the small strongyles (cyathostomes) to become a greater problem. Reports of tapeworms have also increased. The three methods of diagnosis of parasites are direct examination of feces, concentrations of worm eggs by flotation, and culture of feces for infective larva. The direct examination method is quick but not always accurate.

The flotation method for parasite egg concentration is more accurate to determine the type and number of parasites. The culture method is more suitable for laboratory use and research purposes. The effectiveness of any parasite control program can be evaluated by fecal examination. The fecal examination should be done before administration of a particular dewormer and then again 14 days later. The amount of decreases in egg population will determine the effectiveness of the dewormer. Parasite egg counts that remain high after use of a particular dewormer indicate the presence of resistance and a need to change the control program. The three major classes of anthelmintics available for parasite control in horses are the avermectins, benzimidazoles, and pyrantels.

The avermectins have a broad range of activity, are safe and effective at low doses, and control adult and migrating larval nematodes. Deworming of mares immediately after foaling lessens the foal's exposure to parasites in the mare's manure. Avermectins are not effective against tapeworms; however, the combination of ivermectin with praziquantel is effective against tapeworms as well as large and small strongyles, ascarids, pinworms, and bots. The benzimidazoles (oxibendazole, fenbendazole, and oxfendazole) are effective against most nematodes but not against encysted small strongyles or tapeworms. The pyrantels are effective against large and small strongyles, ascarids, and pinworms. Pyrantels kill nematode parasites slowly. Pyrantel is available as a paste (single dose), and as a tartrate salt that can be used as a daily dewormer mixed in the feed; it is effective against tapeworms but not bots.

The avermectins are effective against bot larva and are recommended in the fall after the botfly season. A fourth class of anthelmintics, the isoquinolines, contains praziquantel, a narrow-spectrum drug approved for horses as a cestocide. Praziquantel is available in combination with either ivermectin or moxidectin.

To slow the development of drug-resistant parasites, the focus of most parasite control programs is to reduce selection pressure for resistance by customizing deworming protocols for the farm and individual horses. This strategy includes identifying horses most susceptible to parasites (ie, the high egg shredders) and maximizing refugia (those parasites not exposed to drug selection pressure) by reducing the overall number of anthelmintic treatments administered and by monitoring the efficacy of different classes of dewormers using the fecal egg count reduction test.

An effective deworming protocol for horses should incorporate a cestocide (eg, a praziquantel-containing product or a double dose of pyrantel pamoate) and a boticide (eg, ivermectin or moxidectin) once or twice a year to control tapeworms and bots, respectively, and a larvicidal dose of anthelmintic effective against encysted cyanthostomes (eg, fenbendazole 10 mg/kg/day, PO, for 5 days, or a single dose of moxidectin) during early winter months in northern climates or during early summer in warmer climates.

Foals should be maintained on a regular deworming schedule every 60 days that includes anthelmintics safe and effective against ascarids. Treatments effective against other nematodes (including encysted cyathostomes) and cestodes should be included in the deworming protocols for foals during the first year of life. Effective deworming programs should also include one or more of the following nonchemical methods of parasite control:

1. Avoid overstocking and overgrazing pastures.
2. Keep pasture roughs mowed to a height of 3–8 in.
3. During hot, dry weather, harrow or rake pastures to disperse manure piles and expose larvae to sun. Rest the pasture at least 3–4 wk after harrowing.
4. Cross-graze pastures with other species. Cattle, sheep, and goats serve as biological vacuums for equine parasites.
5. Make at least one cutting of hay off some pastures to help reduce the parasite burden.
6. Plant an annual crop such as winter wheat.
7. Feed hay and grain in raised containers and not directly on the ground.
8. Remove manure from stalls, paddocks, and pastures every 24–72 hr before strongyle eggs have a chance to hatch and develop into infective larvae (5–7 days during optimal conditions).
9. Clean water sources regularly to prevent fecal contamination.
10. Quarantine new arrivals and perform fecal examinations. Use a larvicidal treatment before turning out new arrivals on pastures.
11. Use fecal egg counts, performed at the proper times, to identify and monitor high, medium, and low strongyle egg shedders, to monitor the efficacy of anthelmintics being used, and to evaluate new arrivals.
12. Compost manure. Properly composted manure will kill strongyle larvae and many ascarid eggs.

6

INFECTIOUS DISEASES IN HORSES

BORRELIA BURGDORFERI INFECTION AND LYME DISEASE

Infection with *Borrelia burgdorferi*, the Gram-negative spirochete bacterium that causes Lyme disease, is common in horses residing in regions endemic for *Ixodes* spp. ticks, and infection prevalence is likely on the rise as tick vectors undergo range expansion. While many horses will become infected with *B. burgdorferi* following a tick bite, the percentage of horses that will go on to develop Lyme disease is unknown. Documented syndromes attributed to *B. burgdorferi* include neuroborreliosis, cutaneous pseudolymphoma, and uveitis. Limited evidence exists to document stiffness, lameness, and malaise in horses as a result of *B. burgdorferi* infection, although these signs might be possible. Diagnosis of clinical Lyme disease in horses can be challenging. Ruling out other diseases which present with similar signs should be undertaken. A variety of serological tests exist to assess antibodies to *B. burgdorferi* in horses. These tests must be interpreted cautiously because a positive test result:

1. only indicates exposure,
2. does not prove that any clinical signs are due to B. burgdorferi infection, and
3. does not mean that the horse will experience disease in the future.

Routine serological testing of healthy horses is not recommended, nor is the treatment of seropositive but otherwise clinically healthy horses.

Definition

Borrelia burgdorferi, a gram-negative motile spirochete, is believed to be the predominate cause of Lyme disease in horses.

Clinical signs

At this time, documented syndromes attributed to *B. burgdorferi* include neuroborreliosis (ataxia, atrophy, cranial nerve deficits, stiff neck, cutaneous hyperesthesia), cutaneous pseudolymphoma (dermal masses at the site of tick bite), and uveitis (blepharospasm, epiphora, yellow-green fibrinous aqueous flare). Limited proof exists for non-specific syndromes including lameness, poor performance, arthritis, and body soreness, but these signs might be possible as the organism preferentially resides in synovial membranes and close to blood vessels and nerves in connective tissue. Lyme disease, which is caused by the bacteria *Borrelia burgdorferi* and transmitted through the bite of a tick, affects domestic animals and humans.

At least 3 known species of ticks can transmit Lyme disease. However, the great majority of Lyme disease transmissions are due to the bite of a very tiny tick commonly called the deer tick, or black-legged tick. *Ixodes pacificus* is the species found the west coast of the US; -*Ixodes scapularis* is the species involved in disease transmission elsewhere. It is important to note that ticks themselves do not cause Lyme disease; they merely harbor and transmit the bacteria that cause it. Lyme disease occurs much more frequently in dogs than in other animals.

Although horses have tested positive for exposure to the disease-causing bacteria, it is unclear whether there is a relationship between the exposure and any signs of infection such as lameness, fever, loss of appetite, fatigue, or difficulty breathing. It is best to consult with your veterinarian regarding the cause if any of these signs appear, particularly in areas where Lyme disease is common (including the northeastern and mid-Atlantic states, the upper Midwest, and Pacific Coast in the United States). Antibiotics are required for treatment. The best protection against Lyme disease is to avoid exposing your horses to the ticks that transmit the *Borrelia burgdorferi* bacteria.

Keep pastures mowed and remove areas where rodents nest. Ask your veterinarian to recommend an appropriate tick repellent for your horse. Daily grooming away from stalls or exercise areas can remove ticks resting on your horse's coat. If possible, capture and properly dispose of any ticks you find; otherwise they may reattach themselves to another horse or other animal. Remove any ticks by using fine-pointed tweezers to grasp the head of the tick (right where it enters the skin). Pull the tick straight off, making sure not to grasp or squeeze its body.

Treatment

Several options exist for treatment of horses with suspected Lyme disease, and a gold standard protocol has not yet been developed. Tetracycline antimicrobials are commonly administered for 7 to 30 days (oxytetracycline 6.6 mg/kg IV q24h; or doxycycline 10 mg/kg PO q12h; or minocycline 4 mg/kg PO q12h). It should be noted that tetracycline antimicrobials exert anti-inflammatory effects through their inhibition of matrix metalloproteases, which may contribute to improvement in clinical signs during treatment independently of any effects on *B. burgdorferi*. Accordingly, relapse of clinical signs following treatment should not necessary be interpreted as failure to clear the organism, as the improvement may have been due to the medication's anti-inflammatory properties alone.

Ceftiofur has also demonstrated in-vitro efficacy against *B. burgdorferi*, with MIC values falling within the range of expected serum and tissue concentrations following administration of ceftiofur crystalline-free acid (Excede®).

Titers should not be used alone to assess response to treatment or as deciding factors for prolonged therapy, as many treated horses maintain positive titers for months to even years.

Prognosis

The prognosis for *B. burgdorferi* infection is generally good as most exposed horses do not show clinical disease. The prognosis for neuroborreliosis and *B. burgdorferi* uveitis is guarded to poor.

Prevention

Tick control through environmental avoidance and diligent removal from horses remains the mainstay of preventing exposure and infection with *B. burgdorferi*.

- Tick repellants: Multiple spray and spot-on tick repellent products are available. These products may contain a combination of cypermethrin, permethrin, pyrethrins, or piperonyl butoxide, and demonstrate variable efficacies and durations of action.
- "Tickscaping": Environmental tick populations can be reduced by removal of leaves and woody debris, pasture mowing, and maintaining dry, well-lit paddocks whenever possible.

Vaccination

While no Lyme vaccines are licensed for use in horses, there is reasonable evidence to suggest that vaccination with canine recombinant OspA vaccine or whole-cell vaccines are at least partially protective. Specific vaccination protocol and protective antibody levels have not been established.

Zoonotic Potential

No known zoonotic potential from horses to humans. Humans participating in outdoor activities in endemic regions are at risk for *B. burgdorferi* infection and Lyme disease if bitten by *Ixodes* spp. ticks.

BOTULISM (CLOSTRIDIUM BOTULINUM)

Botulism is a rapidly fatal disease with motor paralysis. It is commonly caused by eating food contaminated with the toxin (a type of poison) produced by *Clostridium botulinum* bacteria. This organism grows rapidly in decomposing animal tissue and sometimes in plant material. It results in rapid death due to the paralysis of vital organs. Botulism is not usually an infection but a poisoning.

The frequency of botulism in animals is not known with accuracy, but it is low in horses. There are seven types of *Clostridium botulinum* toxins; the C_1 toxin is seen in most animal species, although type B is most common in North America and Europe. The usual source of the toxin is decaying carcasses or vegetable materials such as decaying grass, hay, grain, or spoiled silage.

Toxins of all types have the same action. The signs of botulism are caused by muscle paralysis. They include paralysis that becomes progressively more severe, disturbed vision, difficulty in chewing and swallowing, and overall weakness. Death is usually due to paralysis of the lungs or heart. Diagnosis of this condition is difficult, and it is often made by excluding any other possible causes of paralysis and by association with a likely source of the toxin. Botulism may also originate in two other ways. *Clostridium botulinum* has occasionally been found to grow in the gastrointestinal tract and produce toxins there.

When the toxins are released, they cause typical botulism. This occurs in foals usually less than 4 weeks old and results in the shaker foal syndrome. Foals may be found dead without previous signs, but most often, foals show signs of paralysis that slowly progresses. Stilted gait, muscle tremors, and the inability to stand for more than 4 to 5 minutes are key signs. Other signs include difficulty swallowing, constipation, dilated pupils, and frequent urination. As the disease progresses, labored breathing with extension of the head and neck, rapid heart rate, and respiratory arrest occur.

Death occurs most often 1 to 3 days after signs are first noted. Botulinum antitoxin has been used for treatment, with varying success. Early administration to foals, before they can no longer stand, is reported to be successful. Full supportive care is also important. In endemic areas, such as Kentucky, vaccination with type B toxoid appears to be effective.

A third form of botulism occurs in humans—and sometimes in adult horses—when the bacterium grows and produces toxin in a wound. This is referred to as wound botulism. Botulism is caused when *Clostridium botulinum* spores are ingested (forage poisoning) or infect a wound (wound botulism) and release a neurotoxin.

Another form of the disease is shaker foal syndrome, which results when spores germinate and produce toxin in foals' intestinal tracts. The toxin blocks the communication between nerves and muscles, resulting in progressive flaccid paralysis and reduced muscle strength. Although rare, it is highly fatal unless treated with antitoxin. Horses are more susceptible to botulism than many other species.

Strains of *C. botulinum* can produce seven neurotoxins (A through G), which are generally linked to different geographic locations. Not all of these neurotoxin types are toxic to horses. Types A, B, and C have been reported in relation to equine illness, although type A toxicity is uncommon. Shaker foal syndrome is due to type B and is primarily of concern in Kentucky and other mid-Atlantic states. Type *C. botulism* is often linked to forage contaminated with an infected animal carcass.

Spores of *C. botulinum* are found in the environment, including in the soil, where they can exist for many years without incident. Poisoning can occur when the spores are in an environment favorable to toxin production - moist conditions with low oxygen, high protein, and low acidity - such as decaying plant matter. Feed contamination can also occur due to animal carcasses or birds carrying animal material from off-site.

Etiology of Botulism in Animals

Botulism in most cases is an intoxication, not an infection, and results from ingestion of toxin in food. There are seven types of *C botulinum*, differentiated by the antigenic specificity of the toxins: A, B, C_1, D, E, F, and G. Types A, B, and E are most important in humans; C_1 in most animal species, notably wild ducks, pheasants, chickens, mink, cattle, and horses; and D in cattle. In horses, the most common type in North America and Europe is type B (>85% of US cases), and in the western US type A has been reported in only two outbreaks, both in humans, known to have been caused by type F. Type G, isolated from soil in Argentina, is not known to have been involved in any outbreak of botulism. The usual source of the toxin is decaying carcasses or vegetable materials such as decaying grass, hay, grain, or spoiled silage.

Toxins of all types have the same pharmacologic action. Like tetanus toxin, botulinum toxin is a zinc-binding metalloprotease that cleaves specific proteins in synaptic vesicles. Motor neuron surface receptors vary for the different botulinum toxins; therefore, some of the species differ in susceptibility to the various toxins. The exact incidence of botulism in animals is not known, but it is relatively low in cattle and horses, probably more frequent in chickens, and high in wild waterfowl.

Probably 10,000–50,000 birds die in most years, with deaths reaching 1 million or more during the great outbreaks in the western US. Most affected birds are ducks, although loons, mergansers, geese, and gulls also are susceptible. Dogs, cats, and pigs are comparatively resistant to all types of botulinum toxin when challenged orally; however, individual case reports mention botulism in dogs.

Most botulism in cattle occurs in South Africa and South America, where a combination of extensive agriculture, phosphorus deficiency in soil, and *C botulinum* type D in animals creates conditions ideal for the disease. The phosphorus-deficient cattle chew any bones with accompanying bits of flesh they find on the range; if these came from an animal carrying type D strains of *C botulinum*, intoxication is likely to result.

Any animal eating such material also ingests spores, which germinate in the intestine and, after death of the host, invade the musculature, which in turn becomes toxic for other cattle. Type C strains also cause botulism in cattle in a similar fashion. This type of botulism in cattle is rare, although a few cases have been reported from Texas under the term loin disease, and a few cases have occurred in Montana. Hay or silage contaminated with toxin-containing carcasses of birds or mammals and poultry litter fed to cattle have also been sources of type C or type D toxin for cattle ("forage botulism").

Big bale silage and haylage seem to be a particular risk and result in botulism problems if fermentation fails to produce a low and stable pH (<4.5). Botulism in sheep has occurred in Australia, associated not with phosphorus deficiency as in cattle, but with protein and carbohydrate deficiency, which results in sheep eating carcasses of rabbits and other small animals found on the range. Botulism in horses often results from forage contaminated with type C or D toxin. In six of eight outbreaks of equine botulism associated with type A, the source of infection was confirmed to be hay or silage. Toxicoinfectious botulism is the term given the disease in which *C botulinum* grows in tissues of a living animal and produces toxins there.

The toxins are liberated from the lesions and cause typical botulism. This has been suggested as a means of producing the shaker foal syndrome. Gastric ulcers, foci of necrosis in the liver, abscesses in the navel and lungs, wounds of the skin and muscle, and necrotic lesions of the GI tract are predisposing sites for development of toxicoinfectious botulism. This disease of foals and adult horses appears to resemble "wound botulism" in humans. Type B toxin is often implicated in botulism in horses and foals in the eastern US. Toxicoinfection is also suggested as a cause of equine grass sickness (equine dysautonomia) and recently in Japan as a cause of botulism in cattle.

Botulism in mink usually is caused by type C strains that have produced toxin in chopped raw meat or fish. Type A and E strains are occasionally involved. Botulism has not been reported in cats but occurs sporadically in dogs. Type C toxin is usually responsible, but there have been reports in which type D was the source.

Clinical signs of botulism

Clinical signs of botulism in horses can include weakness, exercise intolerance, muscle tremors, drooling, and reduced tongue strength. Progressive paralysis can lead to labored breathing and difficulty swallowing. Death can occur from respiratory paralysis and heart failure.

Clinical signs of botulism are caused by flaccid muscle paralysis and include progressive motor paralysis, disturbed vision, difficulty in chewing and swallowing, and generalized progressive paresis. Death is usually due to respiratory or cardiac paralysis. The toxin prevents release of acetylcholine at motor endplates (neuromuscular junction). Passage of impulses down the motor nerves and contractility of muscles are not hindered. No characteristic gross and histologic lesions develop, and pathologic changes may be ascribed to the general paralytic action of toxin, particularly in the muscles of the respiratory system, rather than to the specific effect of toxin on any particular organ.

Epidemics have occurred in dairy herds in which up to 65% of adult cows developed clinical botulism and died 6–72 hours after the onset of recumbency. Major clinical findings included drooling, decreased tongue tone, dysphagia, inability to urinate, and sternal recumbency that progressed to lateral recumbency just before death. Skin sensation is usually normal, and withdrawal reflexes of the limbs are weak. Initially, clinical signs resemble second-stage parturient paresis, but the cows do not respond to parenteral administration of calcium.

Reported clinical signs in horses are very similar, with progressive muscle paresis, recumbency, dysphagia, and decreased muscle tone (tail, tongue, jaw), respiratory distress, and death.

In shaker foal syndrome, foals are usually <4 weeks old. Affected foals may be found dead without premonitory clinical signs; most often, they exhibit signs of progressive symmetric motor paralysis. Stilted gait, muscular tremors, and the inability to stand for >4–5 minutes are salient features. Other clinical signs include dysphagia, constipation, mydriasis, and frequent urination. As the disease course progresses, dyspnea with extension of the head and neck, tachycardia, and respiratory arrest occur. Death ensues most often 24–72 hours after the onset of clinical signs due to respiratory failure. The most consistent necropsy findings are pulmonary edema and congestion and excessive pericardial fluid, which contains free-floating strands of fibrin.

Diagnosis

A botulism diagnosis is challenging and is often primarily based on clinical signs and exclusion of other potential neurological (such as tick paralysis, hypermagnesemia, West Nile virus) and toxicological (such as lead toxicity) causes.

Laboratory assays are often inconclusive due to low circulating levels of the neurotoxin. The available mouse bio-assay requires at least six milliliters of plasma or serum from an affected horse prior to antitoxin treatment. The levels of circulating toxin are often below the detection threshold for this assay.

The most accurate diagnosis comes from being able to identify the bacteria in the horse's feed or environment. This is more likely to be successfully determined in outbreaks, rather than when only one or two horses from a property are affected. Sometimes *C. botulinum* spores can be identified in intestinal contents of horses with clinical signs. Definitive diagnosis has been achieved through the identification of the specific neurotoxin through PCR testing in the feces, gastrointestinal tract or wound. An electrophysiological test (nerve testing) developed for large animals at UC Davis has been successful in strongly supporting botulism as a clinical diagnosis.

The mouse inoculation test is the traditional diagnostic test

Although sporadic cases of botulism are often suspected because of the characteristic motor paralysis; however, it is difficult to establish the diagnosis via detection of the toxin in animal tissues or serum samples or in the suspect feed. Commonly, diagnosis is made by eliminating other causes of motor (flaccid) paralysis. Filtrates of the stomach and intestinal contents should be tested for signs of toxicosis in mice, but a negative result is unreliable. Primary supportive evidence is provided if feeding suspect material to susceptible animals produces similar clinical signs. In peracute cases, the toxin may be detectable in the blood by use of the mouse inoculation tests but usually is not useful in the typical field case in animals on farms. Use of ELISA testing for detection of the toxin makes it feasible to test large numbers of samples, increasing the chances of diagnostic confirmation. In toxicoinfectious botulism, the organism may be cultured from tissues of affected animals.

Treatment and Control of Botulism in Animals

- Control and correction of dietary deficiencies
- Immunization with region-specific type toxoid
- Supportive care
- Sometimes, botulinum antitoxin

Any dietary deficiencies in range animals should be corrected and carcasses disposed of, if possible. Decaying grass or spoiled silage should be removed from the diet. Immunization of cattle with types C and D toxoid has proved successful in South Africa and Australia. Toxoid is also effective in immunizing mink and has been used in pheasants.

Botulinum antitoxin has been used for treatment with varying degrees of success, depending on the type of toxin involved and the species of host. Treatment involves hydration, correcting electrolyte disturbances, and general supportive measures. Treatment of ducks and mink with type C antitoxin is often successful; however, such treatment is rarely used in cattle. Early administration of antitoxin (type B) specific or polyvalent to foals before recumbency (30,000 IU, IV) is reported to be successful. Supportive care in valuable animals is essential; prognosis is poor in recumbent animals. In endemic areas (eg, Kentucky), vaccination with type B toxoid appears to be effective.

CLOSTRIDIAL DIARRHEA/ENTERITIS

Definition

Clostridial diarrhea is caused by the gram-positive, anaerobic, spore-forming bacteria *Clostridium* spp. While the most common isolates are *C. perfringens* and *C. difficile*, multiple others, including *C. septicum*, *C. cadaveris* and *C. sordellii*, have also been associated with enterocolitis.

Clostridial bacteria are present in the environment and in feces. In adult horses clostridial diarrhea has been associated with factors that may alter the balance of the intestinal flora such as the administration of antibiotics, feed changes, and transportation but can occur in the absence of any identifiable risk factors.

Clostridium difficile and *C perfringens* are common causes of enterocolitis in horses and foals. Antimicrobial administration has been associated with *C difficile* diarrhea. Some reports attribute 50% of cases of foal diarrhea to *C perfringens*. *C difficile* produces toxin A and/or toxin B, which cause fluid secretion and lead to intestinal inflammation. It is common for the GI tract of newborn foals to be rapidly colonized by *C difficile*, which can be cultured from feces using sensitive anaerobic techniques. Nontoxin-producing strains are considered commensals. *C difficile* can be isolated from various segments of the small and large intestine and rectum of a large proportion of healthy horses, and from fecal samples of as many as 8% of healthy horses.

Approximately one-third of healthy broodmares and >90% of foals in the general population shed *C perfringens* in their feces; therefore, it is important to determine the presence of a toxin-producing strain. Strains of *C perfringens* are classified by the toxins they produce. However, toxins and toxin-producing strains of *C perfringens* and *C difficile* can be detected in healthy as well as in diarrheic horses and foals. The most common type of *C perfringens* identified is type A, which can be detected in the feces of as many as 8% of healthy horses.

Type C is rarely identified in the feces or environment of healthy broodmares and their foals but is associated with the highest mortality. Antimicrobial use, food deprivation, and other stressors have been suggested to predispose horses to the overgrowth of either or both *C perfringens* and *C difficile*, leading to GI disease. In one report, mares whose foals were being treated with erythromycin developed fatal enterocolitis associated with *C difficile*. Clostridial spores can persist in the environment and can be resistant to many disinfectants; therefore, nosocomial infection can occur in contaminated environments.

Clinical Signs

Clinical signs include sudden death, diarrhea with or without blood, colic, fever, reduced feed intake, and lethargy. Disease can range from subclinical to severe enterocolitis to peracute death before the development of diarrhea. With advanced diagnostic techniques, clostridial infections account for a large proportion of the previously undiagnosed cases known as "colitis-X." Because of the loss of mucosal integrity, bacterial translocation across the GI tract can occur, resulting in bacteremia due to clostridial or other enteric bacterial species. Clinical signs of sepsis or systemic inflammatory response are often present and consistent with other causes of enterocolitis.

Clostridiosis cannot be clinically distinguished from salmonellosis. Foals affected at <3 days of age with *C perfringens*–associated enterocolitis often have bloody diarrhea and colic. Fluid and gas-filled intestine is often identified on ultrasound or radiography. In severe cases, necrotizing enterocolitis occurs with thickening and even intramural gas evident within the wall of the intestine.

Several foals on a particular farm may be affected, but the disease is typically sporadic. The role of *C perfringens* type A in enterocolitis in neonatal foals is less clear; it has been reported that >90% of foals at 3 days of age shed this organism in their feces and that *C perfringens* type A is likely one of the first bacteria to colonize the intestinal tract of newborn foals, irrespective of hygiene protocols.

C difficile has been associated with enterocolitis in newborn foals as well as in adult horses. It has been identified as a nosocomial infection in people, and this may also be seen in horses. The mortality rate associated with *C difficile* and *C perfringens* enterocolitis, especially type C, can be high, even with intensive medical treatment.

- May occur as an individual case or cluster of horses with enterocolitis
- Diarrhea onset may be peracute (with rapid progression to death), acute, or gradual
- Diarrhea is often hemorrhagic, or dark and foul smelling but may have any appearance
- Colic
- Fever
- Reduced appetite or inappetance
- Septic shock
- Sudden death

Risk Factors

Disruption of intestinal flora is thought to induce overgrowth of intestinal toxigenic clostridia, resulting in diarrhea. Factors associated with this include:

- Stress
- Hospitalization
- Surgery
- Administration of antimicrobials
- Sudden dietary changes
- Deworming of horses having a heavy parasite load
- Gastric acid suppression has been implicated in human beings and foals

Transmission

- Fecal-oral
- Environmental

While clostridial bacteria are considered to be part of normal equine gastrointestinal flora, it is prudent to isolate any horse with acute diarrhea and take appropriate hygiene precautions. Outbreaks of clostridial diarrhea among horses and foals at farms and hospitals have been reported.

Diagnosis

Diagnosis is based on identification of toxigenic clostridia from fresh fecal samples, reflux, intestinal contents, or tissue. Blood culture is indicated in foals and adults with severe enterocolitis. Fecal samples for culture and detection of toxins or toxin-producing genes should be delivered directly to the laboratory, or shipped overnight, chilled (not frozen) on ice. Samples for culture must be maintained in an anaerobic environment.

Isolation of clostridial organisms requires anaerobic conditions and, depending on the organism, special growth media. *C difficile* is inherently difficult to culture, hence its name. Communicating to the laboratory that clostridial enterocolitis is a differential diagnosis is critical, because many veterinary laboratories do not routinely culture fecal samples anaerobically unless specifically requested to do so.

Because nonpathogenic serovars are common, a positive culture for *C difficile* or *C perfringens* must be confirmed by identification of toxins or their genes. A PCR test, available at selected laboratories, allows differentiation of *C perfringens* types A, B, C, D, and E based on combinations of α, β, op ε toxins, as well as on identification of the gene coding for the β_2 toxin. Commercially available tests for clostridial toxins include an ELISA for *C difficile* toxin A and *C perfringens* enterotoxin, and a latex agglutination test for *C perfringens* enterotoxin. Toxin tests can be performed in-house, are rapid, and for *C difficile* are both sensitive and specific.

Diagnosis of clostridial enterocolitis is often made at necropsy and is based primarily on identification of intestinal necrosis associated with large gram-positive rods in intestinal smears. Tissue and fecal specimens must be taken immediately after death to avoid degradation of toxins or an overgrowth of clostridial organisms.

Treatment

Treatment with metronidazole (15–20 mg/kg, PO, tid-qid) appears to be beneficial in treating enteric clostridial infections. Pharmacokinetic studies have not been performed in foals, but oral and even IV metronidazole appears generally safe. In some geographic regions, metronidazole-resistant *C difficile* strains have emerged that appear sensitive to vancomycin; however, metronidazole should be used whenever possible. Supportive care is similar to that for other causes of equine enterocolitis, often requiring large volumes of IV polyionic fluids, with supplemental electrolytes (potassium, magnesium, and calcium), plasma or synthetic colloids for low oncotic pressure, anti-inflammatories such as flunixin meglumine, and broad-spectrum antibiotics if the horse is leukopenic and at risk of bacterial translocation across the compromised GI tract.

Polymyxin B may aid in binding systemic endotoxin. Total or partial parenteral nutrition to provide nutritional support can be useful in foals if milk is withheld or decreased to allow gut rest. Foals with colic or profuse diarrhea often benefit from milk withdrawal. Continuous infusion of IV fluids and parenteral nutritional support is optimal but labor intensive and requires separation of the foal and mare. However, the course of diarrhea appears to be dramatically shortened, thus justifying the more intensive approach in some severe cases.

The yeast *Saccharomyces boulardii* has been shown to be protective in clostridial diarrhea in other species, and there is some evidence of beneficial effects in the treatment of horses with colitis. It produces a protease that specifically degrades *C difficile* toxins A and B. Orally administered DTO smectite powder also blinds clostridial toxins and may be useful in horses with diarrhea.

Specific antitoxin for *C perfringens* type C and D has also been used in foals; however, it is not approved for this use. The benefit of type C and D antitoxin in disease associated with type A or β2 toxin is unknown, but based on production methods, the α and β2 toxins are unlikely to be present in high levels in this toxoid.

Prevention

No proven effective biologic products are available to immunize horses or foals against clostridial enterocolitis. When the disease is a problem in multiple foals on a farm, preventive measures have been implemented, but the efficacy and safety of these interventions have yet to be critically evaluated. These measures include vaccinating pregnant mares twice at 2- to 4-wk intervals at least 1 mo before foaling with *C perfringens* type C and D toxoid (bacterin products and those with oil adjuvants should be avoided); using *C perfringens* type C and D antitoxin prophylactically, PO, in newborn foals; and administering antimicrobials (eg, metronidazole) prophylactically to foals for the first 3–5 days of life.

The *C perfringens* type C and D toxoid and antitoxin are not approved for use in horses; however, these products have been used by some owners because of the high mortality rate in foals with clostridial enterocolitis on problem farms. Adverse reactions to the *C perfringens* type C and D toxoid have been reported in broodmares.

The most important strategy for prevention is good farm hygiene. Clostridial spores are extremely resilient in the environment and resistant to many disinfectants. Keeping the foaling area and mare as clean as possible during the perinatal period and ensuring rapid ingestion (by stomach tube if necessary) of colostrum within 1 hr of birth have reduced incidence of disease on some contaminated farms. The mare's hindlegs, tail, and udder can also be washed in soapy water immediately after foaling to decrease ingestion of fecal material by newborn foals. Affected animals should be isolated to limit cross-infection and contamination of pastures and stalls.

EASTERN EQUINE ENCEPHALITIS (EEE)

Eastern equine encephalitis (EEE), also known as sleeping sickness, is a viral disease that causes inflammation of the brain and spinal cord. Wild birds are a natural reservoir for

EEE virus, and mosquitoes that feed on these birds can transmit the virus to mammals, including horses and humans.

Eastern equine encephalitis (EEE) virus is spread to people by the bite of an infected mosquito. Only a few cases are reported in the United States each year. Most cases occur in eastern or Gulf Coast states. Although rare, EEE is very serious. Approximately 30% of people with EEE die and many survivors have ongoing neurologic problems.

There are no vaccines to prevent or medicines to treat EEE. You can reduce your risk of infection with EEE virus by using insect repellent, wearing long-sleeved shirts and long pants, and taking steps to control mosquitoes indoors and outdoors.

Cases are most commonly seen in the southeastern United States, with the mosquito *Culiseta melanura* as the primary vector (although other species of mosquito can also transmit the virus). Infected horses and humans do not have enough virus in their blood to be contagious to other animals or people. As such, infected individuals do not need to be quarantined.

The disease has a high mortality rate in horses and humans, and, as such, is considered one of the most serious mosquito-borne diseases.

The severity of the disease depends on the individual virus. Infections with Eastern and Venezuelan equine encephalitis are generally severe and can progress to death over a short period of time. West Nile virus and Western equine encephalomyelitis are less severe. Not all infected animals develop signs of disease; a horse may be infected with the virus, develop antibodies to it, and eliminate the virus without showing any obvious signs of illness.

Nervous system signs may vary, depending on the type of virus involved. Observable signs can include impaired vision, aimless wandering, head pressing, circling, inability to swallow, irregular gait, weakness and paralysis, convulsions, and death. Many horses have a fever. Horses with West Nile encephalomyelitis may have spinal cord incoordination, muscle contractions, and an abnormal sensitivity to touch. Nearly half of affected horses have a distinctive twitching of the muzzle early in the course of the disease.

A tentative diagnosis is made based on signs and by comparing the location of the affected horse(s) and the season of the year with known data on the insects that carry the disease. Detection of certain blood antibodies (IgM) against the causative virus provides additional support for the diagnosis.

There is no specific treatment for viral encephalitis. Supportive care includes intravenous fluids if the horse is unable to drink, use of appropriate anti-inflammatory agents, and anticonvulsants if necessary. Good nursing care is essential.

Vaccines are currently available for Eastern, Western, Venezuelan, and West Nile encephalomyelitis. Your veterinarian can recommend the appropriate vaccine and booster schedule for your horse depending on the geographic location and current guidelines.

Other preventive measures involve minimizing potential exposure to infected mosquitoes by managing the environment, keeping living areas clear of weeds and organic material (feces), cleaning water tanks and buckets at least weekly, and removing containers that hold stagnant water.

The outlook depends greatly on the specific viral cause. Horses that recover may or may not have permanent neurologic damage. The disorder can be fatal. Deaths occur within 2 to 3 days after signs appear with Eastern equine encephalitis. Signs of West Nile virus infection may wax and wane over several days to weeks.

Risk to People

People can be infected by all of the viruses that commonly cause viral encephalitis in horses. Signs in people vary from mild flu-like symptoms to death. Children, the elderly, and people whose immune systems are suppressed are the most susceptible. People usually develop permanent neurologic impairment. Human disease is reported infrequently and generally follows equine infections by about 2 weeks.

ETIOLOGY & EPIDEMIOLOGY OF ARBOVIRAL ENCEPHALITIDES:

Alphaviruses

North America is home to some of the most pathogenic encephalitic viruses because of the enduring endemic status of alphaviruses of the family Togaviridae. Endemic species in North, Central, or South America include Eastern equine encephalitis virus (EEEV), Western equine encephalitis virus (WEEV), Highlands J virus, Venezuelan equine encephalitis virus (VEEV), Everglades virus, and Una virus. Other alphaviruses associated with equine encephalitis are Semliki Forest virus in Africa and Ross River virus in Australia and the South Pacific. EEEV has two distinct antigenic variants that are separated longitudinally. The North American variant is the most pathogenic and is found in eastern Canada; all States within the USA east of the Mississippi River and in Arkansas, Minnesota, South Dakota, and Texas; and in the Caribbean Islands.

The South American variant is less pathogenic and confined to central and South America and is now called Madariaga virus (MADV). EEE and WEE viruses are separated in North America primarily latitudinally; however, WEEV is relatively heterogeneous, with several subtypes consisting of WEE, Highlands J virus, Sindbis, Aura, Ft. Morgan, and Y 62–33. Several variants have been found in horses.

WEE is found in western Canada, states in the USA west of the Mississippi, and in Mexico and South America. WEE previously isolated in the south and eastern USA has been shown to belong to the Highlands J virus serogroup. VEE has six antigenically related subtypes: subtype I, Everglades, Mucambo, Pixuna, Cabassou, and AG80-663. Subtype I serovars AB and C primarily cause epizootics; subtype I and serovar IE caused a large outbreak in Mexico in 1993. Epizootic strains are not generally found in the USA, although there was an epizootic of VEE in 1971. Sylvatic subtype II (Everglades) has been isolated from people and mosquitoes in Florida; subtype III has been isolated in the Rocky Mountains and northern plains states.

The general life cycle of alphaviruses involves transmission between birds and/or rodents and mosquitoes. In North America, theoretically, EEEV is perpetuated in a sylvatic cycle between avian hosts (passerine birds) and mosquitoes, with primary transmission in this cycle via *Culiseta melanura*. Birds do not develop disease but develop sufficient viremia for transmission to mosquitoes unless the bird belongs to an introduced species that in North America includes European starlings, house sparrows, pheasants, and emus. Field work in Alabama indicates that the northern cardinal is the primary target for *C melanura* feeding; however, other mosquitoes (*C erraticus*) are capable of feeding on a wider variety of birds, including robins, chickadees, owls, and mockingbirds. Mammalian reservoirs may also be important during years of high EEEV transmission. Experimental infection of cotton rats, a marshland rat found throughout the Americas, resulted in viremia just being capable of transmitting EEEV, with juvenile rats developing higher titers and 100% mortality to infection.

Horses and people are clinically affected but do not develop viremia sufficiently high enough to transmit virus to mosquitoes and so are considered "dead-end" hosts. However, young animals are more susceptible to EEEV, and it is not known how important non-neural tissues are for harboring high viral infection. Presumed extraneural sites of infection include cardiac tissue and bone marrow. During epizootics, alpacas, llamas, cattle, swine, cats, and dogs can develop disease. Snakes have been identified as a possible reservoir.

Freshwater hardwood swamps are the most associated enzootic niche for EEEV. In the southern USA, which has the highest number of reported annual cases, reemergence within mammalian hosts is associated with "tree farms" that often function as inland freshwater swamps. Nonetheless, EEEV disease occurs frequently in naive horses in southeastern habitats not associated with sylvatic field ecology, so a full understanding of the epizootic cycle still remains to be elucidated. Intense focal activity has been reported in Michigan, Wisconsin, Ohio, Massachusetts, and New Hampshire. In 2005, Massachusetts experienced a human case affected rate more than five times that of the preceding 10 yr; affected people resided within ½ mile of a cranberry bog or swamp associated with forest habitat.

The principal vectors of MADV belong to *Culex* (*Melanoconion*) spp found in Central and South America. These vectors feed on birds, rodents, marsupials, and reptiles, with rodent reservoirs possibly featuring more importantly in this life cycle. Before the year 2000, comparatively few epizootics of disease caused by MADV in horses were recorded in South America, with minimal disease reported in people. Furthermore, there are notable differences in virulence between EEEV strains in South America vs in North

America. In 2008 and 2009, larger outbreaks occurred in Central and South America. In northeastern Brazil, 229 horses were affected, with a case fatality rate of 73% and disease severity similar to that of EEEV in North America.

WEE, which is found just west of the Mississippi river and throughout the West, is transmitted primarily by *C tarsalis*. This mosquito breeds in sunlit marshes and in pools of irrigation water in pastures. WEE can also be transmitted by the tick *Dermacentor andersoni*. Epizootics of WEE are associated with increased rainfall in early spring followed by warmer than normal temperatures.

Sylvatic VEE viruses are found throughout America in jungle or swampy areas. Two cycles occur with VEEV, the enzootic cycle and the epizootic cycle. The mosquitoes that serve as the primary vectors for the bird- or rodent-mosquito life cycle are members of the subgenus *Melanoconion* (*C cedecci*). Epizootics are associated with a mutation to a subtype I (AB, C, and possibly E), a change in mammalian pathogenesis, and a change to several bridge vectors. The enzootic cycle centers around sylvatic rodents such as spiny and cotton rats, which have high natural infection rates and can develop viremia high enough to transmit VEEV to mosquitoes. Opossums, bats, and shore birds likely contribute to dispersal of the enzootic virus so that constant cycling occurs.

When epizootics occur with mutation of the virus and this change in mosquito vectors, equine infection becomes a predominant feature in the maintenance of epizootic VEE. All mammalian hosts are capable of developing a high-titer viremia of ~106 plaque-forming units/mL for up to 5 days, but the horse is likely to be the most important mammalian host in terms of vector capacity.

Flaviviruses

In general, viruses belonging to the Flaviviridae and Bunyaviridae families are less pathogenic than the Togaviridae; however, viral encephalomyelitis caused by any of these pathogens is a potentially catastrophic illness for any vertebrate host. There are 53 species of flavivirus, and many are clinical pathogens for horses, including Japanese encephalitis, West Nile virus (WNV) encephalitis, Kunjin virus (KUN), and Murray Valley encephalitis virus. Overall, the diseases caused by the Japanese encephalitis serogroup are similar.

All of these viruses are transmitted by a mosquito vector, with *Culex* spp usually the most efficient transmitter. KUN is actually a strain of WNV and is found in Australia, some southeast Asia countries, and New Guinea. Disease in horses caused by Murray Valley fever is geographically restricted to the South Pacific and is sporadic in occurrence.

WNV has the widest geographic distribution of all of the flaviviruses. Prior to 1999, WNV was recognized in Africa, the Middle East, Asia, and occasionally in European countries.

In 1999, WNV infection was first recognized in North America. Since then, the virus has spread throughout the USA and parts of Canada and Mexico. WNV isolated from the outbreak in New York in 1999 appears to be closely related to an isolate recovered from geese in Israel in 1998.

Since 2010, continued worldwide spread and reemergence of many flaviviruses, especially WNV, has occurred. As of 2014, WNV is recognized as having seven lineages, with lineage 1 (sublineage 1a, 1b, and 1c) and lineage 2 affecting people and horses. Lineage 1a activity in the USA and Europe dominated much of the end of the 1990s until the mid-2000s, causing neuroinvasive infections in people and horses in Africa, Europe, Australia, Asia, North and Central America, and the Middle East.

In 2012, a very large epizootic occurred in the USA, with 5,674 human and 690 equine cases reported. New emergences have occurred in Greece and Serbia, and the first lineage 1a case in India was detected in 2012. Lineage 1b viruses are primarily represented by KUN, with Australia undergoing the largest epizootic of arboviral disease in 2011, involving 900 horses. Although multiple pathogens were detected, including KUN, Murray Valley encephalitis virus, and Ross River virus, there was emergence of a new strain of KUN. The 1c viruses are fairly nonpathogenic and found in India.

Lineage 2 strains, long considered African based and inducing mild disease in horses, is also expanding globally with increased neuroinvasive activity. Neuroinvasive disease due to lineage 2 has emerged across Europe in Hungary, Austria, Italy, and Greece, which had at least four epizootic cycles with cases of neuroinvasive disease identified in horses.

Both wetland and terrestrial birds may be involved in the natural cycle of WNV, with migratory birds thought to introduce the virus into a geographic region. However, a wide range of infected birds (~326) have high, sustained viremia and little or no clinical disease (passerines). Fatal infections among corvids (eg, crows, blue jays, and magpies) have been the hallmark of WNV infection in the USA. Ticks have been demonstrated to be infected with WNV, but their role in natural transmission is unknown. Experimentally, transmission has been documented between cohabitating birds and from oral exposure to WNV in drinking water in birds. Oral transmission has been demonstrated experimentally in several types of raptors.

In people, other important routes of infection include blood transfusions, organ donation, breast milk, and across the placenta. Sporadic infections and illness have also occurred in several other mammalian species, including dogs, cats, camelids, sheep, and squirrels. Oral transmission has been demonstrated experimentally in cats. Farmed alligators have demonstrated disease and mortality due to WNV, and there has also been a report of WNV-induced disease in crocodiles. Alligators are susceptible to oral infection. In addition to birds, only alligators have consistently demonstrated high enough viremia (10^4–10^5 plaque-forming units) to amplify virus, serve as reservoir hosts, and transmit virus back to mosquitoes.

Most equine-associated flaviviruses are maintained in an enzootic transmission cycle between wild birds and mosquitoes, although tickborne encephalitis found in Eurasia can cause disease in horses. Many species of mosquitoes can transmit the equine virulent viruses, although *Culex* spp are principal vectors to maintain enzootic activity. *C pipiens* complex and *C tarsalis* are thought to play the largest role in natural transmission in North America. In the eastern and Midwestern regions of the USA, *C pipiens* is one of the major vectors, whereas in the western regions of the USA, *C tarsalis* is thought to be one of the most efficient vectors.

Bunyaviruses

Cache Valley virus (transmitted by mosquitoes and *Culicoides* sp among rabbits), Main Drain virus (transmitted by *Culicoides varipennis* among hares and rodents in the western USA), and snowshoe hare virus (transmitted by *Culiseta* and *Aedes* mosquitoes among rabbits in southern Canada and northern USA) have all been identified, although infrequently, as the cause of encephalitis in horses.

Clinical Findings of Viral Encephalomyelitis in Equids

The initial clinical signs are similar for the arboviruses; progression of clinical signs and severity of disease are the differentiating features. Initially, horses are quiet and depressed, with clinical neurologic signs generally occurring 9–11 days after infection. Compared with WEE and WNV disease, clinical signs of EEEV (and VEEV) encephalomyelitis more frequently include altered mentation, impaired vision, aimless wandering, head pressing, circling, inability to swallow, irregular ataxic gait, paresis and paralysis, seizures, and death. Spinal signs are often symmetric with ataxia in all limbs, rapidly progressing to quadriparesis, along with intensification of forebrain signs. Many horses progress to recumbence within 12–18 hr of onset of neurologic abnormalities. Most deaths occur within 2–3 days after the onset of signs.

WEST NILE VIRUS ENCEPHALOMYELITIS, HORSE

The clinical signs and course of disease are highly variable in WNV disease and other flavivirus encephalomyelitis. Presenting complaints most often include neurologic abnormalities; other common initial complaints include colic, lameness, anorexia, and fever. Initial systemic signs include a mild fever, feed refusal, and depression.

Neurologic signs are highly variable, but spinal cord disease and moderate mental aberrations are most consistent. Spinal cord disease manifests as asymmetric, multifocal or diffuse ataxia and paresis. Severe manifestations of WNV may occur independently in the fore- or hindlimbs, unilaterally, or in a single limb. In all clinical studies published to date, for WNV, >90% of affected horses developed some type of spinal cord signs, whereas 40%–60% developed behavioral changes characterized by periods of hyperesthesia, ranging from mild apprehension to overt hyperexcitability, with fractious reactions to aural, visual, and tactile stimuli.

Fine and coarse tremors of the face and neck muscles are common, described in 60%–90% of horses. Some horses have periods of cataplexy or narcolepsy that may render them temporarily or permanently recumbent. Cranial nerve deficits can be seen in all arbovirus infections of horses; these include most cranial nerves with cell bodies located in the mid- and hindbrains. Weakness and/or paralysis of the face and tongue are most frequent. Horses with facial and tongue paresis can be dysphagic, and overt signs of quidding or even esophageal choke can develop. Many horses with severe mental depression and facial paresis will keep their heads low, resulting in severe facial edema.

Occasionally, head tilt may be seen. Infrequently in WNV disease, urinary dysfunction ranging from mild straining to stranguria has been reported, making differentiation from equine herpesvirus 1 (EHV-1) more challenging.

During the neurologic phase, horses frequently thrash and injure themselves. Sepsis from trauma in recumbent horses also occurs. Prolonged recumbency leads to pulmonary infections, especially in foals, in which a long duration of slinging and treatment may be pursued more frequently than in large, recumbent animals. Dysphagia leads to decreased water and food intake, with renal damage due to concurrent use of anti-inflammatory drugs. Skin and muscle necrosis are common in recumbent horses. Life-threatening trauma can also occur, including a ruptured diaphragm and fractures.

Lesions

All necropsies on horses suspected of viral encephalitis should be performed with all participants wearing personal protective gear (ie, waterproof gown, boots, gloves, N-95 or N-99 mask, face shield, and hair covering). Gross lesions are most common with EEEV and severe VEEV disease and are characterized by widespread and prominent congestion of the meninges. In other infections, gross lesions are rarer and are limited to small multifocal areas of discoloration and hemorrhage throughout the brain and spinal cord. The brain should be examined microscopically for the presence of meningoencephalitis.

In EEEV infection, a severe gliosis with necrosis of the neuropil is seen in the cerebrum and extending through the corona radiata through the hindbrain and cervical spinal cord. Although mononuclear cells are present, neutrophils are widespread and diffusely distributed. The gliosis is less nodular than in WNV, and when there are accumulations of cells, there is extensive necrosis and often frank microscopic hemorrhage within and around lesions. In milder cases and in WNV infections, microscopically there is a non-necrotizing lympho-histiocytic poliomeningoencephalitis.

Slight to severe inflammation, characterized by perivascular cuffing of lymphocytes and monocytes, is usually present. In more severe cases, there can be extravasation of fluid and red blood cells from vessels. Often the distribution of lesions is multifocal, with more severe lesions present in grey matter. In the neuropil, dying neurons often are surrounded by microglial cells. The most severe gliosis and perivascular cuffing is often in the midbrain (thalamus, hypothalamus) and hindbrain (pons and medulla), extending into the cerebellum. Lesions can be multifocal in the spinal cord and can be more severe in the lumbar cord.

Diagnosis

No consistent changes in clinical pathology have been found in equine viral encephalitis. With EEEV and WNV in horses, peripheral lymphopenia is common. Horses are frequently azotemic, likely from decreased food and water intake.

In general, no pathognomonic signs distinguish flavivirus infection in horses from other CNS diseases, and a full diagnostic evaluation should be performed. Confirmation of flavivirus infection with encephalitis in horses begins with assessment of (1) whether the horse meets the case definition based on clinical signs; (2) whether the horse resides in an area in which flavivirus has been confirmed in the current calendar year in mosquitoes, birds, people, or horses; and (3) lack of appropriate vaccination.

In terms of antemortem diagnostic testing, analysis of CSF can be a valuable adjunct to presumptive clinical assessment. CSF analyzed from horses with acute EEEV infection typically shows a neutrophilic pleocytosis with markedly increased total solids. Horses infected with EEEV that are partially immune may have predominantly mononuclear cells, but nondegenerate neutrophils are still present. Although WNV-infected horses can have normal CSF, if the CSF is abnormal, there is a mononuclear pleocytosis with moderately to markedly increased total solids. In a few horses with acute infections, virus may be isolated from the CSF.

By the time neurologic signs are seen, viremia has ended and detection of virus in the plasma of clinically affected horses is of no value. Serology is the key to antemortem diagnosis of recent alphavirus and flavivirus infection in horses showing clinical signs. IgM antibody rises sharply and is increased in 85%–90% of horses with clinical arboviral encephalitis. Thus, the IgM capture ELISA is the test of choice to detect recent exposure to these viruses. Neutralizing antibody titers (primarily IgG) develop slowly during this time and stay increased for several months.

Although neutralizing antibody tests will differentiate between subtypes of these viruses, and are thus considered the gold standard for confirmatory serology, paired serum samples are essential to detect recent exposure and to differentiate antibody response due to field infection from vaccine responses for any of these viruses. Because virus-neutralizing antibodies appear at the end of viremia and may precede appearance of neurologic signs, paired samples may not show a 4-fold increase in horses while demonstrating neurologic signs.

In horses that succumb without premortem and postmortem testing, paired samples from febrile herdmates may be necessary to confirm presence of arbovirus activity within a locale. Maternal antibodies may interfere with neutralizing responses in young foals.

This response is confounded by recent vaccination. The most common neutralizing antibody test formats are the classic plaque reduction neutralization test (PRNT) and a microwell format test. Practical application of the microwell vs the PRNT indicates that the endpoint titer in the microwell test can be several logs higher than in the PRNT, so results cannot be compared between samples. Several postmortem diagnostic assays are available and, although specific, they vary in sensitivity, depending on the virus.

The midbrain and brain stem have the highest concentrations of encephalitic viruses, including rabies virus. Immunohistochemistry and PCR testing for EEEV and EHV-1 are relatively straightforward compared with that for WNV. Diagnostic testing continues to confirm the unreliability of detection of virus, even by PCR, because of the low viral load in WNV infection. Often, only a single neuron in one or two sections may yield positive virus staining in the horse by immunohistochemistry.

When tested by PCR, the limited viral load dictates accurate testing of appropriate tissues consisting of several locations, including thalamus, hypothalamus, rostral colliculus, pons, medulla, and anatomically identified spinal cord. Viral isolation is still important for molecular epidemiology. Infectious and noninfectious causes of brain and spinal cord diseases should be considered as differential diagnoses. Infectious causes include alphaviruses, rabies, equine protozoal myeloencephalitis, and EHV-1; less likely causes are botulism and verminous meningoencephalomyelitis (eg, *Halicephalobus gingivalis*, *Setaria* spp, *Strongylus vulgaris*). Noninfectious causes include hypocalcemia, tremorigenic toxicities, hepatoencephalopathy, and leukoencephalomalacia.

Treatment

Treatment of viral encephalitis is supportive, because there are no specific antiviral therapies. Management is focused on controlling pain and inflammation, preventing injuries associated with ataxia or recumbency, and providing supportive care. Intervention does not appear to significantly affect the outcome of most fulminate EEEV infections. For WNV, flunixin meglumine (1.1 mg/kg, IV, bid) early in the course of the disease decreases the severity of muscle tremors and fasciculations within a few hours of administration.

Recumbent horses that are mentally alert frequently thrash, causing self-inflicted wounds and posing a risk to personnel. Responses to tranquilizers and anticonvulsant medications are variable, depending on the virus and severity of disease.

A sling and hoist may be used to assist horses that are recumbent and have difficulty rising; however, recumbent horses with EEEV generally are too comatose to sling. Dysphagic horses require fluid and nutritional support. Until equine protozoal myeloencephalitis is excluded, prophylactic antiprotozoal medications may be instituted. Other supportive measures (eg, oral and parental fluids and nutrition for dehydrated and dysphagic horses) are also important. Broad-spectrum antibiotics should be given for treatment of wounds, cellulitis, and pneumonia.

Horses with intermittent or focal neuropathies have a better prognosis than those with complete flaccid paralysis or that appear comatose. Efficacy of specific antiviral agents for treatment of naturally occurring WNV or EEEV infection is unknown, even in people. Recent work with passive immunotherapy indicates possible benefit after the onset of clinical signs in WNV models.

Prognosis

Mortality of horses showing clinical signs from EEEV is 50%–90%, from WEEV 20%–50%, from VEEV 50%–75%, and from flavivirus infections 35%-45%. Horses with clinical neurologic signs from alphavirus infection that recover have a high incidence of residual neurologic deficits, whereas many horses that recover from WNV disease have been reported to have no residual neurologic deficits. In EEEV infection, death is frequently spontaneous. With WNV disease, horses are euthanized for humane reasons, but spontaneous death does occur. In EEEV, most surviving horses exhibit longterm neurologic signs.

In WNV disease, overt clinical signs in horses that recover can last from 1 day to several weeks; improvement usually occurs within 7 days of onset of clinical signs. Although 80%–90% of owners report that the horse returns to normal function 1–6 mo after disease, at least 10% of owners report longterm deficits that limit athletic potential and resale value. Deficits include residual weakness or ataxia in one or more limbs, fatigue with exercise, focal or generalized muscle atrophy, and changes in personality and behavioral aberrations.

Prevention

Vaccination against alphaviruses and flaviviruses as core annual vaccines are considered the standard of care for all horses in the USA as endorsed by the American Association of Equine Practitioners. Formalin-inactivated whole viral vaccines for EEEV, WEEV, and VEEV are commercially available in bi- and trivalent forms, usually formulated with tetanus toxoid; several now include WNV. Nonvaccinated adult horses require the label priming two injections. For adult horses in temperate climates, an annual vaccine within 1 mo before the start of the arbovirus season is recommended.

However, for horses that travel between northern and southern areas affected by the virus, injections should be given two or even three times yearly in active arbovirus seasons. Mares should be vaccinated 1 mo before foaling to induce colostral antibody. If a pregnant mare is naive, the full priming series starting 2 months before foaling is recommended. However, some mares do not produce colostral antibody if vaccinated for the first time during gestation.

In foals that have received adequate colostrum from vaccinated dams, vaccination should begin at 5–6 mo of age; foals should receive two additional vaccinations at 30 and 90 days after the first one. It is unclear whether maternal antibody interferes with vaccine responses in foals; however, epidemiologic evidence strongly indicates that horses between 4 mo and 4 yr old are highly susceptible to EEEV.

If there is early spring (March) activity in the southeastern USA, horses may require three injections throughout the year, especially in horses <5 yr old and in horses that have recently arrived in the southeastern USA. In foals born to nonvaccinated or minimally vaccinated mares, maternal immunity may wane, and vaccination should be performed at 4, 5, and 6 mo of age. In Florida, where the highest numbers of EEEV cases occur, horses of all ages should be vaccinated in January and again in April before the peak of the season. A third vaccination should be administered late in the summer if the season is particularly active. The frequency of vaccination may be minimized to once or twice per year in climates that have short mosquito seasons and in which limited activity has historically been reported.

Currently, several whole inactivated virion vaccines, one recombinant inactivated vaccine, and a canarypox-vectored vaccine are licensed for prevention of WNV viremia in most of the Americas, including the USA and Canada, and Europe. An inactivated virus vaccine is readily available against Japanese encephalitis virus. There is experimental evidence that the canarypox WNV lineage 1 vaccine provides cross-protection against WNV lineage 2 infection. WNV challenge studies indicate that ~10% of properly immunized horses do not produce neutralizing antibodies to WNV and that 2.3%–3% of equine WNV cases seen in the field are in fully vaccinated horses. The duration of immunity from vaccination with the killed, adjuvanted WNV vaccine is unknown.

Protection of horses from arboviruses must also include efforts to minimize exposure to infected mosquitoes. Mosquito mitigation includes applying an insect repellent that contains permethrin on the horses at least daily during vector season, especially at times of day when mosquitoes may be most active. Environmental management is also essential and includes keeping the barn area, paddocks, and pastures cleared of weeds and organic material, such as feces, that might harbor adult mosquitoes. Cleaning water tanks and buckets at least weekly will reduce mosquito breeding areas. Removal of other containers such as flower pots and used tires that may hold stagnant water is essential for reducing the number of mosquitoes in the area.

Options for control of arbovirus infection in other animals emphasize reduction of exposure. Few arbovirus infections have been documented in dogs and cats; however, exposure to EEEV and WNV is detected in both species during arbovirus seasons. In active years, young dogs have been reported to be susceptible to EEEV infection.

Keeping dogs and cats indoors or in a screened area, especially during the time when mosquitoes are most active, reduces exposure. Disposal of dead birds or other small prey that might be eaten may reduce oral exposure.

Clinical cases of both of these diseases have also been recorded in other domestic and exotic animals during active seasons. Emus are exceptionally susceptible to EEEV.

These animals are used for the commercial food industry, and infection results in high viremia and high amounts of virus shedding rectally, orally, and in regurgitated material. Vaccination will prevent viremia, shedding, and disease. Camelids are susceptible to WNV, and numerous reports of disease and pathology were recorded as the virus spread across North America. The killed, adjuvanted vaccine marketed for use in horses has been used in camelids without any reports of major adverse effects, and animals have demonstrated production of neutralizing antibody.

Zoonotic Risk

The reporting of these diseases (or suspicion of such) on an international and national basis is a basic duty of all veterinarians to ensure the health and safety of horses and people. As such, a thorough diagnostic investigation to confirm these infections is imperative, irrespective of state resources available for subsidized testing.

People may be infected by most of the arboviruses that commonly cause viral encephalitis in horses. Clinical signs in people vary from mild flu-like symptoms to death. Children, the elderly, and those who are immunosuppressed are the most susceptible. People with neurologic disease due to arboviruses usually have permanent neurologic impairment after recovery. Human disease is reported infrequently and generally follows equine infections by ~2 wk. Veterinarians should be aware of the possibility of human infection and use repellents and other procedures to protect themselves from hematophagous insects when working in sylvatic virus habitats or handling viremic horses. In addition, waterproof clothing (gown, boots, gloves), respirator (N-95 or N-99 mask), face shield, and hair covering are recommended during all necropsies performed on horses suspected of having encephalomyelitis.

The initial clinical signs are similar for the arboviruses; progression of clinical signs and severity of disease are the differentiating features. Initially, horses are quiet and depressed, with clinical neurologic signs generally occurring 9–11 days after infection. Compared with WEE and WNV disease, clinical signs of EEEV (and VEEV) encephalomyelitis more frequently include altered mentation, impaired vision, aimless wandering, head pressing, circling, inability to swallow, irregular ataxic gait, paresis and paralysis, seizures, and death. Spinal signs are often symmetric with ataxia in all limbs, rapidly progressing to quadriparesis, along with intensification of forebrain signs. Many horses progress to recumbence within 12–18 hr of onset of neurologic abnormalities. Most deaths occur within 2–3 days after the onset of signs.

EQUINE CORONAVIRUS (ECOV)

Coronaviruses are known to cause illness in a variety of species and tend to attack specific organ systems such as the respiratory or gastrointestinal tracts. Genetically, equine coronavirus (ECoV) appears to be a close relative of bovine coronavirus. There is currently no evidence that equine or bovine coronaviruses are likely to be infectious to humans. However, it is always advisable to follow basic biosecurity protocols when handling sick animals.

Historically, ECoV was thought to occur only in foals, but it has been increasingly reported in adult horses. It is highly contagious and transmitted between horses through exposure to contaminated fecal material. Equine coronavirus is most commonly diagnosed in the winter.

Equine Coronavirus (ECoV) is an important cause of enteric disease in adult horses. Reported worldwide with increasing incidence, it is a single-stranded RNA virus in the beta coronavirus family. The role of ECoV as a cause of diarrhea in foals is still unclear as the virus can be detected in both healthy and sick foals.

Prevalence

Unknown, but likely low. In a study of horses presenting for gastrointestinal disease, ECoV was isolated by PCR from only 1/258 fecal samples. In a study investigating seroprevalance, 9.6% of adult healthy horses from the United States tested seropositive to ECoV. Geographic region (Mid-West), breed (Draft horses) and specific uses of horses (ranch/farm and breeding use) were all statistically significant risk factors for seropositivity. ECoV infections have predominantly been reported in adult horses since 2010 with increasing frequency of positive cases reported by diagnostic laboratories.

Clinical signs

Clinical disease is generally mild, but mortality from necrotizing enteritis and hyperammonemic encephalopathy has been reported. Miniature horses appear to be at higher risk of complications from ECoV infection. ECoV cases occur year round, with a large proportion diagnosed during the winter months.

- May occur as an individual case or outbreak.
- Fever up to 105° F (40.5° C).
- Leukopenia characterized by neutropenia and lymphopenia (can be severe).
- Inappetance.
- Lethargy.
- Diarrhea is an inconsistent finding.
- Scant fecal production.
- Colic.

Complications that occur in rare cases:

- Hypoproteinemia, electrolyte and metabolic derangements secondary to intestinal inflammation.

- Hyperammonemic encephalopathy (lethargy, obtundation, wandering, ataxia, seizures).
- Death secondary to septicemia.

Risk Factors

- Exposure to clinical and subclinical horses shedding ECoV in feces.
- Co-mingling with horses of unknown infection status.

Transmission

Fecal-oral

- During farm outbreaks, clinically unaffected horses may shed virus
- Transmission can occur directly between horses as well as through environmental contamination.
- Fomite transmission is possible, especially via contaminated stalls, muck forks, manure spreaders, thermometers, hands, and clothing.

Diagnostic Sampling, Testing, and Handling

A diagnosis of ECoV infection relies on the presence of clinical signs compatible with ECoV infection, the exclusion of other infectious agents, and the detection of ECoV in feces. A consistent hematological abnormality observed in horses infected with ECoV is leukopenia due to neutropenia and/or lymphopenia. Laboratory support of ECoV infection should be based on the molecular detection of ECoV in feces via PCR.

Post-mortem diagnosis of ECoV can be achieved by PCR on feces or small intestinal contents collected at post-mortem examination.

In outbreak situations, the testing of in-contact healthy horses may help determine the extent of the outbreak and confine ECoV shedding from subclinically infected horses.

Shedding of Virus

Under natural conditions, fecal shedding of ECoV has been reported to range from 3 to 25 days. In a small experimental infection study, horses shed from days 3 to 15 following infection. Horses with no clinical signs of the disease can shed the virus.

Carrier status

Carrier status is currently unknown but subclinical horses (horses with no clinical signs) have been found to shed the virus in feces, and likely serve as silent reservoirs for infection.

Treatment

Treatment for ECoV involves supportive care based on the clinical signs. Severe cases may require hospitalization for intravenous fluid treatment, colloid support, and/or correction of electrolyte and metabolic derangements.

Prognosis

Good. Exposure to the virus can result in up to 85% infection rate but most animals do not show clinical signs. Mortality is generally low.

Environmental Persistence

Unknown, however greater survival and viability of ECoV is to be expected in colder weather and is one possible explanation for the apparent higher prevalence of virus positive fecal samples and clinical disease during cooler weather.

Prevention

There are currently no vaccines for ECoV. Prevention involves minimizing contact between at-risk horses, maintaining high standards of sanitation in all equine facilities and carefully disposingl of manure where it cannot contaminate pastures, paddocks or drinking water.

Biosecurity

ECoV should be suspected in any horse with fever and no evidence of respiratory illness. Horses positive for ECoV should be isolated and strict biosecurity measures and manure management instituted to prevent the spread of infection to other horses in the vicinity. Other horses on the property should be monitored for fevers and/or leukopenia. Personnel working with infected horses should use disposable gloves and personal protective equipment (gowns, boot covers) and wash hands thoroughly with liquid hand soap and water followed by 70% ethanol hand sanitizer after handing sick animals.

EQUINE HERPESVIRUS (EHV-1 AND EHV-4)

Equine herpesviruses are DNA viruses that are found in most horses all over the world. Almost all horses have been infected with the viruses and have most of the times no serious side effects. It is currently unknown what causes some infected horses to develop the serious neurological forms associated with EHV1 that may be fatal.

In its most common form, EHV-1 causes respiratory disease in foals, yearlings and young horses in training. They show variable signs that include elevated temperature, watery nasal discharge, enlarged glands under the jaw and coughing. Some cases may progress to secondary pneumonia. In horses in training, symptoms may be mild but 'epidemic' loss of performance may occur. EHV-1 can cause single or multiple abortions ('virus abortion') in mares during mid to late pregnancy. Also, infected foals may be prematurely born alive but soon fade and die while others are born dead at full term. Disastrous epidemics ('abortion storms') can occur in susceptible pregnant mare populations. Also, the virus can also cause paralysis, in horses of all ages and types, often first involving weakness of the hind limbs but then progressing to involve all four limbs and resulting in death or a requirement for euthanasia.

EHV-2 does not usually cause disease on its own but is believed to cause suppression of the horse's immunity to other viral infections and allows them to cause signs of disease, usually respiratory infection, i.e., elevated temperature, watery nasal discharge, enlarged glands under the jaw and coughing.

EHV-3 causes 'coital exanthema' that is an infection of the external genital region (vulva in mares, penis and scrotum in stallions) characterized by numerous small blisters or spots, sometimes called 'the pox'. The blisters burst and become secondarily infected by skin colonizing bacteria and then heal leaving white (de-pigmented) skin spots. The infection spreads venereally usually from carrier mare to stallions and then to other mares. It has no direct effect on the fertility of stallions or mares but natural mating must be stopped to allow the disease to take its natural course (usually 10 days to 2 weeks to complete healing) and to prevent further spread of infection.

EHV-4 is a common cause of coughing and loss of performance in racehorses. Usually the respiratory disease is not severe but the disruption to training and performance programs and consequent economic losses can be very significant. Rarely, EHV-4 is a cause of isolated abortions in mares.

Etiology and Epidemiology

Equine herpesvirus 1 (EHV-1) and equine herpesvirus 4 (EHV-4) comprise two antigenically distinct groups of viruses previously referred to as subtypes 1 and 2 of EHV-1. Both viruses are ubiquitous in horse populations worldwide and produce an acute febrile respiratory disease upon primary infection, characterized by rhinopharyngitis and tracheobronchitis. Outbreaks of respiratory disease occur annually among foals in areas with concentrated horse populations. Most of these outbreaks in weanlings are caused by strains of EHV-4. The age, seasonal, and geographic distributions vary and are determined by immune status and horse population. In individual horses, the outcome of exposure is determined by viral strain, immune status, pregnancy status, and possibly age. Infection of pregnant mares with EHV-4 rarely results in abortion.

Mares may abort several weeks to months after clinical or subclinical infection with EHV-1. The neurologic form of EHV-1 has demonstrated increasing morbidity and mortality in the documented outbreaks since 2000 and appears to be evolving in virulence and behavior. Therefore, the USDA has designated neuropathic EHV-1 as a potentially emerging disease. The natural reservoir of both EHV-1 and EHV-4 is the horse. Latent infections and carrier states are seen with both virus types. Transmission occurs by direct or indirect contact with infectious nasal secretions, aborted fetuses, placentas, or placental fluids.

Clinical Findings

The incubation period of EHV is 2–10 days. Susceptible horses develop fever of 102°–107°F (38.9°–41.7°C), neutropenia and lymphopenia, serous nasal discharge, malaise, pharyngitis, cough, inappetence, and/or submandibular or retropharyngeal lymphadenopathy. Horses infected with EHV-1 strains often develop a biphasic fever, with cell-associated viremia coinciding with the second temperature peak. Secondary bacterial infections are common and manifest with mucopurulent nasal exudate and pulmonary disease. The infection is mild or inapparent in horses immunologically sensitized to the virus.

Mares that abort after EHV-1 infection seldom display premonitory signs. Abortions occur 2–12 wk after infection, usually between months 7 and 11 of gestation. Aborted fetuses are fresh or minimally autolyzed, and the placenta is expelled shortly after abortion. There is no evidence of damage to the mare's reproductive tract, and subsequent conception is unimpaired. Mares exposed late in gestation may not abort but give birth to live foals with fulminating viral pneumonitis. Such foals are susceptible to secondary bacterial infections and usually die within hours or days.

Outbreaks with specific strains of EHV-1 infection result in neurologic disease. Clinical signs vary from mild incoordination and posterior paresis to severe posterior paralysis with recumbency, loss of bladder and tail function, and loss of skin sensation in the perineal and inguinal areas. In exceptional cases, the paralysis may progress to quadriplegia and death. Prognosis depends on severity of signs and the period of recumbency.

Lesions

The pathogenetic mechanisms of EHV-1 and EHV-4 differ significantly. EHV-4 infection is restricted to respiratory tract epithelium and associated lymph nodes; EHV-1 strains develop cell-associated viremia and have a predilection for vascular endothelium, especially the nasal mucosa, lungs, placenta, adrenal, thyroid, and CNS. The neuropathic strain of EHV-1 produces a viremic load 10- to 100-fold higher than that of non-neuropathic strains.

Gross lesions of viral rhinopneumonitis are hyperemia and ulceration of the respiratory epithelium, and multiple, tiny, plum-colored foci in the lungs. Histologically, there is evidence of inflammation, necrosis, and intranuclear inclusions in the respiratory epithelium and germinal centers of the associated lymph nodes. Lung lesions are characterized by neutrophilic infiltration of the terminal bronchioles, peribronchiolar and perivascular mononuclear cell infiltration, and serofibrinous exudate in the alveoli.

Typical lesions in EHV-1 abortion include interlobular lung edema and pleural fluid; multifocal areas of hepatic necrosis; petechiation of the myocardium, adrenal gland, and spleen; and thymic necrosis. Intranuclear inclusions are found in lung, liver, adrenal, and lymphoreticular tissues.

Horses with EHV-1–associated neurologic disease may have no gross lesions or only minimal evidence of hemorrhage in the meninges, brain, and spinal cord parenchyma.

Histologically, lesions are discrete and comprise vasculitis with endothelial cell damage and perivascular cuffing, thrombus formation and hemorrhage, and in advanced cases, areas of malacia. Lesions may occur at any level of the brain or spinal cord.

Diagnosis

Equine viral rhinopneumonitis is difficult to clinically differentiate from equine influenza (see Equine Influenza), equine viral arteritis (see Equine Viral Arteritis), or other equine respiratory infections solely on the basis of clinical signs. Definitive diagnosis is determined by PCR or virus isolation from samples obtained via nasopharyngeal swab and citrated blood sample (buffy coat) early in the course of the infection.

In cases of suspected EHV-1 abortion, definitive diagnosis is based on PCR, virus isolation, and characteristic gross and microscopic lesions in the aborted fetus. Lung, liver, adrenal, and lymphoreticular tissues are productive sources of virus. Serologic testing of mares after abortion has little diagnostic value. Diagnosis of neuropathic EHV-1 is determined by real-time PCR on samples obtained from nasal secretions, CSF, or neural tissue to detect the neuropathic strain of EHV-1. A presumptive diagnosis can be based on clinical signs and CSF analysis (xanthochromia, albuminocytologic dissociation). Necropsy reveals characteristic perivascular cuffing and hemorrhage in the CNS.

Treatment

There is no specific treatment for EHV infection. Rest and nursing care are indicated to minimize secondary bacterial complications. Antipyretics are recommended for horses with a fever >104°F (40°C). Antibiotic therapy is instituted upon suspicion of secondary bacterial infection evidenced by purulent nasal discharge or pulmonary disease. Most foals infected prenatally with EHV-1 die shortly after birth despite intensive nursing and antimicrobial medication. If horses with neuropathic EHV-1 remain ambulatory or are recumbent for only 2–3 days, the prognosis is usually favorable. Valacyclovir (30 mg/kg, PO, bid) has shown promise in the treatment of affected horses and in prophylaxis during EHV-1 outbreaks. Intensive nursing care is necessary to avoid pulmonary congestion, pneumonia, ruptured bladder, or bowel atony. Recovery may be complete, but a small percentage of cases have neurologic sequelae.

Control

Immunity after natural infection with either EHV-1 or EHV-4 involves a combination of humoral and cellular immunity. Whereas little cross-protection occurs between virus types after primary infection of immunologically naive foals, significant cross-protection develops in horses after repeated infections with a particular virus type. Most adult horses are latently infected with EHV-1 and EHV-4. The infection remains dormant for most of the horse's life, although stress or immunosuppression may result in recrudescence of disease and shedding of infectious virus. Immunity to reinfection of the respiratory tract may persist for as long as 3 mo, but multiple infections result in a level of immunity that prevents clinical signs of respiratory disease. Diminished resistance in pregnant mares allows cell-associated viremia, which may result in transplacental infection of the fetus.

For prevention and control of EHV-4- and EHV-1–related diseases, management practices that reduce viral spread are recommended. New horses (or those returning from other premises) should be isolated for 21 days before commingling with resident horses, especially pregnant mares. Management-related, stress-inducing circumstances should be avoided to prevent recrudescence of latent virus. Pregnant mares should be maintained in a group away from the weanlings, yearlings, and horses out of training. In an outbreak of respiratory disease or abortion, affected horses should be isolated and appropriate measures taken for disinfection of contaminated premises. No horse should leave the premises for 3 wk after recovery of the last clinical case.

Vaccination (EHV-4 and EHV-1) should begin when foals are 4–6 mo old. A second dose is given 4–6 wk later, and a third dose at 10–12 mo of age. Booster vaccinations may be indicated as often as every 6 mo through maturity (5 yr of age). Vaccination programs against herpesviruses should include all horses that travel to high-risk destinations (racetrack, show grounds) and all other horses on the premises. A high-antigen load, inactivated EHV-1 vaccine is recommended to prevent EHV-1 abortion. Vaccine should be administered during months 3, 5, 7, and 9 of pregnancy. Mares are often vaccinated with inactivated EHV-1/EHV-4 at an interval 4–6 wk before foaling. A modified-live EHV-1 vaccine is available to help prevent respiratory disease caused by EHV-1.

Infection by other Herpesviruses

Equine herpesvirus 2 (EHV-2) is ubiquitous in respiratory mucosa, conjunctiva, and WBCs of normal horses of all ages. The pathogenic significance remains obscure. It has been suggested that EHV-2 is the cause of herpetic keratoconjunctivitis and inflammatory airway disease in young horses. Equine herpesvirus 3 (EHV-3) is the cause of equine coital exanthema (see Equine Coital Exanthema), a benign, progenital exanthematous disease.

Equine gamma herpesvirus 5 (EHV-5) has emerged as the pathogen associated with equine multinodular pulmonary fibrosis (EMPF). The role of EHV-5 in EMPF is unclear (precipitating, causative, incidental). Clinical signs include weight loss, cough, fever (variable), and respiratory difficulty. EMPF is seen primarily in middle-aged horses, although it has been reported in young horses. Physical examination findings include tachycardia, tachypnea, increased respiratory effort (inspiratory), and poor body condition. Wheezes and crackles are often ausculted without a rebreathing procedure. In early cases, EMPF may be mistaken as heaves. In addition to EMPF, EHV-5 has been associated with lymphoproliferative disease and lymphoma. One unusual case report describes a 21-yr-old horse with profound pancytopenia and pulmonary fibrosis; EHV-5 was isolated from the bone marrow of this horse.

Diagnostic testing includes routine blood work, thoracic radiographs, and virus-specific PCR testing on pulmonary secretions (bronchoalveolar lavage) or percutaneous lung biopsy sample. CBC reveals neutrophilic leukocytosis with or without hyperfibrinogenemia and anemia. Findings on thoracic radiographics range from a moderate interstitial pattern to a severe reticulonodular pattern. Differential diagnoses of radiographic images include fungal pneumonia and metastatic neoplasia. Fungal pneumonia typically occurs after primary GI disease with neutropenia, and metastatic neoplasia is rare. The most common antemortem diagnostic test is virus-specific PCR of bronchoalveolar lavage fluid. Percutaneous, ultrasound-guided lung biopsy can be performed to confirm the diagnosis and establish a prognosis. The procedure is not without risk in dyspneic horses. Histopathology reveals multifocal granulomas, type II pneumocyte hyperplasia, and intraluminal cellular accumulation. Advanced pulmonary fibrosis indicates a poor prognosis for survival.

The prognosis for survival is ~50%. Horses with granulomatous inflammation have been successfully treated with antiviral therapy. Valacyclovir (30 mg/kg, PO, tid) and/or acyclovir (10 mg/kg, IV, in 1 L of isotonic crystalloid fluid as a constant-rate infusion over 1 hr, bid × 2 days) appear promising, although sensitivity of the virus to these medications has not been documented.

Doxycycline (5-10 mg/kg, PO, once to twice daily) is administered to combat secondary bacterial infection and for its anti-inflammatory properties. Administration of corticosteroids is controversial, although they are commonly used. Corticosteroids (0.08-0.1 mg/kg, IV, every 24–48 hr) may improve disease outcome through reduction of pulmonary cytokines and inflammatory mediators, but they may also cause immunosuppression, which may enhance viral replication and disease severity.

EQUINE INFECTIOUS ANEMIA (EIA)

Equine Infectious Anemia (EIA) is a viral disease affecting only members of the equidae family (horses, ponies, zebras, mules, and donkeys). There is no vaccine or treatment for the disease. Infection is often in-apparent and results in a lifelong carrier state if the horse survives the acute phase of the infection.

EIA is found widely throughout the world. There is no evidence that EIA is a threat to human health. EIA is a reportable animal disease in all states.

Equine infectious anemia (EIA) is a retroviral disease of equids that may be characterized by acute and/or chronic recurring clinical signs including fever, anemia, edema and cachexia in some animals. Many horses have very mild or inapparent signs on first exposure, and carry this virus subclinically.

The owners of these animals are unlikely to realize that they are infected unless serological testing is done. All infected horses, including those that are asymptomatic, become carriers and are infectious for life. Infected animals must either be destroyed or remain permanently isolated from other equids to prevent transmission.

Etiology and Pathogenesis

The causal agent of equine infectious anemia is an RNA virus, classified in the *Lentivirus* genus, family Retroviridae. The virus is readily inactivated by most common disinfectants, such as bleach, ethanol, iodophore disinfectants, phenolic compounds, glutaraldehyde, and formalin. Because bleach-based and ethanol disinfectants are readily inactivated in the presence of organic material, for example manure or soil, contaminated surfaces must first be cleaned thoroughly of such matter using soap and water before treating with a disinfectant. Pressure washing of a soiled surface is contraindicated because of the risk of aerosolization of potentially infectious blood or other body fluids on wall or floor surfaces.

In equids infected with EIA virus, there is a very close relationship between the development of overt signs of disease and the amount of virus present. Virus is found free in plasma or associated with monocytes and macrophages in infected animals. Virus burdens reach their highest levels during febrile episodes, after which they decline. It has been shown that the concentration of EIA virus in tissues must reach a threshold level to trigger a clinical response. The potential of a viral strain to induce disease is largely due to its replicative capacity or pathogenicity in the infected host.

The pathology of EIA-mediated disease is a consequence of macrophage infection that in turn interferes with host-cell gene expression; this leads to increased production of pro-inflammatory mediators or cytokines, in particular TNF-alpha, IL-1, IL-6, and transforming growth factor beta. Aside from the latter activating the arachidonic pathway that results in increased production of prostaglandin E2 and the induction of a febrile response, these cytokines may also cause thrombocytopenia. Increased production of TNF-alpha may also be partly responsible for the anemia that develops in EIA virus-infected equids by virtue of its ability to inhibit erythropoiesis.

Aside from the foregoing role that pro-inflammatory cytokines play in the pathogenesis of EIA, adaptive immune responses are also involved in the pathology of the disease. Platelets from infected horses have significant amounts of bound IgG or IgM, which result in their immune-mediated destruction, contributing to both splenomegaly and hepatomegaly.

There is reason to believe that cell-mediated and not humoral immune responses are responsible for initial control of EIA virus infection. Once acute viral infection has been controlled, the infected individual will remain free of overt signs of disease until a variant virus emerges that can evade the host's immune system.

Epidemiology and Transmission

All equids infected with EIA virus remain lifelong carriers. Such individuals constitute the natural reservoir of the virus and ensure its perpetuation in equid populations over time.

The combination of frequent carriers and mechanical transmission by blood-feeding insects explains why EIA is found in equine populations in a wide range of climatic zones and countries around the world.

Although EIA is usually considered a blood-borne infection, all body fluids and tissues should be regarded as potentially infectious, especially during febrile episodes when viral levels are high. Evidence of EIA virus has even been found in nasal swabs and in swabs taken from the buccal cavity and genitalia. There are limited data to suggest that infectious virus can be present in milk. EIA virus can also be passed to foals in utero. Evidence in support of venereal transmission is questionable; it is unlikely to occur unless semen is contaminated with blood in the case of an infected stallion.

There is circumstantial evidence suggesting that EIA virus may, under exceptional circumstances, also be transmitted via the respiratory route through aerosolization of blood when an infected horse is bleeding from the nostrils.

Transmission of EIA by biting flies is purely mechanical; the virus does not replicate in the insect. The chances of transmission of EIA among horses in close proximity to one another has been shown to be directly proportional to the volume of blood retained on the mouthparts of an insect after feeding. Based on this, horse flies, deer flies, and to a lesser extent, stable flies, are the most efficient vectors of the virus. It is also because the bites are irritating and trigger host defensive behavior that interrupts the flies' feeding routine and results in their seeking out another susceptible host to complete their blood meal.

EIA transmission is influenced by the number and species of flies, density of the horse population, level of viremia in the host, and quantity of blood transferred. Infections are especially common in hot, humid countries of the world with very large biting fly populations. Symptomatic, febrile horses are more likely to transmit the disease than animals with inapparent infections.

Aside from the natural transmission of EIA by blood-feeding insects, the disease can also be readily transmitted iatrogenically through the re-use of blood-contaminated syringes and needles, surgical instruments, dental equipment, and IV sets and by the transfusion of infective blood or blood products. The virus is purported to persist for up to 96 hours on contaminated hypodermic needles. The importance of iatrogenic spread of EIA cannot be overstated. It has become increasingly common in some countries among a certain element of the equine industry that is indifferent to the inherent risks involved and the potential for dissemination of the virus.

Clinical Findings

The clinical findings and course of infection with equine infectious anemia virus are variable, depending on the virulence of the virus strain, viral dose, and susceptibility of the horse. After an incubation period of 15–45 days or longer in naturally acquired cases of infection, classic cases of the disease have been described as progressing through three clinical phases. An initial or acute episode lasting 1–3 days is characterized by fever, depression, and thrombocytopenia. Because these signs can be mild and transitory, they are often overlooked or misdiagnosed. Typically, this initial phase is followed by a prolonged period associated with:

- Recurring episodes of fever
- Depression
- Thrombocytopenia
- Increased heart and respiration rates
- Anemia
- Jaundice
- Petechiation on mucous membranes
- Epistaxis
- Dependent edema
- Muscle weakness
- Loss of condition

The interval between episodes can range from days to weeks or months. In most cases, the episodes of clinical disease subside within a year, and infected horses become inapparent carriers and reservoirs of EIA virus. Many of these horses remain clinically normal. However, some chronically infected horses may continue to experience recurrent episodes varying from fever and thrombocytopenia to many of the extensive range of clinical signs that have been described. Such episodes are frequently associated with intercurrent infections and other sources of stress.

Although the foregoing represents the most commonly described clinical course of the disease, some outbreaks of EIA can be associated with peracute infection in which the primary viral infection is uncontrolled; this can result in a very high fever, severely reduced platelet counts, and infrequently acute depression and epistaxis leading to death. In view of the wide variation in response seen in natural cases of infection, it is not possible to confirm a diagnosis of EIA based solely on clinical grounds.

Although clinical signs can differ in range and severity between individuals, cases of EIA can present with many or most of the following:

- Fever
- Depression
- Low platelet count

- Anemia
- Increased heart and respiration rates
- Jaundice
- Hemorrhages on mucous membranes
- Epistaxis
- Dependent edema
- Muscle weakness
- Muscle atrophy

Lesions

Gross lesions frequently seen in acute cases of EIA include enlargement of the spleen, liver, and abdominal lymph nodes; dependent edema; and mucosal hemorrhages. Chronic cases of infection are characterized by emaciation, pale mucous membranes, petechial hemorrhages on internal organs, especially spleen and kidney, enlargement of the spleen and abdominal lymph nodes, and dependent edema of the limbs and ventral abdominal wall. Thrombosis of blood vessels has also been reported.

Histopathologically, there is a nonsuppurative hepatitis and, in some cases, a glomerulonephritis, periventricular leukoencephalitis, meningitis, or encephalitis. Ocular lesions may be seen in chronically infected animals. Proliferation of reticuloendothelial cells is evident in many organs, especially in the liver, where there is also accumulation of hemosiderin in Kupffer cells. Perivascular accumulation of lymphocytes can be found in various organs.

Diagnosis

Diagnosis is based on serologic tests

The clinical signs of acute equine infectious anemia are often nonspecific and not definitive of the disease. Accordingly, a provisional clinical diagnosis must be confirmed by demonstration of antibodies to the virus in blood. Laboratory confirmation of a suspect case of EIA needs to be pursued without delay. A wide range of infectious and noninfectious diseases can clinically resemble and be confused with EIA. These include:

- Equine viral arteritis
- Purpura hemorrhagica
- Piroplasmosis
- Leptospirosis
- Severe strongyliasis or fascioliasis
- Phenothiazine toxicity
- Autoimmune hemolytic anemia

Although the internationally accepted serologic test is the agar gel immunodiffusion or Coggins test, there is increasing acceptance of a variety of ELISA tests, either competitive or synthetic antigen-based, because they can provide rapid results. Because ELISA tests can give a higher rate of false positives, all positive ELISA results must be confirmed by the Coggins test. When used in combination, ELISA and agar gel immunodiffusion tests provide the highest level of sensitivity combined with specificity. The Western blot is a supplemental test that can be resorted to in cases of conflicting results with other diagnostic tests.

A problem with available serologic tests is that they can give negative results when testing sera collected within the first 10–14 days of infection. Whereas the vast majority of horses infected with EIA virus will have seroconverted by 45 days, there have been exceptional cases in which the interval has been e"90 days.

Virus detection assays such as reverse transcription PCR are not routinely used to diagnose EIA. Notwithstanding their sensitivity, they may not detect virus in carrier horses with very low viral loads. Although the animal inoculation test is highly sensitive for detection of EIA virus, for logistic and economic reasons, it is no longer in vogue as a means of diagnosis of EIA.

Treatment

No treatment is available

There is no antiviral treatment or cure for equine infectious anemia. Because confirmed cases of the disease are lifelong carriers of the virus, they are usually euthanized. The alternative to euthanasia is permanent isolation and quarantine of the infected animal at a distance of at least 200 yards from all other equids on a premises. Advocating supportive care under such circumstances is irrelevant.

Prevention and Control

No safe and effective vaccine is available for equine infectious anemia. Without the benefit of prophylactic vaccination, it is recommended that horse owners implement an EIA control plan for their premises. An integral part of such a program should be annual testing of all horses. More frequent testing may be indicated in areas that previously experienced a high incidence of EIA. All equines introduced to a herd should have a negative EIA test before arrival or be isolated while tests are pending. Horses competing in shows or performance events should be accompanied by proof that they have been tested for EIA within a specific period of time.

Vector control practices should be a part of any EIA prevention and control program. These should include routine application of insecticides and repellants as well as the implementation of insect control measures.

Any control program for EIA must emphasize awareness of how readily the causal virus can be transmitted indirectly from an infected individual to other equids on a premises through the re-use of contaminated needles, syringes, surgical or dental instruments, or other equipment. Strict observance of the principles of good hygiene and disinfection is essential if iatrogenic transmission of EIA is to be prevented.

Specific measures to prevent/control EIA can be summarized as follows:

- Infected horses become lifelong carriers and pose a risk of infection to other horses. Management options for an EIA-positive horse are euthanasia or lifetime quarantine, with permanent isolation at least 200 yards away from noninfected horses.
- Prevention is key to stopping the spread of EIA.
- Use a sterile needle, syringe, and IV set for all injections or treatments.
- Disinfect dental, tattoo, surgical equipment, lip chains, and bits thoroughly between horses. Remove all debris and blood with soap and water before disinfection.
- Only administer commercially licensed blood or blood products.
- Keep open wounds clean and covered, if possible.
- Use a sterile needle and syringe each time when puncturing a multidose medication bottle.
- Use sterile technique when drawing up and administering medications.
- Require proof of a recent negative EIA test upon introduction of a horse onto a premises for the first time.
- Practice good fly control by regular mucking out of stalls, proper disposal of manure away from horse stabling areas, and using fly sprays or natural predators to minimize fly presence.

Zoonotic Risk

There is no evidence that EIA virus is a zoonotic agent and transmissible to humans.

EQUINE INFLUENZA (EIV)

Equine influenza is a highly contagious respiratory disease of horses and other equidae. It is caused by two subtypes of the influenza A virus, which are related to, but distinct from, influenza viruses in other species. Equine influenza virus spreads easily through contact with infected horses and via contact with infected clothing, equipment, brushes, tack, etc.

Some horses do not show any outward signs of infection, but can shed the virus and infect susceptible horses. Outbreaks result in significant economic losses to the equine industry, and are more likely to occur where large groups of horses gather, such as shows, races and events. Increased transportation of horses across state lines and between countries facilitates the spread of the virus.

Two types of influenza virus routinely circulate and cause seasonal flu epidemics in people: influenza A (which has multiple sub-types) and influenza B. Influenza A viruses are also found in animals and occasionally cross species barriers, causing serious illness and acting as the source of pandemics.

Strains of influenza A virus are named with H's and N's. H stands for hemagglutinin and N for neuraminidase. Both are proteins on the surface of the virus (antigens) that help it invade cells. There are 18 different H subtypes and 11 N subtypes, resulting in 198 possible combinations. Sometimes the strains trade genetic information, taking on new characteristics that our immune systems have never seen. This can lead to severe illness, and even death. Recent cross-species flu outbreaks include H5N1 "bird flu" and H1N1 "swine flu", transmitted from birds to humans and pigs to humans, respectively.

Equine influenza sub-types are H7N7, which is thought to be extinct, and the current H3N8, which is spread widely throughout the world. The H3N8 subtype is further broken down into sublineages, with the Florida sublineage currently circulating. Clades 1 and 2 of this sublineage circulate in Europe. Clade 1 commonly circulates in North America. The H3N8 strain of equine influenza is not known to infect humans. This is partly due to the fact that there is minimal evolutionary pressure to generate strains with higher virulence, so the equine influenza virus evolves slowly in comparison to other influenza viruses.

Clinical Signs

Clinical signs vary in their severity depending on the age and immune status of the horse, and asymptomatic infection is possible. Clinical signs are more common and often more severe in younger horses; ages 1-5yo. Older horses generally have milder disease.

- Fever, up to 106F (41.1C), depression, malaise, anorexia, muscle pain/weakness
- Dry, harsh cough (sometimes paroxysmal) usually precedes fever. The dry, harsh cough is a frequent clinical sign in EI while it is less common with EHV infection. Cough can last up to 6 weeks after all other clinical signs have abated. Can take up to 6 months to regain previous athletic abilities
- Mild enlargement of retropharyngeal lymph nodes
- Serous nasal discharge that frequently progresses to mucopurulent with onset of secondary bacterial infections
- Secondary bacterial infections are very common in influenza-affected horses
- Rarely, clinical signs may include distal limb edema and cardiomyopathy.

Similar to herpesviruses and *Streptococcus equi* subspecies *equi* (agent of strangles), greater incidence of infection is observed in colder months. Abrupt onset of clinical signs is common, and they usually last less than 3 days. Sick horses can exhibit fever, nasal discharge, cough, lethargy, loss of appetite and weakness. A cough is one of the most notable signs of equine flu. The virus causes destruction of cells in the throat and lungs, which take 3 weeks to regenerate. As a result, horses are particularly susceptible to secondary infections such as bacterial pneumonia during the first 2-3 weeks after infection.

May be more severe in donkeys and mules.

Incubation Period

The period between exposure to EIV and appearance of clinical signs is frequently as short as 24 hours and may be up to 3 days.

Risk Factors

- Age: horses 1-5 years of age
- Areas of high comingling of horses such as racetracks, show grounds, veterinary hospitals
- Immunosuppression from traveling, hospitalization, training and showing
- While vaccination reduces the risk of clinical disease, vaccinated horses can still become infected and shed virus (subclinical shedding)

Transmission

- Respiratory transmission occurs most commonly through inhalation of infective droplets from coughing and snorting horses. The distance these droplets may spread through the air has not been definitively established, but may be as far as 50 yards.
- Indirect transmission can occur and can be an important means of spread. This includes transmission of the virus on contaminated clothing, equipment, brushes, shared water buckets, hands, etc.
- Respiratory shedding typically lasts for 7-10 days post infection in naïve animals; much shorter shedding periods occur in partially immune (previously vaccinated) horses.

Diagnostic Sampling, Testing and Handling

Virus isolation from nasopharyngeal swabs

- Samples should be collected within 24-48 hours after onset of clinical signs.
- Swabs should be submitted in viral isolation transport media (NOT bacterial transport media). If no viral transport media is available, place swabs in a red top tube with a few sterile saline drops (enough to moisten the tip of the swab). Ship overnight on ice.
- Nasopharyngeal swabs are a superior alternative to nasal swabs, in that these collect about 10 times as much virus as nasal swabs which reduces the possibility

of a false-negative diagnostic test result. These are also safer in that there is no chance that a horse movement plus inhalation might cause the swab to be lodged inaccessibly within the nasal meatus.

- Nasopharyngeal swabs are typically 40cm long, with Rayon gauze tips similar to nasal swabs but larger. These are commercially available from Medline Inc. or Birchwood Laboratories Inc.
- Nasopharyngeal swabbing technique: Holding the swab at least 10 cm from the gauze tip to avoid contamination, insert the swab into the nostril, angling inwards and down so as to avoid the dorso-medial blind pouch inside the nostril, then pass the swab as far as possible down the ventral nasal meatus to the nasopharynx, (about 25 cm for an adult horse, 20 cm for a pony, and 15-20 cm for a foal). Rotate 3-4X, then remove. The gauze tip will need to be cut off with scissors to fit within the transport tube. That transport tube should contain enough viral transport media (or sterile normal saline) to completely immerse the gauze tip.

EQUINE PARVOVIRUS-HEPATITIS VIRUS (EQPV-H)

A novel viral etiology for equine serum hepatitis (Theiler's Disease) has been identified as equine parvovirus-hepatitis (EqPV-H). Two epidemiological presentations of EqPV-H are recognized in adult horses; cases either present 4-12 weeks after administration of an equine biologic product (such as tetanus antitoxin or equine plasma) or the cases may occur as small outbreaks lasting 1 or more weeks during warmer months where no biologics were administered. EqPV-H is hepatotropic and pathogenic but the great majority of recently infected horses (within 4-12 weeks) have non-clinical hepatitis with 2 or more weeks of elevated serum liver enzymes.

Clinically affected horses may represent only 1-2% of the infected horses and typically present with clinical signs of lethargy, anorexia, and jaundice, or neurologic symptoms characteristic of hepatic encephalopathy. Mortality of clinically affected horses is nearly 50%. The epidemiology behind equine serum hepatitis outbreaks where no biologics have been administered remains under investigation by Drs. Thomas Divers, Joy Tomlinson and Gerlinde Van de Walle at Cornell University. In addition to transmission by infected blood products, other proposed alternative mechanisms for EqPV-H transfer include insect vector, or possible spread via nasal or fecal shedding from infected horses.

Another recently discovered equine hepatitis virus is non-primate hepacivirus (NPHV), renamed as equine hepacivirus (EqHV). EqHV is phylogenetically the closest known virus to the human hepatitis C virus. EqHV may cause subclinical disease in adult horses with transient mild elevations in liver derived serum enzymes.

Equine serum hepatitis, formerly referred to as Theiler's Disease, is caused by infection with equine parvovirus-hepatitis virus (EqPV-H). EqPV-H is a hepatotropic single-stranded DNA virus capable of causing hepatitis in infected horses. Two distinct etiologies of EqPV-H infection are recognized: biologic transmission and non-biologic transmission. Asymptomatic infection is common, and only a small percentage of infected horses will develop clinical signs of liver disease.

Prevalence

Surveillance studies suggest the prevalence of EqPV-H infection in equine populations varies from 3-17%, most of which are asymptomatic. Although seroprevalence up to 54% has been reported on farms with clinical cases of serum hepatitis, it is estimated that only 2% of horses infected with EqPV-H develop clinical disease.

Transmission

Two modes of transmission are recognized in horses:

- Biologic transmission occurs through the administration of biologic products containing EqPV-H. To date, EqPV-H has been identified in tetanus antitoxin (TAT), botulinum antitoxin, Streptococcus equi antiserum, pregnant mare's serum, allogenic stem cell preparations and equine plasma products. Cases generally present 4-13 weeks after receiving equine biologic products.
- Non-biologic transmission occurs sporadically in horses with no history of receiving biologic products. Herd outbreaks are possible, and while the mechanism for this type of infection has not yet been elucidated, seasonal incidence in late summer to early fall (when insects are active) suggests an insect-borne mode of transmission. This is an area of ongoing research.

Incubation Period

Clinical signs of liver disease occur 4-13 weeks after administration of an EqPV-H infected biologic. The incubation period for non-biologic transmission cases is unknown, but is likely also approximately 4-13 weeks.

Risk Factors

- Administration of allogeneic biologic products that have not been tested for EqPV-H by PCR
- Sharing of needles across multiple horses
- Introduction into herds with confirmed cases of serum hepatitis, especially during late summer to early fall months.

Clinical Signs

Horses infected with EqPV-H may develop a wide range of clinical signs, varying from asymptomatic to mild illness to fulminant liver failure. The factors that determine host response to infection have not yet been elucidated.

Asymptomatic infection: Most horses infected with EqPV-H remain asymptomatic. Some may develop evidence of subclinical hepatitis characterized by transiently elevated serum liver enzyme activities that return to normal concentrations within 1-4 weeks without any clinical signs or long-term health effects.

Clinical hepatitis: It is estimated that approximately 2% of infected horses will develop clinical liver disease, ranging from mild illness to acute fulminant liver failure. Clinical signs in affected horses may include one or more of the following:

- Lethargy
- Anorexia
- Jaundice
- Neurological signs associated with hyperammonemic encephalopathy (altered mentation, maniacal behavior, head pressing, blindness, staggering)
- Discolored urine (secondary to hemolysis and/or bilirubinurea)
- Colic
- Recumbency
- Death usually within 72 hours

Horses with clinical hepatitis will have serum biochemical profiles that reflect acute liver dysfunction and sometimes failure. Specific abnormalities may include:

- Elevated serum liver enzyme activities (GGT, AST, SDH, GLDH) (Elevated GGT is the most commonly observed abnormality)
- Abnormal liver function assays (bile acids)
- Elevated blood ammonia
- Hyperbilirubinemia (both direct and indirect)
- BUN may be elevated or decreased
- Blood glucose may be decreased

Diagnostic Sampling, Testing, and Handling

EqPV-H should be suspected in horses with signs of illness and/or liver disease and a history of receiving biologic products in the preceding months. A definitive diagnosis of EqPV-H is achieved using PCR, and current recommendations are to submit fresh liver, fixed liver and serum for concurrent testing. EqPV-H PCR testing is currently performed at the Animal Health Diagnostic Center (AHDC) at Cornell University. Fresh tissue and blood samples should be shipped chilled in insulated containers for overnight delivery.

Blood

- Serum (removed from clot) is the preferred blood sample, but EDTA whole blood or EDTA plasma may also be used.
- Samples from EqPV-H viremic horses will be PCR positive.

Liver tissue (biopsy)

- Liver tissue from EqPV-H infected horses will be PCR positive
- Acceptable samples include fresh, frozen, or formalin-fixed liver
- Histopathologic findings include varying degrees of centrilobular hepatitis and hepatocellular necrosis. Lymphocytic/plasmacytic infiltration of the periportal area is common with a fewer number of neutrophils. Remaining hepatocytes may be vacuolated.
- Histology results are useful for identifying additional causes of liver disease that may be contributing to clinical signs, such as chronic pyrrolizidine alkaloid toxicosis, hepatic fibrosis, etc.

Note: Liver mass may be severely reduced in fulminant hepatitis cases and ultrasound guidance is recommended to determine if a biopsy is possible.

Post-Mortem Findings

Hepatic lesions in EqPH-H infected horses will vary depending on severity of disease. Asymptomatic or subclinically affected horses may have grossly normal livers with histologic findings of mild centrilobular to midzonal hepatocellular necrosis and mild lymphocytic/plasmacytic periportal infiltration. Livers from horses with fulminant hepatitis are often discolored and markedly reduced in size, with a flaccid texture and 'dish-rag' appearance. Histologic findings in severely affected horses include widespread, severe, centrilobular to mid-zonal hepatocellular necrosis with hemorrhage and lymphocytic/plasmacytic periportal infiltration.

Additional Hepatotropic Viruses

The recently discovered hepatotropic virus, equine hepacivirus (EqHV), can also infect horses and cause transient mild elevations in liver enzyme activities, however, clinical illness has not been reported as a result of EqHV infection. Equine pegivirus (EPgV) and Theiler's Disease Associated Virus (TDAV) are also hepatotropic viruses known to infect horses, but neither are associated with known clinical disease. Donkeys have been shown to be infected with EqPV-H and EqHV but disease manifestations and clinical course are unknown.

Treatment

There is no specific treatment for EqPV-H infection. Asymptomatic horses do not require any treatment, although serial monitoring of serum biochemistry may be helpful for monitoring elevations in liver enzyme activities. Treatment of clinically affected horses relies primarily on supportive care and treatment of liver dysfunction. Referral to an intensive care facility may be required for severely ill horses.

Virus Shedding

Viremia detectable by PCR generally occurs 1-4 weeks after exposure, and viral loads may continue to increase for an additional 2-4 weeks before decreasing. In experimental infection, virus has been found in nasal secretions and feces. It is important to note that experimental infection is achieved using very high viral challenge doses, and it is not currently known whether nasal and fecal shedding occurs under natural infection conditions. Some horses will continue to have persistent low-level viremia detectable by PCR, but it is unclear whether this lowlevel viremia is associated with chronic viral shedding.

Carrier Status

Horses clinically or subclinically infected with EqPV-H can remain asymptomatically infected for long periods of time. This chronic low-level viremia (as determined by quantitative PCR) has not been associated with clinical signs of chronic liver disease. The percentage of horses that become chronic carriers is unknown, however, carrier horses may serve as reservoirs for infection to others. The mechanism and likelihood of transmission from a chronic carrier to a healthy horse is unknown at this time.

Prognosis

The prognosis for asymptomatic infections is excellent. Cases of subclinical hepatitis (no clinical signs, transient elevations in liver enzyme activities) generally return to normal within 1-4 weeks with no long-term health effects. Prognosis for horses with acute fulminant hepatitis is guarded to poor with a mortality rate of 50-90%.

Prevention

- There is no vaccine for EqPV-H.
- At this time, the only means of preventing EqPV-H in horses is to administer autogenous biologics and/or USDA licensed biologics that have been PCR tested and confirmed free of the virus.
- Any biologic donor horses should be routinely tested for EqPV-H and other potential blood borne pathogens. The optimal frequency of donor testing is not currently known.

Zoonotic Potential

None known.

EQUINE PROTOZOAL MYELOENCEPHALITIS (EPM)

Equine protozoal myeloencephalitis is caused by infection of the central nervous system with the protozoan parasites *Sarcocystis neurona* and, less commonly, *Neospora hughesi*. It is often a progressively debilitating disease and can affect any part of the nervous system, from the front of the cerebrum to the end of the spinal cord. Equine protozoal myeloencephalitis is considered the most prevalent cause of neurologic disease of horses.

The range of the opossum, the definitive host of *S. neurona*, defines the geographic range of clinical EPM in horses. In areas where the opossum is common, approximately 50% of horses are seropositive (have antibodies to the parasite in the blood), indicating exposure to the organism. Opossums shed the infective sporocysts (egg-like stages of development) in their feces. Horses become infected by ingesting food or water that has been contaminated with opossum feces containing the infective sporocysts.

In <1% of cases, the sporocysts ingested by a horse migrate from the intestinal tract into the bloodstream and cross the blood/brain barrier, causing disease by attacking the horse's central nervous system. *S. neurona* cannot be transmitted from one horse to another. A few cases of EPM are associated with *N. hughesi*, another protozoal parasite. The life cycle, natural host(s), and modes of transmission of this organism are poorly understood.

Affected horses may not show any clinical signs, or may show clinical signs consistent with those caused by *S. neurona*. Infection with *N. hughesi* has also been associated with abortions and neuromuscular disease. Transmission from *N. hughesi*-infected broodmares to their offspring has been reported, but not all offspring developed neurologic signs.

Although clusters of cases have been noted, EPM usually occurs sporadically and often only involves one horse on a given property. Cases occur in horses of all ages, with greater frequently in young athletes, and no sex or seasonal biases have been observed.

Etiology and Epidemiology

Most cases of equine protozoal myeloencephalitis are caused by an apicomplexan protozoan, *Sarcocystis neurona*. Horses are infected by ingestion of *S neurona* sporocysts in contaminated feed or water. The organism undergoes early asexual multiplication (schizogony) in extraneural tissues before parasitizing the CNS. Because infectious sarcocysts are only rarely formed, the horse is considered an aberrant, dead-end host for *S neurona*. Like other *Sarcocystis* spp, *S neurona* has an obligate predator-prey life cycle. The definitive (predator) host for *S neurona* in the USA is the opossum (*Didelphis virginiana*).

Opossums are infected by eating sarcocyst-containing muscle tissue from an infected intermediate (prey) host and, after a brief prepatent period (probably 2–4 weeks), infectious sporocysts are passed in the feces. Nine-banded armadillos, striped skunks, raccoons, sea otters, Pacific harbor seals, and domestic cats have all been implicated as intermediate hosts; however, the importance in nature of each of these species is unknown. Sporadic cases of EPM are associated with *Neospora hughesi*, an organism closely related to S *neurona*. The natural host(s) of this organism have not yet been identified. Transplacental protozoal transmission with the birth of infected foals has been documented for *N hughesi* but not for S *neurona*.

Clinical signs of EPM

Clinical signs due to *S. neurona* infection are dependent on the area of the central nervous system that contains the parasite and the type of damage caused. The onset of the disease may be slow or sudden. Spinal cord involvement can manifest in gait abnormalities, incoordination, ataxia (inability to control voluntary muscle movement), spasticity in all four limbs, and muscle atrophy, whereas brainstem involvement may manifest in lethargy, behavioral changes, and cranial nerve paralysis (facial nerve paralysis, tongue paralysis, difficulty swallowing). Signs may not be the same on both sides of the horse (asymmetrical).

Some horses may stand with their feet splayed or lean against walls or other supports. In some cases, the clinical signs stabilize and then relapse days to weeks later. Factors that influence the progression to severe neurologic disease are not well understood.

Cases of EPM due to *N. hughesi* can have a wide range of clinical signs, including hind limb ataxia and hind limb weakness that progress to more generalized weakness and recumbency. Clinicians at UC Davis have mainly noticed gait abnormalities and ataxia, and that cases diagnosed with EPM due to neosporosis often have concurrent diseases (metabolic conditions, bacterial or viral infections).

Diagnosis

Definitive diagnosis of EPM relies on postmortem examination of neural tissue. No test in the live horse is currently considered definitive. Therefore, EPM is diagnosed based on a combination of (1) a thorough neurologic examination, (2) evaluation of serum and/or cerebrospinal fluid (CSF) for the presence of antibodies to *S. neurona* and/or *N. hughesi*, and (3) the elimination of other neurological disorders.

Diagnostic tests look for the presence of antibodies to the EPM protozoal parasites in serum and/or CSF. A positive blood test only determines that the horse has been exposed to the parasite and does not mean that the horse will develop clinical signs or that the neurological deficits are caused by the protozoal parasite. There is currently no gold standard for EPM diagnostic testing other than necropsy.

Western immunoblot test (WB) – based on the detection of *S. neurona*-specific antibodies in the blood and/or cerebrospinal fluid (CSF). This test is good at ruling out EPM caused by sarcocysts in horses when the prevalence of infection is low or moderate. Although it detects the presence of *S. neurona*-specific antibodies in the serum or CSF, approximately 30% to 60% of clinically normal horses in many parts of the United States have antibodies to *S. neurona* without having EPM. Additionally, contamination of cerebrospinal fluid with even minute quantities of peripheral blood can produce a false positive result if the horse has antibodies in the blood.

Indirect fluorescent antibody test (IFAT) – provides a quantitative result so that the titer is associated with a calculated probability of disease. The SarcoFluor® IFAT is used to diagnose *S. neurona* antibodies and the NeoFluor® IFAT detects antibodies to *N. hughesi*. The SarcoFluor® test offers increased sensitivity and specificity for identifying infected horses compared with the Western immunoblot test. Results are truly quantitative, thereby allowing improved interpretation of the likelihood of active EPM infection and disease rather than simply an indication of exposure. The higher the IFAT antibody titer, the more likely that EPM is the cause of the horse's neurologic signs. These tests are less sensitive to blood contamination of CSF, resulting in fewer false-positive results, and they are faster, less labor-intensive, and less expensive than the Western immunoblot test. Increased accuracy towards supporting a diagnosis of EPM should include the testing of CSF for specific antibodies to *S. neurona* and/or *N. hughes*i. A positive result often indicates the production of intrathecal (the space in the spinal canal that holds the CSF) antibodies and supports the clinical diagnosis of EPM.

ELISAs – SAG ELISAs are quantitative tests of *S. neurona* surface antigens, which are highly expressed in the parasite. Some of these tests are based on antigens that are not expressed by all strains of *S. neurona*, limiting their usefulness for EPM diagnosis. Although several studies have compared some of these newer tests to WB and IFAT, they have not all been evaluated. An ELISA test for a *N. hughesi* surface antigen is available but has not been validated for EPM diagnosis due to the small number of known EPM cases caused by this parasite. Greater accuracy of the ELISAs has been determined by using CSF or calculating a serum to CSF ratio, indicating intrathecally derived antibodies to the specific parasites.

Treatment

Treatment to control infection should include an FDA-approved anticoccidial drug (Ponazuril, Diclazuril, Sulfadiazine/Pyrimethamine). Additional treatments should be provided as needed based on the severity of the clinical signs and any associated complications. NSAIDs (i.e. phenylbutazone or banamine) may be given to moderately to severely affected horses during the first week of antiprotozoal treatment in an effort to prevent worsening of neurological deficits. In diagnosed horses that show brain involvement, or are in danger of falling, a short course of corticosteroids and dimethyl sulfoxide may reduce the inflammatory response.

Vitamin E is sometimes used as an antioxidant treatment in infected horses, but the benefits of this practice, if any, have yet to be established experimentally. Length of treatment depends on the duration and resolution of the clinical signs. Duration of treatment for the FDA approved products is approximately one month, although some products may require treatment for 3-9 months. Treatment duration is mostly dependent on the clinical improvement (i.e. treat as long as there is improvement noted). Because of safety and efficacy concerns, compounded antiprotozoal drugs should not be used in horses with suspected EPM.

Prognosis

If left undiagnosed and untreated, EPM can cause devastating and lasting neurological deficits. The success rate for treated horses is high. Many will improve and a smaller percentage will recover completely, but 10-20% of cases may relapse within two years. A prompt, accurate diagnosis is important and treatment should be started immediately to maximize the chance for recovery.

Prevention and Control

No proven preventive is available. A conditionally approved vaccine was marketed, but the license lapsed in 2008, and the vaccine is no longer offered. There is interest in using antiprotozoal drugs for prevention, and it has been shown that daily diclazuril prevents foals from seroconverting against *S neurona* and *N hughesi.*

Evidence-based protocols for preventive use of antiprotozoal drugs are not yet available. The source of infective sporocysts is opossum feces, so it is prudent to prevent access of opossums to horse-feeding areas. Horse and pet feed should not be left out; open feed bags and garbage should be kept in closed galvanized metal containers, bird feeders should be eliminated, and fallen fruit should be removed. Opossums can be trapped and relocated.

Because putative intermediate hosts cannot be directly infective for horses, it is unlikely that control of these populations will be useful in EPM prevention.

Biosecurity Issues for Receiving Animals

Horses with EPM do not present a biosecurity risk to other animals because the disease is not transmissible between horses. Opossums, the only known definitive hosts for *S. neurona.* Therefore, horses imported from other countries to the Americas should have no previous exposure to *S. neurona* and should be seronegative. However, horses exported from the Americas to other countries might have been exposed previously to *S. neurona* or be actively infected; in both scenarios the horse is likely to be seropositive. These seropositive horses do not pose a risk to other animals but could individually succumb to disease after export.

Disinfection

Horses with EPM are not contagious and do not pose a risk to neighboring horses. Disinfection is not necessary for areas or objects in contact with affected horses.

Zoonotic Potential None

Humans are not susceptible to *S.neurona* or *N. hughesi.*

EQUINE VIRAL ARTERITIS (EVA)

Equine Viral Arteritis (EVA) is a contagious viral disease in horses caused by Equine Arteritis Virus (EAV). Infection can go undetected by horse owners/breeders and in herds that were previously unexposed (naïve) abortion rates in pregnant mares can reach up to 70%. Most horses infected with EAV will show minimal if any clinical signs and recover without incident although stallions can become carriers and lifelong shedders of the virus.

There is a vaccine available that has been shown to prevent infection with EAV. Vaccination should be performed at least 21 days prior to the start of breeding season to provide adequate levels of immunity. EVA has not been shown to be zoonotic. Equine viral arteritis (EVA) is an economically important, contagious, viral disease of equids caused by equine arteritis virus (EAV).

Exposure to EAV may result in clinical or more frequently, asymptomatic infection, depending on the virus strain, host genetic factors, and various management and environmental factors. EAV infection can cause abortion, respiratory illness, establishment of a carrier state in stallions, and interstitial pneumonia and death in young foals. Diagnosis of EVA is based on virus detection in body secretions or fluids, whole blood, or tissues by virus isolation, RT-PCR and in situ hybridization; identification of viral antigen in tissues; and detection of viral-specific antibodies by serology. The treatment of EVA is general supportive care during the acute phase of infection.

There is no treatment to eliminate persistent infection in stallions. Attenuated and inactivated vaccines are available in North America and Europe, respectively, for prevention and control. Although equine arteritis virus (EAV) infection is restricted almost exclusively to equids (horses, donkeys, mules, and zebras), limited data suggest the host range may also extend to alpacas and llamas. EAV is known to be present in equine populations in many countries worldwide, with the notable exceptions of Japan, Iceland, and New Zealand, which successfully eradicated the disease. The prevalence of infection varies widely both between countries and among breeds in the same country. It is frequently highest in Standardbreds and Warmbloods.

Despite the widespread global distribution of EAV, laboratory-confirmed outbreaks of equine viral arteritis (EVA) are relatively uncommon. However, this situation appears to be changing in more recent years, with an increase in the number of verified occurrences of the disease being reported. A major factor contributing to this change is the continued escalation in the volume of international horse movements and trade in equine germplasm.

Etiology and Pathogenesis of Equine Viral Arteritis

Equine arteritis virus is a small, enveloped, positive-sense, single-stranded RNA virus. EAV has been reclassified as a member of the subfamily *Equarterivirinae,* genus *Alphaarterivirus,* in the order *Nidovirales,* and renamed as *Alphaarterivirus equid.* The viral genome is approximately 12.7 kb and contains at least 10 open reading frames (ORFs). ORFs 1a and 1b encode two polyproteins that are processed into 13 nonstructural proteins. The remaining ORFs 2a, 2b, 3, 4, 5a, 5b, 6, and 7 encode seven envelope structural proteins (E, GP2, GP3, GP4, ORF5a protein, GP5, and M) and the nucleocapsid N protein. The major neutralization determinants of the virus are located in the N-terminal ectodomain of GP5.

Phylogenetic analysis based on partial ORF5 sequences segregates EAV isolates from around the world into North American (NA) and European (EU) lineages, with each of these lineages further subdivided into two North American (NA-1 and NA-2) and European (EU-1 and EU-2) clades. Although, there is only one known serotype of EAV, the prototype Bucyrus strain, genomic and antigenic variation exists among temporally and geographically different strains of the virus. EAV ûeld strains have been shown to differ in their virulence, pathogenicity and neutralization phenotypes. Thus, some field strains of EAV are capable of causing moderate to severe clinical signs whereas others only induce mild clinical disease. EAV is readily inactivated by lipid solvents and by common disinfectants and detergents. The virus survives 75 days at 4°C, 2–3 days at 37°C, and 20–30 minutes at 56°C.

EAV can maintain infectivity in tissues and various body fluids, including semen, for years when stored at -70°C or below. After respiratory exposure, EAV invades the upper and lower respiratory tract and multiplies in nasopharyngeal epithelium and tonsillar tissue and in bronchial and alveolar macrophages. Infected $CD14^+$ monocytes and a small subpopulation of $CD3^+$ T lymphocytes transport EAV to the regional lymph nodes (eg, bronchial lymph node), where it undergoes a further cycle of replication before being released into the bloodstream. The cell-associated viremia that follows ensures dissemination of EAV throughout the body.

By day 6–8, the virus localizes in the vascular endothelium and medial myocytes of the smaller blood vessels, especially the arterioles, and causes a panvasculitis. It can also be found in the epithelium of certain tissues, particularly the adrenals, seminiferous tubules, thyroid, and liver. Vascular lesions include endothelial swelling and degeneration, neutrophilic infiltration, and necrosis of the tunica media of affected vessels.

These lesions give rise to edema and hemorrhage, which are believed to result from activation of the proinflammatory cytokines IL-1 beta, IL-6, IL-8, and possibly TNF-alpha. Maximal vascular injury occurs by about day 10, after which lesions begin to resolve. Except in certain infected stallions that become carriers of the virus, EAV is no longer detectable in tissues and body fluids beyond day 28 after primary infection. The virus causes abortion in pregnant mares, and abortion rates during natural outbreaks of EVA can vary from <10%–71%.

EAV-induced abortions can occur at any time between 2 and 10 months of gestation without premonitory signs. However, the pathogenesis of fetal infection and the mechanism responsible for abortion is poorly characterized. EAV is vertically transmitted to the fetus as evidenced by the high viral titers and abundance of viral antigen in fetal membranes and diverse fetal tissues. It is speculated that abortion occurs as a consequence of vasculitis of myometrial blood vessels and myometrial necrosis, which leads to placental dysfunction and chorionic detachment.

Following natural EAV infection, 10%–70% of stallions become persistently infected and continuously shed virus in their semen for either a short (ranging from several weeks to <1 year, defined as short-term shedders [STS] or short-term carriers) or a long period of time (> 1year to lifelong; defined as longterm persistently infected [LTPI] shedders or carriers) without adverse effects on semen quality or reproductive capacity. The carrier state has been confirmed in sexually mature intact males, specifically postpubertal colts and stallions, but not in mares, geldings, sexually immature colts, or fillies. The establishment and LTPI of EAV in the reproductive tract of stallions is testosterone-dependent and, therefore, does not cause persistent infection in mares, foals, and sexually immature colts.

The virus persists exclusively in the male reproductive tract despite the presence of high levels of neutralizing and mucosal antibodies, and a moderate to severe inflammatory response. The analysis of multiple tissues from the reproductive tract of EAV carrier stallions unequivocally confirmed the ampullae as the primary site of EAV persistence. EAV infects vimentin-positive fibrocytes and mononuclear cells (T and B lymphocytes and macrophages) but not in the ampullae's glandular epithelium.

It has been demonstrated that the establishment of EAV LTPI correlates with the in vitro susceptibility of a subpopulation of $CD3^+$ T lymphocytes to EAV infection and, consequently, stallions with the $CD3^+$ T lymphocyte susceptibility phenotype are at higher risk of becoming LTPI carriers compared to those that lack this phenotype. Thus, variation in the frequency of the carrier state in certain horse breeds has been shown to be related to the distribution of $CD3^+$ T lymphocyte cell populations susceptible or resistant to infection with EAV. A genome-wide association study demonstrated that these phenotypes are associated with the CXCL16 gene located on equine chromosome 11. Subsequently, studies have identified two allelic variants of CXCL16 (CXCL16S and CXCL16R) that differ by four nonsynonymous nucleotide substitutions in exon 1.

Of the two encoded proteins, the CXCL16S isoform has EAV receptor activity and is associated with the $CD3^+$ T lymphocyte susceptible phenotype and establishment of LTPI in stallions; whereas the CXCL16R isoform lacks receptor activity and results in a $CD3^+$ T lymphocyte resistant phenotype and early viral clearance in stallions (short-term carriers of the virus).

Carrier stallions also serve as the principal means by which genetic diversification of EAV can occur, with potential emergence of novel viral variants. It has been shown that persistent infection is characterized by extensive genome-wide purifying selection mediated by intrahost selective pressures; nucleotide substitutions occurring in nonstructural protein-2 encoding region of ORF1a, ORF3, and ORF5 have been found to be important in the evolution of EAV in carrier stallions over time.

Epidemiology and Transmission of Equine Viral Arteritis

The epidemiology of equine viral arteritis involves virus-, host-, and environment-related factors that include variability in pathogenicity among naturally occurring strains of the virus, modes of transmission, occurrence of the carrier state in stallions, and the nature of acquired immunity to infection. Outbreaks of EVA are most often linked to the movement of infected animals or the shipment of virus-contaminated semen (chilled or frozen) and frozen embryos.

Transmission of EAV can occur by respiratory, venereal, and congenital routes or by indirect means. Spread by the respiratory route is the principal mode of dissemination of the virus during the acute phase of infection. It is primarily responsible for transmission of EAV among susceptible equids kept in close contact. It can also occur through contact with placenta, placental fluids, and tissues of EAV abortions. EAV can also be transmitted venereally during natural or artificial insemination with infective semen from acutely and persistently infected stallions.

Mares can be readily infected by the venereal route after breeding to a carrier stallion either by live cover or artificial insemination with fresh-cooled or cryopreserved semen. There is limited evidence that EAV can be spread through embryo transfer. It is important to emphasize that infection can also be spread through indirect contact with virus-contaminated fomites (eg, breeding shed equipment, buckets, shanks, or twitches) or on the hands, apparel, or footwear of animal handlers.

The carrier stallion is the natural reservoir of EAV and is responsible for its dissemination and persistence in equine populations. Persistently infected stallions shed EAV constantly in the sperm-rich fraction of the semen but not in any other secretions or excretions. Persistent EAV infection clears spontaneously in a variable percentage of stallions, with no evidence of subsequent reversion to a shedding state. Whereas acutely infected stallions may experience a period of subfertility that can last for up to 4 months, existence of the carrier state does not appear to impair the fertility of infected stallions nor otherwise adversely affect their health.

Compared with other equine respiratory viruses, EAV stimulates a stronger, longer-lasting immunity that is protective against development of clinical disease, including abortion and establishment of the carrier state in stallions. High levels of neutralizing antibodies that frequently persist for at least 2–3 years can be stimulated by natural exposure to the virus and by vaccination.

Clinical Findings of Equine Viral Arteritis

Clinical signs of equine viral arteritis vary considerably among individual horses and among outbreaks. Exposure to equine arteritis virus may result in clinical or asymptomatic infection, depending on the relative virulence of the strain involved, viral dose, age and physical condition of the animal, and various environmental factors. Most cases of primary infection are asymptomatic. Onset of the acute phase of EAV infection, whether associated with clinical signs or not, is preceded by an incubation period of 2–14 days, which varies mainly with the route of exposure. The interval can be 2–3 days after respiratory exposure and is usually 6–8 days after venereal transmission of the virus.

Clinical signs can differ in range and severity between outbreaks and between individuals in the same outbreak. Any combination of the following **clinical signs** may be observed:

- Fever (up to 41°c)
- Depression
- Anorexia
- Leukopenia
- Dependent edema (limbs, ventrum, scrotum, prepuce, mammary glands, peri- or supraorbital region)
- Conjunctivitis, with or without lacrimation
- Photophobia
- Serous to mucoid nasal discharge
- Stiffness of gait
- Petechial hemorrhages on oral mucous membranes
- Urticaria or hives (localized on face, neck, pectoral region, or generalized)
- Diarrhea
- Icterus
- Ataxia
- Abortion
- Fatal pneumonitis or pneumoenteritis in neonatal and young foals
- Temporary subfertility in stallions

Strains of EAV can cause abortion throughout much of pregnancy (2 months to more than 10 months). Abortion may occur late in the acute phase or early in the convalescent phase of infection, with or without prior clinical signs of EVA. In natural outbreaks, abortion rates can vary from <10% to as high as 60%. There is no evidence confirming that mares bred with EAV-infective semen will abort later in gestation. Mares that abort from the virus are already pregnant at time of exposure; this occurs primarily by the respiratory route through direct proximity with an acutely infected animal, frequently sharing the same pasture or having across-the-fence contact. Abortion occurs 1–4 weeks later.

Mares exposed very late in gestation may not abort but give birth to a foal congenitally infected with the virus. There is no evidence to indicate that mares that abort from EAV infection are subsequently less fertile. Aborted fetuses may be delivered autolyzed or nonautolyzed and may exhibit interlobular pulmonary edema, pleural and pericardial effusion, and petechial and ecchymotic hemorrhages on the serosal and mucosal surfaces of the small intestine. Stallions with EVA may undergo a period of short-term subfertility during acute infection. This has been observed in individuals that develop a high and/or prolonged fever and significant scrotal edema.

Affected stallions may exhibit reduced libido associated with decreases in total and progressively motile sperm, curvilinear velocity, percentage of live spermatozoa, and percentage of morphologically normal spermatozoa. The changes in semen quality are believed to result from increased intratesticular temperature and not from the direct effect of EAV on spermatogenesis and testicular function. There is strong evidence that fever and scrotal edema can exert independent effects on semen quality. Semen changes can last for 14–16 weeks before returning to normal. No longterm adverse effects on fertility have been seen in fully recovered stallions. The frequency and severity of clinical illness associated with EAV infection tend to be greater in very young, old, or debilitated individuals and under adverse climatic conditions.

Regardless of severity of clinical signs, affected horses invariably make complete recoveries, even in the absence of symptomatic treatment. Mortality in older horses is very rarely encountered in natural outbreaks. However, it can occur in neonatal and in young foals up to a few months of age that succumb from a fulminating pneumonia or pneumoenteritis.

Lesions

The gross and microscopic lesions observed in fatal cases of EVA reflect the extensive and considerable vascular damage caused by the virus; these descriptions are primarily based on experimental infection with the horse-adapted highly pathogenic Bucyrus strain of EAV.

The most significant gross findings include edema, congestion, and hemorrhages, especially in the subcutis of the limbs and abdomen; excess peritoneal, pleural, and pericardial fluid; and edema and hemorrhage of the intra-abdominal and thoracic lymph nodes and of the small and large intestine, especially the cecum and colon.

Gross lesions are usually absent in aborted fetuses; if present, they are limited to an excess of fluid in body cavities and a variable degree of interlobular pulmonary edema.

Pulmonary edema, emphysema and interstitial pneumonia, enteritis, and infarcts in the spleen have been reported in naturally acquired fatal cases of the disease in foals.

The characteristic microscopic lesion seen in cases of EAV infection is a vasculitis, involving primarily smaller arterioles and venules. Histologically, changes can range from vascular and perivascular edema, with occasional lymphocytic infiltration and endothelial cell hypertrophy in mild cases, to fibrinoid necrosis of the tunica media, extensive lymphocytic infiltration, necrosis and loss of endothelium, and thrombus formation in severe cases.

There are no characteristic histologic features of EAV infection in the fetus, but severe necrotizing panvasculitis of small vessels has been observed. Affected muscular arteries show foci of intimal, subintimal, and medial necrosis, with edema and infiltration of lymphocytes and neutrophils. Prominent vascular lesions are also seen in the placenta, brain, liver, and spleen of the aborted fetuses. Lungs of affected neonatal foals have severe interstitial pneumonia.

Fatal cases of EAV infection in young foals are characterized by interstitial pneumonia, emphysema, interlobular edema, congestion and mononuclear cell infiltration in the lungs, and lymphoid depletion and hemorrhage in lymphoreticular tissues. Focal hemorrhages and necrosis of the intestinal mucosa have been described in cases with an associated enteritis.

Diagnosis of Equine Viral Arteritis

- Viral isolation, serology, RT-PCR, or demonstration of viral antigens in tissue

The signs of equine viral arteritis can mimic that of a range of other respiratory and nonrespiratory equine diseases. Thus, the differential diagnosis of EVA includes other viral respiratory tract infections such as equine herpesvirus 1 and 4, equine influenza virus, equine rhinitis A and B viruses, and equine adenovirus. It may also include equine infectious anemia, purpura hemorrhagica, allergy-induced urticaria, and toxicosis due to hoary alyssum (*Berteroa incana).* Furthermore, several foreign animal diseases that should be considered in a differential diagnosis of EVA include Getah virus infection, dourine, and African horse sickness.

Thus, confirmation of a provisional clinical diagnosis of EVA should be pursued without delay in suspected outbreaks of the disease. Abortion caused by EAV must be differentiated from that due to equine herpesvirus 1 or 4. A helpful but not always reliable distinguishing feature is that mares that abort because of EAV may display prior clinical signs of EVA, whereas mares that abort because of equine herpesvirus 1 or 4 seldom exhibit any premonitory clinical evidence of infection. Furthermore, EAV-infected fetuses not infrequently are somewhat autolyzed at time of expulsion and very often, are devoid of any gross and even microscopic lesions.

In contrast, herpesvirus-infected fetuses are invariably fresh and usually display characteristic gross and microscopic lesions. Laboratory confirmation of EVA can be based on virus isolation, detection of viral nucleic acid by standard RT-PCR, real-time RT-qPCR or RT-insulated isothermal PCR (RT-iiPCR), and in situ hybridization (conventional or RNAscope), visualization of viral antigen by immunohistochemical examination, or demonstration of a humoral antibody response by testing paired (acute and convalescent) sera collected 3–4 weeks apart. Of the serologic assays evaluated for detection of antibodies to EAV, the complement-enhanced virus neutralization test continues to be regarded as the most reliable for the diagnosis of acute EAV infection and for seroprevalence studies.

A number of ELISAs have been developed, only one or two of which approximate the sensitivity and specificity of the virus neutralization test. None of the available serologic tests can differentiate antibody titers resulting from natural infection from those due to vaccination. The most appropriate samples for virus isolation and/or detection of viral nucleic acid by RT-PCR are nasopharyngeal swabs or washings and unclotted (citrated or EDTA) blood samples.

To optimize the chances of isolation or detection of virus, samples should be collected as early as possible upon onset of clinical signs or suspicion of EAV infection. After collection, swabs should be transferred directly into viral transport medium and shipped refrigerated or frozen in an insulated container via an overnight delivery service to a laboratory with expertise and experience in testing for this infection. Unclotted blood samples should be transported refrigerated but not frozen.

In suspect cases of EAV-related abortion, virus detection should be attempted from placental tissues and fluids and from fetal lung, liver, lymphoreticular tissues (especially thymus), and peritoneal or pleural fluid. Chorioallantoic membrane and fetal lung are the tissues of choice for recovery of virus.

When EAV is suspected in deaths of young foals or older horses, a wide range of tissue specimens, especially the lymphatic glands in the thoracic and abdominal cavities and related organs, should be collected and submitted for laboratory examination, including viral nucleic acid detection by RT-PCR or virus isolation, together with histologic and immunohistochemical testing. Investigation of the putative carrier status of a stallion is based initially on determining whether the individual is seropositive or negative for antibodies to EAV.

In the absence of a certified history of vaccination, stallions with a virus neutralizing antibody titer >1:4 are considered seropositive and should be regarded as potential carriers of the virus until proven otherwise, based on absence of detectable EAV in their semen. Confirmation of the carrier state is based on demonstration of virus in a semen sample containing the sperm-rich fraction of the ejaculate either by isolation of virus in cell culture or its detection by RT-qPCR. The carrier state can also be determined by test breeding a stallion to two seronegative mares and checking the mares for seroconversion to EAV 28 days after breeding.

Treatment of Equine Viral Arteritis

- Supportive care: There is no specific antiviral treatment currently available for equine viral arteritis. Aside from young foals, virtually all horses naturally infected with EAV make complete clinical recoveries, even in the absence of symptomatic treatment.

Supportive treatment is indicated, however, in moderate to severely affected horses, especially stallions. This supportive treatment should include:

- Antipyretics
- Anti-inflammatory drugs
- Diuretics
- Adequate rest
- Good nursing care
- Gradual return to breeding activity

Prompt symptomatic treatment of stallions with a high or prolonged fever and significant scrotal and preputial edema can reduce the likelihood of short-term subfertility.

There is no effective treatment for EVA-related cases of pneumonia or pneumoenteritis in foals. Because congenitally infected foals are very productive sources of EAV by the respiratory route and their chances of survival are essentially nil, early euthanasia is warranted to minimize the risk of further spread of the virus to any susceptible contacts, especially pregnant mares and young foals.

There is some evidence that temporary downregulation of circulating testosterone by GnRH immunization or through the use of a GnRH antagonist promotes clearance of EAV from the reproductive tract of some but not all treated carrier stallions. Neither strategy has yet been proven to be free from possible adverse effects on the reproductive behavior of treated individuals. The carrier state can be permanently eliminated from a stallion by surgical castration.

Prevention and Control of Equine Viral Arteritis

Vaccination and sound management of breeding populations

The primary focus of current control programs is to restrict the spread of equine viral arteritis in breeding populations and to reduce the risk of outbreaks of virus-related abortion, death in young foals, and establishment of the carrier state in stallions and postpubertal colts. Although EAV has occasionally been responsible for extensive outbreaks of disease at racetracks, shows, sales, and veterinary hospitals, these have been so sporadic that no specific control programs have been developed to prevent such occurrences.

EVA is a manageable and preventable disease that can be controlled by observance of sound management practices together with a targeted vaccination program. Attenuated live and inactivated vaccines are available in North America and Europe, respectively, for prevention and control. The attenuated modified-live vaccine available in North America protects against development of EVA, including abortion, and establishment of the carrier state in stallions.

Annual revaccination of vaccinated horses is recommended to boost the level of protective immunity. Although the vaccine is safe and immunogenic for stallions and nonpregnant mares, the manufacturers do not recommend its use in pregnant mares, especially in the final 2 months of gestation or in foals <6 weeks of age, unless there is a high risk of exposure to natural infection.

Experimental and field studies have shown that there are no adverse consequences to vaccinating pregnant mares up to 3 months before foaling and during the immediate postpartum period. However, there is a low risk of abortion in mares vaccinated during the last 2–3 months of pregnancy.

All seronegative mares being bred to a persistently infected stallion should be vaccinated 21 days prior to natural breeding or artificial insemination. Those previously vaccinated should be given a booster immunization. Minimizing or eliminating direct or indirect contact of unprotected horses with infected animals or with virus-infective semen is critical to the success of any prevention program.

Control programs are predicated on observance of sound management practices similar to those recommended for other respiratory infections. These include isolation of new arrivals on a premises for 3–4 weeks before allowing them to co-mingle with the resident equine population, maintenance of pregnant mares in small isolated groups, identification of carrier stallions, annual immunization of noncarrier breeding stallion populations, and vaccination of colts at 6–12 months of age to minimize their risk of becoming carriers later in life.

Carrier stallions should be managed separately and bred only to naturally seropositive mares or mares vaccinated against EVA. Personnel need to take all appropriate precautions during the breeding or collection of semen from such stallions to ensure that EAV is not accidentally spread to other horses on the premises by indirect means through the use of virus-contaminated fomites.

Because fresh-cooled or frozen semen can be an important source of EAV, it should be tested by a laboratory with appropriate diagnostic expertise to confirm its negative EAV status, especially if imported. When breeding a mare artificially with virus-infective semen, the same precautions apply as if breeding by live cover to a carrier stallion.

Specific **measures to prevent or control EVA on breeding farms** include:

- Identifying any carrier stallions
- Separately managing any carrier stallions
- Vaccinating noncarrier stallions annually
- Restricting breeding carrier stallions to eva-vaccinated mares or mares naturally seropositive for antibodies to eav
- Isolating mares bred with infective semen for the first time from eav seronegative horses for 3 weeks
- Screening semen intended for ai use for virus, particularly if imported
- Observing sound management practices, especially of pregnant mares
- Vaccinating colt (male) foals between 6 and 12 months of age to prevent possible development of a carrier state later in life
- Under circumstances of intensive management and limited facilities, considering vaccination of all at-risk animals

In the event of a suspected outbreak of EVA, relevant animal health authorities, federal, state, or other officials should be promptly notified, with affected and in-contact horses isolated and with restrictions immediately imposed on movement of horses onto and off the affected premises. Appropriate specimens should be collected as soon as possible after onset of clinical signs and submitted for laboratory confirmation of a diagnosis of EVA. Breeding activity should be suspended on breeding farms to minimize risk of further spread of the infection. Stalls and equipment that might have come in contact with infected animals should be thoroughly sanitized. In consultation with a veterinarian, vaccination of the at-risk equine population on a premises should be seriously considered as a means of restricting further transmission of EAV and of expediting control and resolution of an outbreak. Movement restrictions should not be lifted until at least 3 weeks after the last clinical or suspected case of EVA or laboratory-confirmed case of EAV infection.

Release of Animals from Isolation

Release of animals from isolation can be considered 4 weeks after the last case of EVA or confirmed case of EAV infection. Animals can be released if virus detection tests (nasal/pharyngeal swab and blood) are negative. After all animals have been released from isolation, thorough disinfection of the area holding facility should be undertaken.

Zoonotic Potential

None known.

PIGEON FEVER (CORYNEBACTERIUM PSEUDOTUBURBULOSIS)

Pigeon fever is caused by *Corynebacterium pseudotuberculosis*, which is a gram-positive, rod-shaped bacteria. Horses and small ruminants typically get different strains of the infection, but cattle can get both types. In goats, the disease is known as caseous lymphadenitis, and affected animals will have external abscesses (typically found on the head, behind the ears, or on the neck, shoulder or flank). Abscesses also occur in horses and cattle infected with this bacteria.

Natural transmission from horses to goats or *vice versa* is not thought to commonly occur. *Corynebacterium pseudotuberculosis* is a soil organism that can survive for months to years in direct sun. The largest number of cases is typically reported in the dry months of fall and winter. *Corynebacterium pseudotuberculosis* is the causative agent in pigeon fever, and the name is derived from the swelling that often occurs in the pectoral muscles, which resembles a pigeon's breast.

Over the last few years, more states have reported cases of pigeon fever which had not reported in their state previously. *Corynebacterium pseudotuberculosis* "biovar ovis" causes caseous lymphadenitis in small ruminants; and the equine diseases, which include pigeon fever and ulcerative lymphangitis, are caused by the "biovar equi." The natural cross-species transmission does not occur between horses and small ruminants but can occur in cattle and horses.

Cattle have both biotypes. This disease is endemic in the Southwestern part of the US, Australia, and Brazil. There is a seasonal incidence associated with the presence of biting flies, but in this reported case biting flies were not active in NY at the time of infection. It is not contagious between horses, but the abscesses serve as a source of environmental contamination. There is a zoonotic concern for pneumonia and lymphadenitis. *Corynebacterium pseudotuberculosis* causes suppurative abscesses, both internally and externally, and ulcerative lymphangitis.

It may affect any age of the horse, but young horses appear to be more susceptible. Internal abscesses can cause systemic illness and be challenging to diagnose. The abscess material should be cultured aerobically for a definitive diagnosis. Internal abscesses can be diagnosed with the help of a serological SHI test (synergistic hemolysis inhibition) in horses with compatible signs. Many things about this disease in horses are still not completely understood, such as the incubation period.

The incubation period is the time it takes to develop clinical symptoms of the disease after being infected with the bacteria. In horses, the incubation period can vary and ranges from weeks to months. The bacteria can enter the horse through the skin, wounds, or abrasions in the mucous membranes. Horses with pigeon fever may have a poor appetite, fever, lethargy, swelling along the chest or ventral abdomen, and/or lameness. Three forms of the disease can occur in horses: 1) external abscesses, 2) internal abscesses, and 3) ulcerative lymphangitis. Horses with the most common form of pigeon fever will develop external abscesses.

These occur in about 90% of the cases. The disease got its name because abscesses will commonly develop in the pectoral region, which becomes swollen and painful. In addition to the pectorals, abscesses may form on the prepuce, mammary gland, axilla, limbs, inguinal region, head, and other areas. No breed or sex is predisposed to acquire the infection, although young horses may have some increased risk.

Horses with the second form of the disease will have internal abscessation, which has been reported in about 8% of cases. The most common site of internal abscesses is the liver, but they can be associated with other organs as well. The third form found in horses is ulcerative lymphangitis, which is a severe cellulitis that occurs in the fewest number of cases. Clinical cases of ulcerative lymphangitis have severe lameness and swelling of the limb or limbs.

Pathogenesis and Clinical Findings

The onset of ulcerative lymphangitis in horses is variable and usually manifests as painful inflammation, nodules, and ulcers, especially in the region of the lower limb, or lameness and edematous swelling can extend up the entire limb. The exudate is odorless, thick, tan, and blood tinged. Usually, only one leg is involved. If the animal is not treated aggressively with antimicrobials, lesions and swelling usually progress and become chronic with relapses.

C pseudotuberculosis infection in horses occurs at any time of the year. However, peak incidence of disease is during the summer and fall, when flying insects are present. Infection results in abscessation of the pectoral region or ventral abdominal region, with secondary dissemination to internal organs.

Clinical Signs

Three forms have been described in horses: ulcerative lymphangitis or limb infection, external abscesses and internal infection. Ulcerative lymphangitis and internal infection must be treated more aggressively with antimicrobial therapy, while use of antimimicrobials for external abscesses is often unnecessary

Ulcerative lymphangitis is the least common form seen in North America, although this form of disease has been reported worldwide. Ulcerative lymphangitis manifests as a severe limb swelling and cellulitis, with multiple draining tracts following lymphatics. Most commonly one or both hind limbs are affected. Horses often develop a severe lameness, fever, lethargy and anorexia. Aggressive medical therapy (antimicrobial and anti-inflammatory) is necessary or the disease often becomes chronic, resulting in limb edema, prolonged or recurrent infection, lameness, weakness, and weight loss.

External Abscesses are the most common manifestation, and may occur anywhere on the body, but most frequently develop in the pectoral region (swelling resembles a pigeon's breast) and along the ventral midline of the abdomen. Abscesses contain tan, odor-free purulent exudate and are usually well encapsulated. Additional sites for abscess formation are the prepuce, mammary gland, triceps, axilla, limbs, and head. Septic joints and osteomyelitis have been reported. Horses may have a single or multiple abscesses involving different regions of the body. Horses with external abscesses do not usually develop signs of systemic illness, however one-quarter will develop fever. If signs of systemic illness are present, further diagnostics to rule out internal infection are warranted, and antimicrobial therapy should be considered. While there is considerable variation in severity among horses, most straight - forward cases can be treated with lancing and draining the abscesses when mature. The case fatality for horses with external abscesses is very low (0.8%).

Internal infection occurs in approximately 8% of affected horses, which is associated with a high case fatality rate (30 to 40%). Diagnosis can be challenging, and long-term antimicrobial therapy is imperative for successful outcome. In a retrospective study, the organs most commonly involved were liver, kidney, spleen and lungs. Abortion due to placentitis or fetal infection has been reported.

Transmission

The portal of entry of this soil-dwelling organism is thought to be through abrasions or wounds in the skin or mucous membranes. Many insects have been incriminated as vectors for the transmission of the disease to horses, and studies have shown that Haematobia irritans, Musca domestica, Stomoxys calcitrans can act as mechanical vectors of this disease. The regional location of abscesses suggests that ventral midline dermatitis is a predisposing cause of infection. Temporal and special analysis indicated an incubation period of 3 to 4 weeks. Within a geographic area, the disease appeared to be transmitted between 7 and 56 days throughout a 4.3 to 6.5 km distance, strongly suggesting that the disease could be transmitted through horse-to-horse contact or from infected to susceptible horses via insects, other vectors, or contaminated soil. The organism has been shown to survive for up to 2 months in hay and shavings, and more than 8 months in soil samples at environmental temperatures. The incidence of disease fluctuates considerably from year to year presumably due to herd immunity and environmental factors such rainfall and temperature. Disease incidence is seasonal, with highest number of cases occurring during the dry months of the year, which is summer and fall in the Southwestern US, although cases may be seen all year. Horses with internal infection are more frequently seen one to two months following the peak number of cases with external abscesses.

Diagnosis

- Bacterial culture of pus from external abscesses
- Abdominal ultrasound, clinicopathologic evidence of inflammation, and serology for internal infection
- PCR testing of abdominal fluid for Corynebacterium pseudotuberculosis

Isolation of *C pseudotuberculosis* from lesions is necessary to confirm diagnosis of infection. In all forms of lymphangitis in horses, samples for culture include aspirates of abscesses, swabs of purulent exudate beneath crusts associated with folliculitis, and punch biopsies.

Differential diagnoses of *C pseudotuberculosis* infection include:

- pyoderma
- abscesses
- lymphangitis from other bacteria (eg, Staphylococcus aureus, Rhodococcus equi, Streptococcus spp, or Dermatophilus spp)

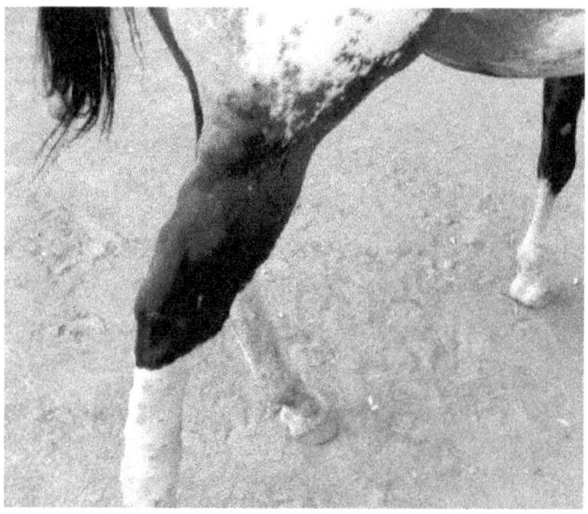

Fig. 1 Ulcerative lymphangitis

- dermatophytosis
- sporotrichosis
- equine cryptococcosis
- North American blastomycosis
- onchocerciasis

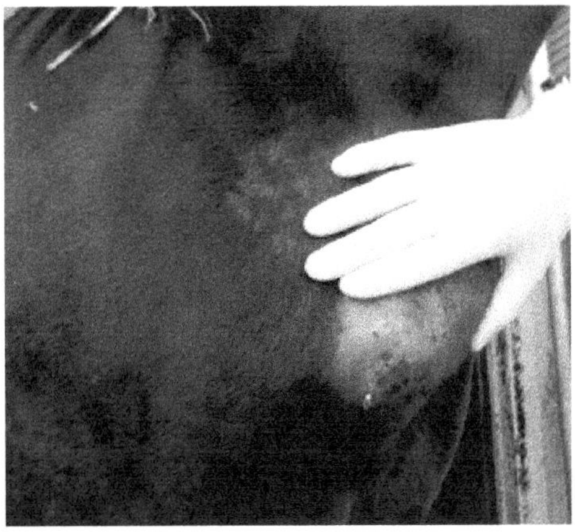

Fig. 2 Typical pectoral abscess with flies attracted to exudates

Ultrasonography of the abdomen and thorax is useful for detection of internal infection of the liver, spleen, kidneys, or lungs. Ultrasonography is also useful for detection and drainage of deep abscesses causing lameness, particularly in the triceps musculature. Transtracheal aspirates are required to confirm pneumonia caused by *C pseudotuberculosis*.

In horses, serologic testing with the synergistic hemolysis inhibition test, which detects IgG to the phospholipase D exotoxin, is a useful adjunct for diagnosis of internal infection in the absence of external infection. Serologic testing should not be used alone for diagnosis of infection.

Treatment

- Lance and drain external abscesses
- Longterm antimicrobial therapy for ulcerative lymphangitis, limb infection, and internal infection
- Fly control

Lymphangitis and internal infection should be treated with longterm antimicrobials (a minimum of 1 month duration or as directed by follow-up ultrasonography). The organism is susceptible to most commonly administered antimicrobials; however, antimicrobial treatment of uncomplicated external abscesses may prolong the disease by delaying abscess maturation. External abscess swellings are treated with hot packs, poultices, or hydrotherapy until they rupture or are drained surgically. Abscesses are lanced and flushed with dilute antiseptic solutions. Deep abscesses in the triceps or quadriceps region require ultrasonography to guide placement of an indwelling drain. Phenylbutazone or flunixin meglumine relieves pain and swelling. General supportive and nursing care is indicated.

If treatment is successful, the swelling gradually recedes over days or weeks. Internal infection may have a 30%–40% mortality rate in horses, even with appropriate treatment.

Severe or untreated lymphangitis cases often become chronic, and fibrosis and induration of the leg occur. Isolation of infected animals, comprehensive fly control including insect growth regulators, and good sanitation are recommended for prevention. A conditionally licensed bacterin/toxoid is currently available for horses.

Biosecurity Management for Receipt of Animals

Once horses are recovered and there is no drainage from abscesses no precautions should be needed to reduce the risk these horses pose for spread of infection. There is no practical way at this time for eliminating the bacteria from soil.

Zoonotic Potential

There exist few reports of human illness through working with infected sheep, mostly in Australian sheep shearers who had open wounds on their hands and developed axillary lymphadenitis. One veterinary student from California developed pneumonia following exposure to an infected horse, presumably from inhalation of the bacteria from a contaminated environment.

POTOMAC HORSE FEVER (EHRITICHIA RISTICCI)

Potomac Horse Fever (PHF) is a non-contagious, infectious equine disease caused by the rickettsial organism *Neorickettsia risticii* (previously known as *Ehrlichia risticii*). The disease can affect any age, breed or sex of horse. PHF cases usually occur in summer and fall, but may occur in any season depending on weather conditions.

Potomac horse fever is an acute enterocolitis syndrome producing mild colic, fever, and diarrhea in horses of all ages, as well as abortion in pregnant mares. The causative agent is *Neorickettsia risticii*. The infection of enterocytes of the small and large intestine results in acute colitis, which is one of the principal clinical signs of PHF. The disease is seen in spring, summer, and early fall and is associated with pastures bordering creeks or rivers. The epidemiology of PHF has been shown to involve a trematode vector.

Sporadic disease caused by *N risticii* has been reported in dogs and cats; cattle appear to be resistant to infection. PHF has been reported in many areas of the USA and Canada using an indirect fluorescent antibody test as evidence of exposure; however, recent studies indicate a high rate of false-positive titers with this test, and the true geographic range of distribution is not known. Isolation or detection of the causative agent from clinical cases of PHF using conventional cell culture or PCR assay has been reported only from California, Illinois, Indiana, Kentucky, Maryland, Michigan, New York, New Jersey, Ohio, Oregon, Pennsylvania, Texas, and Virginia.

Etiology and Pathogenesis

N risticii is a gram-negative obligate intracellular bacterium with a trophism for monocytes. Initial morphologic studies of this organism isolated from cell culture, as well as the serologic responses of *N risticii*, caused this bacterium to be assigned to the genus *Ehrlichia*. However, DNA analyses have shown *N risticii* is most closely related to *N helminthoeca*, the agent of salmon poisoning in dogs, and *Ehrlichia sennetsu*, a disease of people in Japan. The organism is not visible in monocytes in blood films from clinical cases, in contrast to *Anaplasma phagocytophilum*, which is readily identifiable in granulocytes of infected horses.

N risticii has been identified in freshwater snails and isolated from trematodes released from the snails. *N risticii* DNA was detected in 13 species of immature and adult caddisflies (Trichoptera), mayflies (Ephemeroptera), damselflies (Odonata, Zygoptera), dragonflies (Odonata, Anisoptera), and stoneflies (Plecoptera). Transmission studies using *N risticii*-infected caddisflies have reproduced the clinical disease.

One route of exposure is believed to be inadvertent ingestion of hatched aquatic insects that carry *N risticii* in the metacercarial stage of a trematode. The incubation period is ~10–18 days. The causative organism is present in the feces of experimentally infected horses, but the biologic significance of this is unknown. Clinically ill horses are not contagious and can be housed with susceptible horses. Additional studies are needed to determine the exact role of the vector and helminth hosts in the complex maintenance cycle of *N risticii*.

Clinical Signs

Highly variable, including:

- High fever to 107° F (41.6o C) reported. Fevers may occur 7–14 days before signs of colitis develop
- Diarrhea: variable, ranging from absent to severe
- Depression
- Anorexia
- Lethargy
- Laminitis (with or without diarrhea) may progress from mild to severe
- Mild to moderate colic
- Decreased gastrointestinal sounds
- Edema of limbs and ventral body, prepuce of males
- Abortion (by transplacental transmission)

Note: Concurrent infections with Salmonella have been documented.

Incubation Period

Approximately 1–3 weeks

Risk Factors

- Housing near (within approximately 5 miles) a freshwater stream or river or on irrigated pasture in endemic areas
- Nighttime use of barn lights which attract parasitized insects
- Transmission
- Oral ingestion of trematodes present in aquatic insects (caddisflies, mayflies, damselflies and dragonflies)
- Whole blood transfusion from an infected donor
- Transplacental
- Exposure to freshwater or operculate snails

(Note: Affected horses are not considered to be contagious by natural contact with other horses.)

Diagnosis

A provisional diagnosis of PHF often is based on the presence of typical clinical signs and on the seasonal and geographic occurrence of the disease. A definitive diagnosis should be based on isolation or identification of *N risticii* from the blood or feces of infected horses by cell culture or PCR. Serologic testing is of limited value as a diagnostic tool, although many infected horses have high antibody titers at the time of infection. Because of the high prevalence of false-positive titers, interpretation of the indirect fluorescent antibody test in individual horses is difficult.

Rising paired titers can be helpful. Isolation of the agent in cell culture, although possible, is time-consuming and not routinely available in many diagnostic laboratories. A real-time PCR assay that allows detection of *N risticii* DNA within 2 hr is a much more feasible test for routine diagnostic examination. To enhance the chances of detection of *N risticii*, the assay should be performed both on blood and fecal samples, because the presence of the organism in blood and feces may not necessarily coincide.

Treatment

Horses with PHF can be treated successfully with oxytetracycline (6.6 mg/kg, IV, bid), if given early in the clinical course of the disease. A response to treatment is usually seen within 12 hr. This is associated with a drop in rectal temperature, followed by an improvement in demeanor, appetite, and borborygmal sounds. If therapy is begun early, clinical signs frequently resolve by the third day of treatment. Generally, antimicrobial therapy is for no more than 5 days. In animals that exhibit signs of enterocolitis, fluids and NSAIDs should be administered.

Laminitis is more common than in other causes of enterocolitis, and if it develops, is usually severe and often refractory to treatment. The overall case fatality rate is 5%–30%.

Prevention

Several inactivated, whole-cell vaccines based on the same strain of *N ristícii* are commercially available. Although vaccination has been reported to protect 78% of experimentally infected ponies, it has been marginally protective in the field. Vaccine failure has been attributed to antigenic and genomic heterogeneity among the >14 different strains of *N risticii* isolated from naturally occurring cases. Furthermore, vaccine failure may also be due to lack of antibody protection at the site of exposure, because the natural route of transmission has been determined to be oral ingestion of the agent. Minimizing insect ingestion in stabled horses by turning off barn lights at night, which normally attract the insects, has been suggested.

Biosecurity

Issues for Receiving Animals Diarrheic horses should be isolated as a matter of routine until contagious causes can be ruled out and normal feces are produced

Zoonotic Potential

None known.

RABIES

Rabies is a neurologic disease caused by a virus in the genus *Lyssavirus.* All mammals are susceptible to rabies and it has the highest case fatality ratio of any infectious disease.

Wildlife have accounted for >90% of rabid animals in the United States since 1980. The primary reservoir species responsible for maintaining rabies are raccoons, bats, skunks, and foxes. The disease is a significant threat to horses in South and Central America but is not a major cause of death in North America due to successful vaccination efforts.

Rabies infection usually occurs by the bite of a rabid animal but can also be transmitted when fresh saliva from an infected animal contacts a wound or mucous membranes. Encounters between horses and rabid animals are rarely witnessed, and bite wounds, which may be punctures, are difficult to find. Bites often occur on the lower limbs or face and the virus migrates to the spinal cord and brain where it causes fatal inflammation of the brain (encephalitis).

With the increasing urbanization of areas where the disease is regularly found in wildlife populations, the risk of exposure continues to be a concern for veterinarians and horse owners. Horse-to-human transmission is rare, but exposure to nervous and other tissues from horses that may be infected should be avoided.

Clinical Signs

- Highly variable
- In unvaccinated horses, rabies is rapidly progressive with death occurring 5-7 days following the onset of clinical signs.

- Insidious onset is the hallmark of equine rabies. Frequently reported initial clinical signs include lameness, colic, dysuria, priapism, and neurologic abnormalities.
- Physical signs may include:
  - Fever
  - Anorexia
  - Blindness
  - Dysphagia
  - Hyperesthesia – manifest as self-mutilation
  - Muscle twitching
  - Lameness
  - Paresis and/or ataxia
  - Incontinence
  - Paralysis – ascending
  - Sudden death
- Behavioral signs:
  - Dumb form: depression/stupor
  - Furious form: mania – these horses are extremely dangerous

NOTE: Rabies should be included as a differential in all neurologic patients.

Incubation Period

Typically, 2-6 weeks, although longer incubation periods have been reported.

Risk Factors

- Unvaccinated horses
- 24-hour access to pasture
- Resident in endemic area

Causes of Rabies

Rabies is caused by a virus that is present in the saliva of infected animals. The infected animal will transmit the disease through bites or through their saliva getting into an open cut or mucous membrane of another animal. Rabies can be present in a variety of animals, for example skunks, bats, foxes, raccoons, cats, dogs and livestock. The disease can also be spread from an infected animal to a human.

Transmission

Exposure occurs primarily through a bite wound from an infected animal.

Aerosolization of nerve or central nervous system (CNS) tissues during necropsy.

Diagnostic Sampling, Testing and Handling

Correct sampling and testing is imperative for a definitive diagnosis in rabies.

See figures 3 and 4 below for areas to test from the brain.

Saliva and other body tissues become virus positive by the time clinical signs are evident, but there remains no fully reliable ante-mortem diagnostic test for rabies. Personnel involved in the necropsy of a rabies suspect case should be vaccinated against rabies and use appropriate barrier clothing for protection.

Send cross section of brain stem (through the medulla, pons, or midbrain area) and cerebellum (through EACH hemisphere and the vermis).

Many laboratories will not start ancillary testing until negative rabies results have been received. Contact the laboratory for specific policies and procedures.

Post-mortem

Rabies does not present with gross lesions. Self inflicted wounds may be found on the body.

Environmental Persistence

Rabies virus is sensitive to drying, ultraviolet radiation, and detergent. Rabies is inactivated and removed by standard decontamination practices which include washing instruments and environment with common disinfectants including quarternary ammonium compounds. Instruments should be sterilized by autoclaving.

Specific Control Measures

Rabies-suspect cases

- Minimize number of personnel in contact with suspect case.
- When possible, limit personnel to those who have been vaccinated.
- Gloves and protective eyewear must be worn by all in-contact personnel.
- Establish records of all individuals having handled the suspect horse beginning 48 hours prior to onset of clinical signs.
- Suspect horses should remain quarantined for 30 days.

Prevention

Vaccination should be administered to horses annually after an initial series.

Previously vaccinated horses: Post-exposure prophylaxis should be performed promptly once exposure is suspected and the animal observed for 3 to 6 months.

Post-exposure vaccination of previously unvaccinated horses is of dubious value.

Feeding and/or housing of wild animals (as pets) are discouraged.

Release of Animals from Isolation

Any horse exhibiting neurologic signs that has not been vaccinated against rabies should be considered a rabies suspect. Such horses should be handled using contact precautions, with records kept as described above. These precautions should remain in place for 30 days or until such time as an alternative diagnosis for the neurological signs are confirmed.

Biosecurity

Issues for Receiving Animals N/A

Zoonotic Potential

Yes. Identification of potential rabies-suspect cases is essential and should be promptly reported to public health authorities.

RHODOCOCCUS EQUI

Rhodococcus equi is a Gram-positive facultative intracellular pathogen that is a common cause of bronchopneumonia in foals between 3 weeks and 5 months of age. *R. equi* can also cause various extrapulmonary infections (see below). Although *R. equi* can be cultured from the environment of virtually all horse farms, the clinical disease in foals is endemic at some farms and only sporadic at others. Infections are extremely rare in adult horses.

Rhodococcus equi is a bacterium that lives in the soil and can cause pneumonia in young (1 to 6 months old) foals. In rare cases, immunodeficient adult horses and humans can also become infected. Disease prevalence varies by region, farm, and year, but *R. equi* can be detected on most horse farms around the world.

A foal can inhale airborne bacteria into their respiratory tract or ingest contaminated soil. Infection progresses slowly and foals often do not begin to show clinical signs until the disease has become severe. Foals infected with *R. equi* can shed the bacteria in their feces, leading to the pathogen becoming endemic on the breeding farm and causing disease in the foal crop year after year.

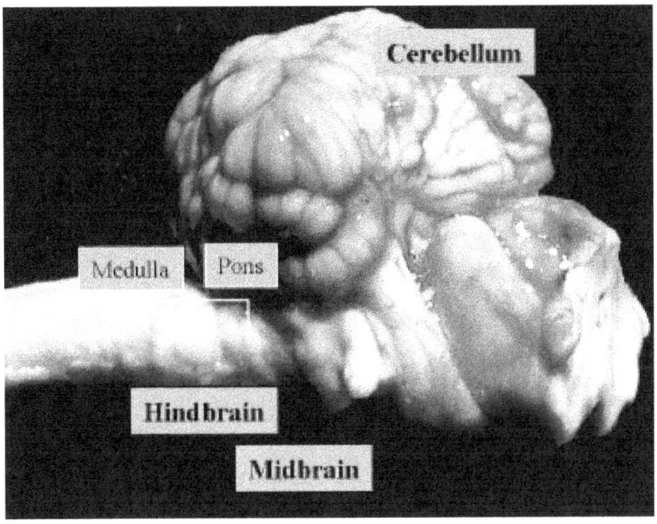

Fig. 3. Lateral view of brain with cerebrum removed to show the extension of brain stem beneath the cerebellum. A rabies diagnosis should include an observation of the cut surface of a cross section of the brain stem (through the medulla, pons, or midbrain area) and the cerebellum (through each hemisphere and the vermis).

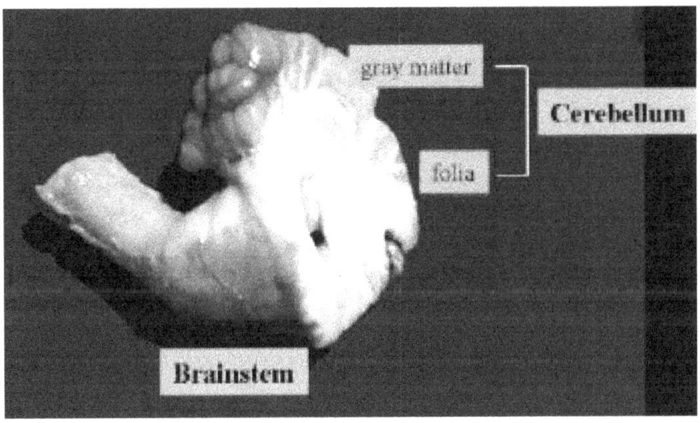

Fig. 4. Surface of cut section through midbrain area showing convoluted gray matter and white foliar regions of the cerebellum, as well as the cerebellar connection to the pons and medulla.

In immunocompromised humans, *R. equi* infection can cause lung infections that result in the formation of abscesses. Mortality can be as high as 50%. Among people with healthy immune systems, infections may only affect a small part of the body and are commonly associated with wound sites.

Biology

R. equi is ubiquitous in soil. Unlike most environmental *R. equi*, isolates from pneumonic foals contain an 80–90 kb plasmid encoding, a surface expressed protein designated virulence-associated protein A (VapA). *R. equi* isolates are often classified as virulent, intermediately virulent or avirulent or based on their ability to replicate in macrophages or to induce disease or death in mice. Virulent *R. equi* isolates contain the large plasmid described above and express VapA. Intermediately virulent *R. equi* isolates contain plasmids encoding VapB or VapN that are related to, but distinct from, VapA. In contrast, avirulent *R. equi* do not express Vap antigens. Intermediately virulent and avirulent isolates are not known to cause naturally occurring disease in horses.

Etiology and Pathogenesis

R equi is a gram-positive, facultative intracellular pathogen that is nearly ubiquitous in soil. Inhalation of dust particles laden with virulent *R equi* is the major route of pneumonic infection. Development of clinical disease is related to immunocompetency of individual foals; foals that produce little to no detectable □ interferon (IFN-□) are at risk of developing pneumonia. Manure from pneumonic foals is a major source of virulent bacteria contaminating the environment. Foals with pulmonary infections swallow sputum laden with *R equi*, which readily replicates in their intestinal tract. The pathogenicity of *R equi* is linked to its ability to survive intracellularly, which hinges on failure of phagosome-lysosomal fusion in infected macrophages and failure of functional respiratory burst upon phagocytosis of *R equi*.

Clinical Findings and Lesions

R equi infection is slowly progressive, with acute to subacute clinical manifestations. Clinical signs of disease are difficult to detect until pulmonary infection reaches a critical mass, resulting in decompensation of the foal. Pulmonary lesions are relatively consistent and include subacute to chronic suppurative bronchopneumonia, pulmonary abscessation, and suppurative lymphadenitis. At the onset of clinical signs, most foals are lethargic, febrile, and tachypneic.

Diarrhea is seen in one-third of foals with *R equi* pneumonia and may be caused by colonic microabscessation.

Cough is a variable clinical sign; purulent nasal discharge is less common. Thoracic auscultation reveals crackles and wheezes with asymmetric/regional distribution. Pulmonary regions with marked consolidation lack breath sounds and exhibit dull resonance on thoracic percussion. In foals with subclinical infections, small to moderate-sized abscesses (<10 cm) may resolve spontaneously.

Immune-mediated polysynovitis (eg, stifle and hock effusion) is often seen in affected foals at presentation. Intestinal and mesenteric abscesses are the most common extrapulmonary sites of infection. Foals with abdominal involvement often present with fever, depression, anorexia, weight loss, colic, and diarrhea. Intestinal lesions are characterized by multifocal, ulcerative enterocolitis and typhlitis involving Peyer's patches with granulomatous or suppurative inflammation of the mesenteric and/or colonic lymph nodes. The prognosis for foals with abdominal forms of *R equi* is less favorable than for those with pulmonary disease.

Septic physitis and osteomyelitis are less common extrapulmonary sites of infection. Vertebral osteomyelitis may result in pathologic vertebral fracture and spinal cord compression and is a devastating manifestation of *R equi* osteomyelitis. Panophthalmitis, guttural pouch empyema, sinusitis, pericarditis, nephritis, nonseptic uveitis, and hepatic and renal abscessation with *R equi* have been reported.

Incubation Period

The incubation period following experimental intrabronchial challenge varies from approximately 9 days after administration of a heavy inoculum to approximately 2–4 weeks when a lower inoculum is administered. However, the incubation period under field conditions is unknown and likely varies depending on several factors including the number of virulent bacteria in air samples in the environment, the age of the foal, and host defense mechanisms.

Transmission

Inhalation of virulent *R. equi* is the major route of pulmonary infection in foals. Ingestion of the organism is an important route of exposure, and likely of immunization, but rarely leads to hematogenously acquired pneumonia unless a foal has multiple exposures to extremely large numbers of bacteria.

Diagnosis

Routine laboratory evaluation of CBC and serum chemistry reveals nonspecific abnormalities consistent with infection and inflammation. Neutrophilic leukocytosis and hyperfibrinogenemia are common, and the severity of these findings relates to prognosis. Thoracic radiographic evaluation may reveal a pattern of perihilar alveolization, consolidation, and abscessation. The presence of nodular lung lesions and mediastinal lymphadenopathy in foals 1–4 mo old is highly suggestive of *R equi*. Bacterial culture of transtracheal wash samples is required for definitive diagnosis. Cytologic evaluation of transtracheal wash samples reveals intracellular coccobacilli, indicating that appropriate antimicrobial therapy should be started pending culture results.

Treatment and Prognosis

The combination of erythromycin (25 mg/kg, PO, qid; esters or salts) and rifampin (5–10 mg/kg, PO, bid) has historically been the treatment of choice for *R equi* infection in foals. These antimicrobials may be bacteriostatic, but their activity is synergistic, and the combination has markedly improved survival of foals with *R equi* pneumonia. Rifampin is lipid soluble (able to penetrate abscess material) and is concentrated in phagocytic cells.

Erythromycin is concentrated in granulocytes and alveolar macrophages; however, its antimicrobial activity is somewhat inhibited by intracellular pH. Adverse reactions are relatively common in foals treated with the erythromycin-rifampin combination.

Diarrhea, idiosyncratic hyperthermia, tachypnea, anorexia, bruxism, and salivation can occur with erythromycin administration, and antimicrobial resistance of *R equi* to erythromycin-rifampin has been reported. Clarithromycin is the macrolide of choice for foals with severe disease, given the most favorable minimum inhibitory concentration against *R equi* isolates obtained from pneumonic foals (90% of isolates are inhibited at 0.12, 0.25, and 1 mcg/mL for clarithromycin, erythromycin, and azithromycin, respectively).

In foals with *R equi* pneumonia, the combination of clarithromycin (7.5 mg/kg, PO, bid) and rifampin is superior to erythromycin-rifampin and azithromycin-rifampin. Foals treated with clarithromycin-rifampin have improved survival rates and fewer febrile days than foals treated with erythromycin-rifampin and azithromycin-rifampin. Reported adverse events of clarithromycin-rifampin include diarrhea in treated foals. The duration of antimicrobial therapy typically is 3–8 wk.

Supportive therapy includes provision of a clean, comfortable environment and highly palatable, dust-free feeds. Judicial IV fluid therapy and saline nebulization facilitates expectoration of pulmonary exudates. NSAIDs should be administered as needed to maintain rectal temperature <103.5°F (39.7°C). Nasal insufflation with oxygen is necessary in foals with severe respiratory compromise. Bronchodilator therapy may or may not improve arterial oxygenation. Prophylactic antiulcer medication is indicated in foals stressed by respiratory difficulty, pain, frequent handling, hospitalization, and transportation.

The survival rate of *R equi* pneumonia is ~70%–90% with appropriate therapy. The case fatality rate without therapy (or with inappropriate antimicrobial therapy) is ~80%. Parameters for discontinuation of medical therapy include clinical signs, serum fibrinogen concentration, and radiographic resolution of pulmonary consolidation and abscessation. Life-threatening, antibiotic-induced enterocolitis, due to *Clostridium difficile*, has been seen in the dams of nursing foals treated with all macrolide preparations.

Prevention

There are several strategies to decrease the incidence of *R equi* pneumonia on endemic farms: early detection of clinical cases, enhanced passive immunity for neonatal foals, and enhanced nonspecific immunity for neonatal foals. Foals should be maintained in well-ventilated, dust-free areas, avoiding dirt paddocks and overcrowding. Pneumonic foals should be isolated and their manure composted. Herd surveillance programs for early detection of pneumonic foals on endemic farms include twice weekly physical examination and auscultation and monthly CBC and fibrinogen concentration.

Foals with a WBC count >14,000 cells/μL should be further evaluated via ultrasonographic examination for *R equi*. Administration of hyperimmune plasma might reduce the incidence and severity of *R equi* within the herd, but it is not completely effective in preventing disease. Hyperimmune plasma (1 L) is administered IV within the first week of life, followed by a second liter at ~25 days of age. Foals with low IFN-γ production in the first month of life appear more susceptible to development of clinical disease. Administration of a nonspecific immunostimulant may enhance IFN-γ production and protect this susceptible population. Mass treatment of foals with subclinical infection has resulted in marcolide- and rifampin-resistant strains and should be avoided.

Environmental Persistence

R. equi is ubiquitous in soil.

Specific Control Measures

In the absence of an effective vaccine, control and prevention of the disease at farms endemic for infections caused by *R. equi* have relied on passive immunization and screening to promote earlier recognition of the disease.

Administration of hyperimmune plasma (HIP)

Intravenous administration of commercially available and licensed plasma containing antibody against *R. equi* is recommended as an aid for preventing pneumonia caused by *R. equi* at endemic farms. Although the data are conflicting, and not all controlled clinical trials have shown a statistically significant reduction in the cumulative incidence of *R. equi* pneumonia, most studies have demonstrated reduction of relative risk, suggesting some benefit of HIP. The optimal amount of plasma to be transfused and the optimal age at which transfusion should occur remain to be determined. There is experimental evidence that administration of HIP before infection is important. Therefore, it is commonly recommended that foals receive transfusion of at least 1 L of HIP no later than the 2nd day of life. Because early administration may result in the decline of passively transferred antibody to a non-protective level at a time when foals are still susceptible to *R. equi* and when environmental challenge is high, it is a common practice to administer a 2nd dose of HIP at 2–4 weeks of age. Currently, there is insufficient information to recommend one brand of licensed antibody product over another. Transfusion of HIP is not completely effective and therefore does not eliminate the need for careful monitoring of foals at risk.

Screening

R. equi pneumonia is often not recognized until it is well advanced and, therefore, difficult to treat. The rationale for screening is the assumption that detecting foals in the early stages of disease along with appropriate treatment of affected foals will improve outcome. It is important to emphasize that screening methods are not diagnostic tests. A useful screening test is one in which the probability of disease is high with a positive test result (high positive predictive value) and very low with a negative test result (high negative predictive value). A variety of screening techniques have been described including visual inspection of foals for clinical signs of pneumonia, monitoring rectal temperatures, measurement of hematological variables or acute phase proteins, serology, and thoracic imaging using ultrasonography. Systematic comparisons of these tests have not been performed but studies indicate that serology to detect antibodies against *R. equi* and measurement of fibrinogen or serum amyloid A concentrations are not useful screening tests.

Over the past 10–15 years, control of *R. equi* infections at many farms where the disease is endemic has relied on early detection of subclinical pulmonary disease using thoracic ultrasonography and initiation of treatment with antimicrobial agents prior to development of clinical signs.

Ultrasonography of the chest offers several advantages over other screening tests:

1. Results are specific for the presence of pulmonary pathology
2. Results are available immediately
3. The procedure allows for assessment of lesion severity and response to therapy

Although controlled studies are lacking periodic ultrasonography of the chest appears to have decreased mortality due to *R. equi* pneumonia at some farms relative to historical data. However, recent double blinded randomized placebo controlled studies at an endemic farm documented that the majority of foals with small pulmonary lesions (sum of lesion diameters [or abscess score] of 1-10 cm) recover without antimicrobial therapy.

In addition, antimicrobial treatment of foals with small ultrasonographic lesions did not significantly hasten lesion resolution compared to administration of a placebo. In contrast, studies performed at the same farm showed that treatment of foals with lesion scores > 10 cm provided a significant benefit over administration of a placebo. The extent to which these results might be extrapolated to other farms is unknown.

Because it is impossible to know which specific foals might recover spontaneously from subclinical disease, and because *R. equi* infections can cause severe disease, many breeding farms elect to treat all foals with ultrasonographic lesions.

This approach has resulted in an increased number of foals treated for presumptive *R. equi* pneumonia. The temporal association between this widespread use of macrolides and rifampin because of ultrasonographic screening and emergence of macrolide and rifampin resistance has been documented at some farms. Additional studies are needed to determine the risks and benefits of treating subclinically affected foals.

Release of Animals from Isolation

There are no isolation requirements for foals with this disease.

Biosecurity Issues for Receiving Animals

Foals with pneumonia caused by *R. equi* shed higher numbers of *R. equi* in their feces than healthy foals or foals with subclinical lesions. Therefore, pneumonic foals might be an important source of contamination of the environment with virulent *R. equi* but there is no evidence that *R. equi* infection is contagious among foals and exposure to virulent *R. equi* is widespread in the environment of foals.

Thus, currently no environmental management practice or biosecurity measure has sufficient evidence on which to base recommendations for controlling and preventing *R. equi* pneumonia.

Zoonotic Potential

R. equi can occasionally cause severe pulmonary or systemic infections in immunosuppressed people. Infections with *R. equi* are extremely rare and typically less severe in immunocompetent individuals.

ROTAVIRUS

Equine rotavirus damages the lining of the intestines, inhibiting digestion and absorption of food. It is one of the most common causes of diarrhea in foals less than six months of age. Foals become infected when they ingest materials or lick surfaces contaminated with infected feces.

Rotavirus destroys the enterocytes on the tip of the villi in the small intestine, which results in malabsorption. Lactase becomes deficient, so lactose passing into the large intestine induces an osmotic diarrhea. Diagnosis is made by identification of virus in the feces by electron microscopy or commercial immunoassay kits designed for detection of human rotavirus. Requesting that the laboratory test specifically for rotavirus, collecting feces early in the course of disease, and sampling several foals improve the chances of virus detection.

Treatment is generally supportive. Certain farm management practices and disinfection techniques have effectively limited the spread of rotavirus during outbreaks. Sick foals are highly contagious and should be isolated in the stall in the barn in which the foal originally became ill or moved to a designated isolation facility. Personnel should wear disposable gloves and cleanable boots and wash their hands with soap before and after handling diarrheic foals.

Foot dips containing phenolic disinfectants outside the stalls of sick foals should also be used. Specific stall-cleaning equipment should be designated only for cleaning the stalls of diarrheic foals. Once the stall has been vacated, it should be cleaned of particulate material, washed with detergent, and then disinfected with phenolic compounds that meet EPA standards.

Bleach, chlorhexidine, and quaternary compounds do not appear to be effective disinfectants for rotavirus. Fecal material of sick foals removed from stalls should not be spread on pastures used for horses and foals, and care should be taken to avoid fecal contamination of alleyways. All stall-cleaning equipment should be disinfected. Stalls with dirt floors are difficult to adequately clean and disinfect. Removal of the top layers of dirt may be required.

Clinical Signs

- May occur as an individual case or as a rapidly spreading diarrhea outbreak involving the entire foal crop.
- Signs are generally more severe in foals less than one week of age.
- Diarrhea can range from watery to cow-pile consistency. Hemorrhagic feces is not a characteristic of uncomplicated rotaviral diarrhea cases.
- Lethargy
- Decreased nursing
- Dehydration and electrolyte imbalances with severe diarrhea
- Signs of weight loss
- Fever is an inconsistent finding
- Lactose intolerance may be present during disease and in the convalescent period
- Some cases may be very mild

Incubation Period

12 to 24 hours.

Risk Factors

- Foals born to mares not vaccinated with the rotavirus vaccine
- Inadequate colostral transfer of immunoglobulins
- Prior occurrence of disease on farm due to environmental persistence
- Inadequate biosecurity in foaling barns (overcrowding, poor hygiene and inadequate cleaning and disinfection protocols)
- Exposure of new foals and mares to established herds without appropriate quarantine measures

Transmission Fecal-oral

- Environmental contamination
- Fomite spread: contamination of personnel and utensils
- During farm outbreaks, clinically unaffected foals may shed virus

Diagnostic Sampling, Testing, and Handling

Fecal samples should be submitted for both virus and bacteriological testing. Consult laboratory for testing capabilities and sample/shipping requirements prior to submitting samples.

In general, the minimum sample is 1-3 grams of feces. It is best to obtain fresh fecal samples (free catch or rectal.)

Many commercially available diagnostic assays are available to detect VP6 (virus protein 6) which is a group-specific inner capsid protein. These tests allow stallside identification of the viral antigen. Examples include a variety of ELISA tests, both plate and lateral flow card types.

More sensitive detection of virus is available by using polymerase chain reaction (RT-PCR), however generally requires submission of samples to a diagnostic laboratory.

These tests are best used to confirm ELISA test results, or if genetic analysis of the virus is a consideration.

Identification of virus is a critical element of control to prevent contamination of the environment or additional cohort foals.

Viral load in feces is variable and in outbreak situations three consecutive negative tests are warranted to confirm negative status of individuals.

Other Tests Include:

- Latex agglutination
- Immunochromatographic assay
- RT-LAMP
- Electron microscopy– lacks sensitivity

Shedding of Virus Following Resolution of Clinical Signs

On average, three days.

Environmental Persistence

Can persist in the environment for up to nine months in most climatic conditions.

Specific Control Measures

Routine isolation and disinfection guidelines should be followed, including proper disposal of manure. Bedding and manure should never be spread on pastures.

Because rotavirus is a non-enveloped virus, many disinfectants are ineffective. Accelerated hydrogen peroxides and some phenolic disinfectants can inactivate the virus in 5% organic matter (read disinfectant label for details). Bleach of appropriate concentration can be used as a disinfectant on clean, hard, nonporous surfaces.

Hand hygiene: Wear disposable gloves to minimize hand contamination, and wash hands after disposing the gloves. Hands contaminated with organic matter (feces, soil, etc.) should be washed with liquid hand soap and water prior to using a hand sanitizer such as 70% ethanol. Chlorhexidine is not effective.

All diarrheic animals should be considered as shedding contagious, and potentially zoonotic organisms.

Vaccination of pregnant mares. Due to variation in antigenicity of field strains compared to commercially available vaccines, disease may occur despite a comprehensive vaccination program.

Release of Animals from Isolation

Three days after resolution of diarrhea and any other clinical signs, foals could be released from isolation.

Biosecurity Issues for Receiving Animals

Use strict isolation measures to reduce the risk of disease spread. Considering the environmental persistence of this virus, manure from isolation facilities housing diarrheic foals up to six months of age should not be spread on pastures.

Use disposable gloves and personal protective equipment (gowns, boot covers); wash hands thoroughly with liquid hand soap and water, followed by 70% ethanol hand sanitizer after handing sick animals.

Because of the high concentration of virus shed in diarrheic feces, thoroughly clean and disinfect all equipment after use. Separate equipment should be used in stalls of sick animals and not used with other horses.

Zoonotic Potential

No known zoonotic potential. However, standard hygiene precautions and use of personal protective equipment should be utilized with any diarrheic patient due to risk of coinfection with zoonotic agents.

SALMONELLOSIS IN HORSES

Salmonellosis is one of the most commonly diagnosed infectious causes of diarrhea in adult horses. Clinical manifestations range from no abnormal clinical signs (subclinical carrier) to acute, severe diarrhea and even death. The disease is seen sporadically but may become an epidemic, depending on the virulence of the organism, level of exposure, and host factors. Infection can occur via contamination of the environment, feed, or water or by contact with animals actively shedding the bacteria. Stress appears to play an important role in the pathogenesis—a history of surgery, transportation, or change in feed; concurrent disease, particularly GI disorders (colic); or treatment with broad-spectrum antimicrobial drugs often precedes the diarrhea.

Salmonella enterica of the serogroup B includes *S enterica* serovar Typhimurium and *S enterica* Agona, two of the most frequently isolated serovars from horses with clinical disease. Knowing the serovar and antibiogram can help track or monitor the type of serovar of salmonellae affecting any given group or population of horses (eg, tracking nosocomial spread within a veterinary hospital). The emergence of multidrug-resistant *S enterica* isolates is concerning both in dealing with nosocomial infections and zoonosis.

Clinical Findings

Three forms of salmonellosis have been recognized in adult horses. One is the subclinical carrier, which may or may not be actively shedding the organism but has the potential to transmit the bacteria to susceptible animals either by direct contact or by contamination of the environment, water, or feed sources. Multiple fecal cultures may be necessary to identify carriers, because the organism is shed in the feces intermittently and in small numbers. If stressed, the carrier may develop clinical disease. The national prevalence of fecal shedding of *S enterica* by normal horses in the USA is estimated to be <2%; however, the proportion of hospitalized horses shedding is much higher (~8%).

The most common serovars identified among the general population of horses were *S enterica* Muenchen and *S enterica* Newport (both serogroup C2). The second form of the disease is characterized by a mild clinical course, with signs of depression, fever, anorexia, and soft but not watery feces. Affected horses may have an absolute neutropenia.

Clinical disease may last 4–5 days and usually is self-limiting, and *S enterica* can be isolated from the feces. Recovered horses may continue to excrete the organism in their feces for days to months; therefore, isolation of the shedding horse and thorough cleaning and subsequent disinfection of the contaminated area are recommended. The third form of salmonellosis is characterized by an acute onset of severe depression, anorexia, profound neutropenia, and frequently abdominal pain.

Diarrhea develops 6–24 hr after the onset of fever; feces are fluid and foul smelling. Affected horses dehydrate rapidly, and metabolic acidosis and electrolyte losses occur as the horse deteriorates. Clinical signs of sepsis and hypovolemic shock can progress rapidly. There may be signs of abdominal discomfort, straining, or severe colic secondary to ileus, gas distension, and colonic inflammation and possible infarction.

Protein-losing enterocolopathy can occur with plasma protein concentrations becoming dangerously low (albumin <2 g/dL) after a few days of diarrhea. These horses can become bacteremic because of bacterial translocation of enteric organisms, and coagulation abnormalities resulting in disseminated intravascular coagulation can occur. If untreated, this form of salmonellosis is often fatal.

Clinical Signs

Clinically normal horses can transiently shed Salmonella, with shedding more common during:

- Concurrent illness: antibacterial usage, physiological disturbance
- Stress: transportation, social, nutritional
- Gastrointestinal disturbance: motility (especially colic), feed change

- Diarrhea (soft feces to projectile, watery diarrhea) is most common, however, horses may have normal feces
- Fever (patient may have normal temperature, especially if treated with NSAIDs)
- Lethargy
- Anorexia
- Colic
- Localized infection (e.g. joint or bone infection)
- Sepsis/septic shock
- Laminitis is a common sequel to enterocolitis
- Abortion with infection by Salmonella serovar abortus-equi (does not occur in the United States of America)

Foals are commonly more seriously affected when compared to older horses, with profound systemic illness including

- Hemorrhagic diarrhea
- Pneumonia
- Meningitis
- Physitis
- Septic arthritis

Incubation Period

>12 hours; varies 1–5 days.

Variation

in onset affected by

- Amount and virulence of organism ingested
- Immunocompetence of host
- Presence of other variables potentially disturbing resistance to intestinal colonization

Risk Factors

- Antibacterial administration
- Feed change
- Concurrent illness
- Increased horse density: overcrowding, overgrazing, poor pasture management (fecal build-up), hospitalization
- Gastrointestinal disturbance, colic, or other illness

- Recent surgery: anesthesia may disturb gastrointestinal motility
- Transportation
- Environmental stressors: hot weather
- Wet barn floors
- Proton pump inhibitor usage for gastric ulcer treatment and prophylaxis may be associated with onset

Transmission

- Fecal-oral spread
- Ingestion of contaminated material (pasture, roughage, feed or water)
- Fomites are a significant means of indirect transmission of infection
- Intermittent shedding by subclinically infected horses
- Aerosol transmission has been suspected in other species; evidence of this route in horses is lacking

Diagnostic Sampling, Testing, and Handling

Fecal culture

- Request Salmonella specifically, along with serotyping and antibiotic susceptibility testing of isolated organism(s)
- A definitive sampling protocol has not been established. A practical schedule for an individual case would be collecting up to 5 samples at 12- to 24-hour intervals due to intermittent shedding
- If several animals are affected, submit samples from as many animals as possible
- Very watery fecal material may be less likely to yield positive cultures due to decreased organism concentration PCR testing
- Testing in conjunction with microbiological culture may provide more rapid identification of the presence of Salmonella spp

Sample Submission

- Feces in a leak proof container for PCR or aerobic culture
- Feces in bacterial transport or specialized enteric transport media (contact diagnostic laboratory for requirements)

Environmental Persistence

- Withstands freezing temperatures and can potentially survive for years under adverse environmental conditions
- Multiplies in temperatures ranging from 44.6–111°F (7–45°C)

- Viable organisms have been recovered from soil after 300 days, water after 9 months, and dried feces up to 30 months
- Susceptible to chemical disinfection on thoroughly cleaned surfaces, however the organism can persist on porous surfaces and difficult to clean areas (e.g. drains, corners, beneath rubber matting) where it can act as a persistent reservoir of infection.

Specific Control Measures

- Quarantine horses that develop diarrhea and/or fever. If a separate stall or paddock is not available, establish barrier precautions at their current location
- Isolate horses following significant colic episodes, impactions (notably small colon), or colic surgery to reduce environmental contamination and potential exposure of other horses should Salmonella subsequently be recovered on fecal culture
- Prevent horses that have come in contact with known infected or clinical cases from mixing with the general population
- Contaminated stall and equipment should have all organic material removed. Dispose of organic matter in a manner which prevents contamination of the facility (do not spread on pastures). Disinfection can be performed after all organic matter has been removed and the surfaces cleaned. Pressure washers or hoses should not be used as they can aerosolize Salmonella, potentially contaminating other parts of the facility or infecting a susceptible horse or human
- No commercially available validated vaccine is currently marketed

Release of Animals from Isolation

For animals with positive cultures while clinically ill:

- Before removing restrictions, following resolution of clinical signs, conduct a series of fecal cultures (see Diagnostic Sampling, Testing and Handling) to determine if all negative
- Where culture is not performed, isolation up to 30 days may be required to minimize risk of exposure of other horses from convalescent shedding of previously infected horses following the cessation of clinical signs (fever, diarrhea)

Zoonotic Potential

All *Salmonella* serotypes which cause disease in horses are potentially contagious to people and can cause serious disease or death.

Immuno-compromised individuals and children should be kept away from any animal with clinical disease, suspected or confirmed to be caused by *Salmonella* spp. and from any clinically normal animals suspected or confirmed to be shedding the bacterium.

STRANGLES (STREPTOCCOCUS EQUI)

Strangles is a highly contagious upper respiratory infection of horses caused by the bacteria *Streptococcus equi* subspecies *equi* (*S. equi*). It is transmitted by inhalation of respiratory particles or direct contact with contaminated surfaces (for example horses sharing water buckets). The bacteria settle in the horse's tonsils and pharynx (back of the throat) within hours of infection, and then infect the lymph nodes under and behind the jaw, resulting in abscesses forming in these structures days later. Horses develop a fever initially, but are typically not contagious during the initial 48-72 hours.

Rarely, infection spreads to other parts of the body resulting in abscesses in other organs such as the intestines, kidneys, lungs, spleen or liver. This is often called "bastard strangles" or metastatic abscessation. A few horses may develop a hypersensitivity reaction to the bacteria with repeated exposure, either in the form of infection or vaccination, otherwise known as purpura hemorrhagica. Horses that develop classic clinical signs and are not treated with antibiotics can develop immune protection from the disease for up to five years.

Etiology and Pathogenesis:

S equi equi is highly contagious and produces high morbidity and low mortality in susceptible populations. Transmission occurs via fomites and direct contact with infectious exudates. Carrier animals are important for maintenance of the bacteria between epizootics and initiation of outbreaks on premises previously free of disease. Survival of the organism in the environment depends on temperature and humidity; it is susceptible to desiccation, extreme heat, and exposure to sunlight and must be protected within mucoid secretions to survive. Under ideal environmental circumstances, the organism can survive ~4 wk outside the host. Under field conditions, most organisms do not survive 96 hr.

Clinical Findings

The incubation period of strangles is 3–14 days, and the first sign of infection is fever (103°–106°F [39.4°–41.1°C]). Within 24–48 hr of the initial fever spike, the horse will exhibit signs typical of strangles, including mucoid to mucopurulent nasal discharge, depression, and submandibular lymphadenopathy. Horses with retropharyngeal lymph node involvement have difficulty swallowing, inspiratory respiratory noise (compression of the dorsal pharyngeal wall), and extended head and neck.

Older animals with residual immunity may develop an atypical or catarrhal form of the disease with mucoid nasal discharge, cough, and mild fever. Metastatic strangles ("bastard strangles") is characterized by abscessation in other lymph nodes of the body, particularly the lymph nodes in the abdomen and, less frequently, the thorax. *S equi* is the most common cause of brain abscess in horses, albeit rare.

Clinical Signs

- Fever, usually preceding other clinical signs by 24–48 hours
- Pharyngitis leading to reluctance to eat and drink. Palpation of the larynx will often elicit pain
- Soft non-productive cough that is often associated with eating
- Mucopurulent nasal discharge that can be unilateral or bilateral
- Lymphadenopathy +/- abscessation (retropharyngeal and submandibular lymph nodes are most commonly involved), but any lymph node may be involved
- Upper airway stridor secondary to pharyngeal compression by the lymph nodes or neuropraxia causing laryngeal hemiplegia
- Guttural pouch empyema is a frequent sequela to previous lymph node abscessation
- Metastatic infection including: Abdominal abscessation, meningitis, Lymphangitis, Purpura hemorrhagica, myositis, and immune mediated myopathies

Clinical signs are age and immune status related, with older horses typically exhibiting milder signs of shorter duration. However, every horse is at risk if the dose and frequency of the challenge is significant.

Incubation Period

Translocation to the mandibular and retropharyngeal lymph nodes occurs within hours of exposure with clinical signs beginning 3–14 days after exposure.

Nasal shedding usually begins 2 to 3 days after the onset of pyrexia.

Risk Factors

Commingling with many horses of unknown origin and medical history.

Transmission

Direct: horse-to-horse contact

Indirect: contaminated fomites which may include water troughs, veterinary equipment, twitches, blankets, grooming tools, buckets, handlers, tack, etc.

Transmission can occur from horses with no clinical signs who are incubating the disease or have developed a persistent subclinical shedder status.

Diagnostic Sampling, Testing and Handling

Given the low numbers shed in the nasal secretion early in the course of the disease, PCR may be the best test in horses that are pyrexic but not yet draining an infected abscess. For practicality an endoscope-directed guttural pouch lavage may provide the best sample for PCR and allow visualization of the pharyngeal inflammation and examination of the guttural pouches for chondroids or purulent material.

PCR in combination with culture is the test of choice to determine the status of exposed and recovered animals. It is more sensitive than culture in detecting small amounts of bacterial DNA but does not differentiate live bacteria from dead. Samples collected early in the course of clinical disease (within 48 hours of onset of fever) may yield negative results on culture. If signs are consistent with Strep equi infection, repeat testing at weekly intervals. If several animals are affected, submit single samples from as many animals as possible.

The SeM Antibody ELISA cannot differentiate antibodies due to natural infection from those induced by vaccination, and is therefore of limited use in managing disease outbreaks. Its value is limited to screening animals that may react to vaccination, (>1:3200) to support a diagnosis of purpura hemorrhagica or metastatic disease (>1:12,800). It is not a measure of protection from disease or an indication of an active infection.

Environmental Persistence

S equi was shown to survive less than 24 hours when cultured onto surfaces exposed to direct sunlight. After aggressive cleaning and disinfection, surfaces should be allowed to dry thoroughly. Special attention should be paid to community surfaces such as water, hay, and feed containers.

There is no evidence for prolonged survival of *S equi* on pastures. However, it is frequently recommended to allow the pastures enough "rest" time to allow for the bacteria to denature. That interval is likely dependent on the environmental moisture, heat, and sunlight.

Biosecurity Issues for Receiving Animals

Limiting exposure is the best method of prevention of an outbreak on a farm.

Quarantine of new arrivals for should also include screening for *S equi*. Isolation with monitoring of rectal temp and endoscopy of the guttural pouch may help to identify infected and sub-clinical shedding individuals.

On a farm currently managing an outbreak. Incoming animals should be quarantined in a "clean" area and screened for infection and sub-clinical status.

If the farm is not instituting risk-based tier management, turning "clean" horses out into infected herds or pastures is likely to perpetuate the outbreak.

Vaccination

While it may be advisable to recommend vaccination, specific vaccination decisions should remain in the purview of the attending veterinarian.

Titers can be measured before vaccination with the goal to identify individuals at risk of developing complications from vaccination. Titers against SeM do not indicate protection. Vaccinating with modified live bacteria can lead to confusion when instituting testing to clear horses. Testing by PCR may cause false positives up to 30 days after vaccinating. Positive vaccine cultures may occur for up to 36 hours post IN vaccine.

Zoonotic Potential

Human cases have been reported, but are uncommon. Immuno-compromised individuals should take precautions to avoid exposure.

VENEZUELAN EQUINE ENCEPHALITIS (VEE)

Arboviral diseases are diseases spread by biting insects and may affect many different species, including horses, water birds and on rare occasions, humans. Arboviral diseases associated with Murray Valley encephalitis (MVE) virus, West Nile virus (Kunjin strain) and Ross River virus are known to occur in Victoria.

As transmission relies on the bite of infected mosquitoes, humans are not at risk of infection from direct contact with infected animals.

Arboviruses (arthropod-borne viruses) of significance to the equine population are:

- Eastern Equine Encephalitis (EEE)
- Western Equine Encephalitis (WEE)
- Venezuelan Equine Encephalitis (VEE)
- West Nile Virus (WNV)

EEE, WEE, and VEE are alphaviruses in the family Togaviridae. West Nile virus is a flavivirus in the family Flaviviridae and is unrelated to the alphaviruses.

Alphaviruses

- Eastern Equine Encephalitis (EEE) virus: In the United States, the highest number of cases occur in the Southeast states, but cases have occurred in all states east of the Mississippi River and as far west as Texas. Mosquito vectors for EEE include Aedes spp., Coquillettidia perturbans, and Culiseta melanura.
- Western Equine Encephalitis (WEE) virus: Cases have principally occurred in the western US and very infrequently in parts of the Midwest. While large equine outbreaks have occurred historically, no equine cases have been reported in the last two decades. The most important mosquito vector of this disease is Culex tarsalis.

- Venezuelan Equine Encephalitis (VEE) virus: geographic distribution is restricted predominantly to northern South America as well as Central America and southern Mexico. The epidemic subtypes of the virus IAB and IC emerge usually in Venezuela or Colombia. The disease last occurred in the US (Texas) in 1971. There is a continuing risk of the introduction of VEE. Several efficient vectors have been identified and include members of the genera, Aedes, Anopheles and Culex spp.

Clinical Signs

Highly variable; none pathognomonic

- Moderate to high fever 102.5–104.5?F (39.17–40.28?C)
- Inappetence
- Diarrhea (VEE only)
- Dysphagia
- Head pressing
- Circling
- Blindness
- Dementia
- Seizures
- Rapid behavioral changes: somnolence, hyperexcitability, mania, selfmutilation
- Cranial neuropathy: nystagmus, facial nerve paralysis, and weakness of the tongue and pharynx
- Coma
- Death

Mortality

EEE: 75–95% (usually within 2–3 days of onset of signs)

WEE: 20–40% (WEE affects horses less severely than EEE)

VEE: 40–90%

Survivors: Alphavirus infection can result in long-term neurologic deficits.

Horses can exhibit abnormal mentation and/or residual spinal cord abnormalities. Horses affected by EEE and VEE are most likely to exhibit these signs.

Incubation Period

- EEE: 3–7 days
- VEE: 2–4 days
- WEE: 2 days–3 weeks Transmission

Indirectly, through bites from mosquitoes which become infected with virus following feeding on a viremic animal, most often an avian host. Multiple animal species (including snakes) may seroconvert with or without the appearance of clinical signs. However, only those that develop a viremia of sufficient magnitude and duration can be considered amplifying hosts.

- EEE/WEE: Birds and some snakes develop high-level viremia, leading to infection of feeding mosquitoes which then transmit the virus. Horses (and humans) become infected when high numbers of viremic birds and mosquitoes result in spillover to bridge vectors (mosquitoes that feed on birds as well as humans and horses). Infected horses do not develop viremia of significant magnitude for transmission and are therefore dead-end hosts. Humans can become exposed during necropsy procedures and handling of infected tissues. Appropriate precautions should be taken whenever handling suspect material.
- VEE: In contrast to EEE and WEE, horses infected with VEE develop viremia high enough to transmit to mosquitoes. Because they are amplifying hosts, horses play an important role in the epidemiology of the disease in both horses and humans.

Diagnostic Sampling, Testing and Handling

IgM-capture ELISA: Single serum sample (red top tube) shipped refrigerated to laboratory by overnight courier. Results of e" 1:400 are confirmatory in horses exhibiting clinical signs consistent with EEE/WEE. Detection of IgM in CSF (if available) is even more conclusive, but death may occur in EEE cases prior to an intrathecal antibody response.

Virus neutralizing antibody titers in paired serum samples in horses that survive: Acute and convalescent samples (red top tubes) collected 2–4 weeks apart and shipped refrigerated to laboratory by overnight courier. Four-fold increase in titers between samples is considered confirmatory in horses exhibiting clinical signs consistent with EEE or WEE and not having been recently vaccinated.

Environmental Persistence

Alphaviruses are enveloped, but are susceptible to drying, ultraviolet light, and detergent.

Specific Control Measures

Vaccination

- Infection is preventable with vaccination. Although WEE and VEE have not occurred recently in the US, vaccination should continue as risk of re-emergence exists
- After an initial vaccination series (per manufacturer's instructions), administer an annual booster 2–4 month prior to mosquito season. In endemic areas,

booster at 4-month intervals during mosquito season. Immunity is short lived (4–6 months), thus requiring frequent boosters

- Pregnant mares should be vaccinated one month prior to foaling to increase colostral protection.

Release of Animals from Isolation

No restrictions need to be placed on recovered animals.

Biosecurity Issues for Receiving Animals

No.

Zoonotic Potential

Human risk of exposure is via bite of infected mosquitoes that acquired virus from birds (not horses; exception: VEE) or through handling CNS tissue and/or fluids of infected animal. Precautions are indicated when performing necropsy examinations of neurologic horses.

VESICULAR STOMATITIS (VS)

Vesicular Stomatitis (VS) is a contagious disease that afflicts horses, livestock, wildlife and even humans. The disease is caused by a virus, which although rarely life threatening, can have significant financial impact on the horse industry. Vesicular Stomatitis is a reportable disease; in a suspect case, state and federal animal health authorities will be contacted by your veterinarian. When a case of vesicular stomatitis is confirmed, your state veterinarian's office will quarantine the affected farm or ranch. In an effort to minimize risk of spread of the disease, horses and other susceptible species will be confined to that location for at least 14 days from the onset of the last case on that property.

Equestrian event organizers may also choose to cancel horse shows, rodeos, and other equestrian activities in the surrounding area. Interstate and international movement of horses may also be restricted.

Etiology

Vesicular stomatitis viruses are members of the family Rhabdoviridae and genus *Vesiculovirus*. They are the prototypes of the *Vesiculovirus* genus. They are bullet shaped and generally 180 nm long and 75 nm wide. The genomic structure is a single strand of negative-sense RNA composed of five genes (N, P, M, G, and L, representing the nucleocapsid protein, phosphoprotein, matrix protein, glycoprotein, and the large protein, which is a component of the viral RNA polymerase).

Although there are many members of the *Vesiculovirus* genus, the New Jersey and Indiana serotypes are of particular interest in the Western hemisphere. These two viruses are similar in size and morphology but generate distinct neutralizing antibodies in infected animals.

Clinical Signs

- Vesicle formation that rapidly progresses to ulceration.
- Ulcerative stomatitis, with the tongue being most severely affected area.
- Ulceration of the mucocutaneous junction of the lips
- Crusting of the muzzle and nares
- Excessive salivation
- Difficulty prehending and masticating feed.
- Coronitis

Less frequent clinical signs:

- Lesions on the udder or prepuce.
- Crusting lesions of the internal ear pinna
- Slow healing wounds secondarily infected with vesicular stomatitis virus.

Transmission

Vesicular stomatitis is seen sporadically in the USA. Outbreaks historically occurred in all regions of the country but since the 1980s have been limited to western states and occur seasonally, usually May through October, with some outbreaks overwintering and continuing into a subsequent year or years.

Vesicular stomatitis viruses are endemic in South America, Central America, and parts of Mexico but have not been seen naturally outside the Western hemisphere.

The virus can be transmitted through direct contact with infected animals with clinical disease (those with lesions) or by biting insects. Black flies (Simulidae), sand flies (*Lutzomyia),* and biting midges (*Culicoides spp)* have been shown to be competent vectors, but other insects may act as mechanical vectors as well.

Exposure to insects that carry the virus is often associated with nearby moving water sources such as creeks or rivers or irrigation of pastures.

Experimental studies have shown that feeding of infected insects on mucosal surfaces and nonhaired areas of the body were more often associated with development of lesions at those sites than if insects fed on haired areas of the body.

The prevalence of clinical cases in a herd is generally low (10%–20%), but seroprevalence within the herd may approach 100%. Viremia has not been detected in livestock species that exhibit clinical signs of vesicular stomatitis, although experimental studies have shown transmission of virus, presumably via lymphatics, between co-feeding black flies on cattle.

Virus is routinely isolated from active lesions in affected animals, and these lesions serve as a source of virus spread by direct contact and contamination of shared feed and water stations.

Many vertebrate species have serologic evidence of exposure, but no definitive reservoir or amplifying host of vesicular stomatitis viruses has been identified.

Prevention

By observing the following guidelines you can help prevent the occurrence of VS:

- Healthy horses are more disease resistant so provide good nutrition, regular exercise, deworming and routine vaccinations.
- Isolate new horses for at least 21 days before introducing them into the herd or stable.
- Observe your horse closely. Immediately isolate any horse that shows signs of infection and contact your veterinarian.
- Implement an effective insect control program. Keep stabling areas clean and dry. Remove manure and eliminate potential breeding grounds (standing water, muddy areas) for insect vectors.
- Use individual rather than communal feeders, waterers, and equipment.
- Clean and disinfect feed bunks, waterers, horse trailers and other equipment regularly.
- Be sure that your farrier and other equine professionals who come into direct contact with your animals exercise due care so as not to spread the disease from one horse or facility to the next.
- On farms where VS has been confirmed, isolate any animals with lesions away from others and handle healthy animals first, ill animals last. Handlers should then shower, change clothing and disinfect equipment to prevent exposing others.
- Anyone handling infected horses should implement proper biosafety methods, including wearing latex gloves and washing hands after handling animals with lesions.
- If you are sponsoring an event during an outbreak, require a more recent health certificate on every horse entering the venue and consider having a veterinarian visually inspect all horses at check-in. Work with your event veterinarian to establish isolation and response procedures that can be implemented quickly if a suspect case is identified at the venue.

Diagnostic Sampling, Testing and Handling

Laboratory testing is required to confirm VSV infection. Diagnosis is made through serologic testing and/or virus identification from samples of lesions. Suspected VS cases are required to be reported to state/federal animal health officials and samples must be submitted the National Veterinary Services Laboratories (Ames, IA or Plum Island, NY) or to an approved National Animal Health Laboratory Network laboratory that has been specifically activated during an outbreak. Practitioners performing necropsies in the field are encouraged to contact one of these VS-approved veterinary diagnostic laboratories in order to be certain they collect appropriate samples and handle them in a manner that will maximize the probability of a definitive diagnosis.

Vaccines And Disinfectants

Vaccines have been developed experimentally to help combat vesicular stomatitis, but none are currently approved for use in horses. There is considerable debate over the efficacy of vaccination in preventing or reducing the severity of an outbreak. The period of protection is thought to be fairly limited and once vaccinated, animals will test positive for long periods of time thereby incurring travel restrictions.

Sunlight and heat are known to quickly destroy the virus that causes vesicular stomatitis. Commercial disinfectants such as chlorine bleach (0.645%), Wescodyne (4 %), Roccal (1:200), Septisol (1:50), and cresylic acids (1 %) are also effective.

Protection from Insect Exposure

Protecting horses from insect exposure during outbreaks of VS may reduce the risk of clinical disease.

- Housing horses indoors or access to a covered shed during the daylight and dusk periods when insect vectors most active
- Promote air circulation in stables (fans)
- Regular application of insect repellants to the horse including the inner surface of the ears (location black flies may feed)

Requirements for New Arrivals to Facility or Event During VS outbreaks, additional requirements for horses that have been in regions where disease has been recognized may reduce risk of introduction of VSV.

- Certificate of veterinary inspection (CVI) with statement related to potential exposure to VSV
- Inspection of newly arriving horses including an oral examination to detect vesicles or ulcers. Wear disposable examination gloves and personal protective clothing. Change between horse examinations.

Release of Animals from Isolation

Determined by state or federal animal health officials. Release of VS cases and their herd mates is based on a specified number of days after onset of lesions in the last affected animal on the premises.

Biosecurity Issues for Receiving Animals

Once horses are released from quarantine no additional precautions should be required.

Zoonotic Risk

The vesicular stomatitis viruses are zoonotic and may cause self-limiting influenza-like disease (headache, fever, myalgia, and weakness) lasting 3–5 days in people working in close contact with the virus (eg, laboratory exposure, direct contact with lesions in infected animals). Rarely, people can develop vesicles on the buccal and pharyngeal mucosa, lips, and nose. More severe signs, including encephalitis, are rare. Personal protective equipment should be used when handling lesioned animals to avoid contact with the virus present in the lesions.

WEST NILE VIRUS (WNV)

A mosquito-transmitted virus causes most cases of West Nile infection. Most people infected with West Nile virus either don't develop signs or symptoms or have only minor ones, such as a fever and mild headache. However, some people develop a life-threatening illness that includes inflammation of the spinal cord or brain.

Mild signs and symptoms of a West Nile virus infection generally go away on their own. But severe signs and symptoms — such as a severe headache, fever, disorientation or sudden weakness — need immediate attention.

Exposure to mosquitoes where West Nile virus exists increases your risk of getting infected. You can lower your risk by protecting yourself from mosquitoes by using mosquito repellent and wearing clothing that covers your skin.

Clinical Signs

- Depression and anorexia without fever during initial viremia
- Mild, low-grade fever (101.5–103.5° F or 38.6–39.7° C) in about 25% of affected horses
- Inappetence
- Lethargy/somnolence
- Neurologic signs
    - Onset of neurologic disease is frequently sudden and progressive
    - Periods of hyperexcitability, apprehension and/or somnolence
    - Fine tremors and fasciculations of the face and neck muscles
    - Cranial nerve paralysis; facial paralysis and weakness of the tongue are very common
    - Head tilt, droopy lip, muzzle deviation

- Weakness, ataxia, and dysmetria in one or all limbs
- Complete paralysis of one or more limbs
- Colic
- Recumbency
- Death

Expect clinical signs to be most severe in the very young and very old.

About 30% of WNV cases experience an increase in severity of clinical signs within 7–10 days of onset, sometimes after initial clinical signs have abated.

Incubation Period

7–10 days

Risk Factors

- Unvaccinated or not up to date on WNV vaccination
- Residence in endemic area
- Pasture turnout during dawn and dusk
- Lack of mosquito control

Transmission

Primarily by mosquitoes

- Reservoir: Only birds appear to develop significant levels of viremia to serve as a source of infection
- A horse affected with WNV encephalitis is not contagious and poses no risk to other horses, or birds
- Peak transmission in Western Hemisphere is July to October, but in sub-tropics it is year-round
- Excessive moisture and increased temperatures increase mosquito activity

Diagnostic Sampling, Testing and Handling

IgM antibody capture ELISA (MAC-ELISA): Single serum sample (red top tube)

- Positive test: WNV-specific IgM titer e" 1:400. Increases in IgM rarely occur after vaccination Plaque Reduction Neutralization Test (PRNT) paired serum antibody titers
- Collect samples 2–4 weeks apart (red top tube)
- Four-fold or greater rise in PRNT titers between samples is considered confirmatory in a horse exhibiting clinical signs consistent with WNV and which has not been vaccinated recently

- Send serum overnight on cold packs to a laboratory competent to test for WNV infection CSF Analysis: elevated mononuclear cell count and/or high total protein
- CSF WBC Count: Highly variable range, when abnormal, CSF WBC is usually > 7 cells/ul
- Protein Level: Highly variable range, when abnormal, CSF protein is usually > 70 mg/dl RT-PCR can be attempted on CSF of clinically affected horses.

Note: CSF fluid should be evaluated immediately. If cytological evaluation cannot be performed, a direct smear can be made, and the CSF and slide sent to a laboratory overnight on cold packs.

Viral isolation may be attempted on CSF, whole blood, or serum.

Histopathology: Fix at least part of the brain for histopathology. Fresh brain should be submitted for virus detection by virus isolation, PCR and/or immunohistochemical examination. Note: Fresh cerebellum and spinal cord must be submitted for rabies testing. D

Environmental Persistence

This enveloped RNA virus is susceptible to drying, ultraviolet light, and detergent.

Specific Control Measures

Vaccination—killed or recombinant:

- Initial injection of either vaccine is followed in 4 to 6 weeks with a booster. The primary series must be administered to elicit optimal antibody production. Vaccination should be initiated before onset of the mosquito season to allow time for development of the neutralizing antibodies. The initial series should not be expected to provide longterm protection beyond one year.
- Follow vaccine manufacturer recommendations regarding initial immunization series and annual boosters. More frequent boosters (i.e. twice yearly) are recommended in areas with year-round mosquito seasons and in endemic areas.

Vector management

- Use insect repellents frequently; re-apply after rain
- Keep horses in at night when possible, and apply insect repellant
- Eliminate or minimize standing water
- Stock tanks or ponds with mosquito-feeding fish
- Eliminate brush piles, gutters, old tires and litter
- Remove all equipment in which standing water can collect

Release of Animals from Isolation

No restrictions need be placed on affected or recovered animals.

Biosecurity Issues for Receiving Animals

None.

Zoonotic Potential

While not a source of virus for insect vectors, an equine case of WNV may be an early warning signal to humans that there are transmitting mosquitoes in an area.

7

EQUINE PHYSICAL THERAPY AND REHABILITATION

INTRODUCTION

Physiotherapy (called physical therapy in some countries) or PT is an important allied health profession where physiotherapists contribute an essential part to the care of individuals. The profession addresses a broad range of conditions in the young to the aged and from the severely debilitated to the elite athlete. Depending on the country, the legally protected title varies and includes physiotherapist, physical therapist and chartered physiotherapist.

PT is an established, independent profession with an excellent reputation for evidence-based practice. Veterinarians have embraced PT and rehabilitation across the world and the last decade has witnessed the development of a close working relationship between veterinarians and physiotherapists.

The American College of Veterinary Sports Medicine and Rehabilitation is a specialist college where veterinarian diplomates have an excellent working knowledge of the benefits of working with PTs in a multidisciplinary team to care for the sports horse during competition and rehabilitation following injury or disease.

Since most PTs in most countries need to work via veterinary referral and veterinarians and their clients understand and are demanding the unique skills base of a professional animal PT, the veterinarian-PT multidisciplinary team has become the gold standard in equine sports medicine and rehabilitation.

HISTORY OF PHYSIOTHERAPY

PT is believed to have been practiced by physicians like Hippocrates and Galen from around the 5th century BC who advocated massage, manual therapy and hydrotherapy to treat people. In the subsequent centuries, the benefits of remedial exercise, hydrotherapy and massage were known and practised by relatively few. The earliest documented origins of PT as scientifically based profession date back to Per Henrik Ling, 'Father of Swedish Gymnastics' who founded the Royal Central Institute of Gymnastics (RCIG) in 1813 for massage, manipulation, and exercise. In 1887, PTs were given official registration by Sweden's National Board of Health and Welfare.

Other countries soon followed including Great Britain which founded its first professional PT society in 1894, and was awarded its Royal Charter in 1920[2](the Chartered Society of Physiotherapy), Australia in 1906, with the formation of The Australian Physiotherapy Association and the United States in 1917 following both an outbreak of poliomyelitis and the first world war and the subsequent need for rehabilitation. The profession was established as The American Physical Therapy Association (APTA) in 1921.

As PT has progressed so has the database of information and journals specific to the area. The profession has its own PT evidence database (PEDro[4]) of over 31,000 randomised trials, systematic reviews and clinical practice guidelines in physiotherapy. Of relevance to animal PT is that much of the human research has been developed based on animal models, especially the cat (for example, spinal cord injury and rehabilitation models), dog (for example, electrotherapies) and pig (for example, back pain models).

The profession is now represented internationally by the World Confederation for Physical Therapy (WCPT)that 'believes every individual is entitled to the highest possible standard of care . . . underpinned by sound clinical reasoning and scientific evidence 'The WCPT currently has twelve internationally recognised subgroups, the: Acupuncture Association of Physical Therapists; Association of Physical Therapists in Animal Practice (IAPTAP); Confederation of Cardiorespiratory Physical Therapists; Society for Electrophysical Agents in Physical Therapy; Federation of Orthopaedic Manipulative Physical Therapists; Organization of Physical Therapists in Mental Health; Neurological Physical Therapy Association; Association of Physical Therapists working with Older People; Organisation of Physical Therapists in Paediatrics; Private Physical Therapy Association; Federation of Sports Physical Therapy; and Organization of Physical Therapists in Women's Health.

World IAPTAP members include the following members:

- Animal Physiotherapy Group (Australia)
- Animal Rehabilitation Division (Canada)
- Finnish Association of Animal Physiotherapists (Finland)
- Fachkommission Tierphysiotherapie (Germany)
- Chartered Physiotherapists in Veterinary Practice (Ireland)
- South African Association of Physiotherapists in Animal Therapy SAAPAT (South Africa)

- Legitimerade Sjukgymnaster inom Veterinärmedicin LSVET (Sweden)
- Schweizerischer Verband für Tierphysiotherapie SVTPT (Switzerland)
- Association of Chartered Physiotherapists in Animal Therapy ACPAT (United Kingdom)
- Animal Rehabilitation Special Interest Group AR SIG (U.S.A.)

DEFINITION OF PHYSIOTHERAPY

Encompassing the range of disciplines within the profession, PTcan be broadlydefined as the restoration of movement and function. PT involves using a professional assessment and reasoning process to select appropriate interventions or treatments for individual patients looking at physical, psychological, emotional and social wellbeing. The profession of PTuses an evidence-based, clinical reasoning process to underpin its management approaches.

The clinical reasoning processes for PT are the same as those practised by veterinarians, although the overall aim is different. The physiotherapist's aim is to reach a functional diagnosis. That is, identification of existing or potential impairments, activity limitations, participation restrictions, environmental influences or abilities/disabilities. In contrast, the veterinary approach is usually to reach a pathoanatomical diagnosis (what pathological processes are occurring and where they are located).

Animal PT is an extension of evidence-based practice in the human field and is not merely the technical application of one or more treatment modalities (e.g. massage, heat, cold, electrotherapy).The difference in aims for PT is important as it dictates the treatment and rehabilitation options used. PT treatments are selected to manage sensory and motor disturbances and provocative factors in work or sport for functional improvement and activity-specific performance rehabilitation.

Animal PTs use physical interventions, such as manual therapies, specific motor retraining, exercise prescription and electrophysical agents, in conjunction with education and advice to restore function and quality of life. Selection of the appropriate combination of techniques is based on clinical reasoning, assessment and reassessment of the patient, with reassessment of improvement following treatment dictated by objective outcome measures.

REGULATIONS AND THE TEAM APPROACH

The titles 'physiotherapist' and 'physical therapist' are protected by law in most countries and regulated by its respective Act or equivalent and as such may only be used by individuals who are registered with the respective government body.

In some countries PT or single modalities (e.g. massage, hydrotherapy, Bowen therapy) are also practised at a technical level by technicians. However, it is important that veterinarians understand the difference between technical and professional training. This is particularly the case in the those countries where referral to a physiotherapist by a veterinarian is required before PT is undertaken on animals, meaning the veterinarian is still professionally responsible for the animal throughout its treatment.

There are many advantages to utilising a professionally medically trained physiotherapist. The medical training allows PTs to have highly developed manual skills, based on their training with verbal feedback from their human patients. For many equine musculoskeletal disorders, there will also be an impact of the rider and the ability of the PT to professionally assess the rider as well as the horse cannot be underestimated. With the skills of clinical reasoning, evidence-based practice and the ability to translate knowledge between species, the PT is an ideal partner in the veterinarian-PT relationship.

Finally, the medically experienced PT is trained to work with and very often is the key facilitator of a multidisciplinary team which ensures the horse receives the most appropriate treatment. Within the equine environment the multidisciplinary team predominantly consists of veterinarian, farrier, saddler, trainer, PT and rider. The wider team can also include nutritionist, veterinary nurse, handler, owner, osteopath, and chiropractor. The professional PT is trained in being part of this team approach and understands the dynamics of these resources, and how to make best use of them in relation to their own clinical practice.

CORE PRINCIPLES OF EQUINE PHYSIOTHERAPY

As for the definition of PT, the core principles of equine PT revolve around clinical reasoning and evidence-based practice to inform assessment, treatment and rehabilitation. During the course of rehabilitation, assessment and reassessment using objective outcomes measures are essential to direct progress and allow for modification of treatments.

Musculoskeletal physiotherapy is the predominant sub-discipline in equine PT, encompassing poor performance, back pain syndromes, other musculoskeletal disorders and some neuromuscular disorders. Underpinning musculoskeletal physiotherapy are the sciences of functional biomechanics, neuromotor control, and the sensori-motor system in joint function.

Equine PT also, importantly, must involve the interaction of the rider and horse, as well as the tack and training aides used. Functional biomechanics is reviewed in a subsequent chapter of this issue, so the focus in this section is on the principles of neuromotor control and the sensorimotor system in the spine, pelvis and peripheral joints, and the horse -rider interaction.

NEUROMOTOR CONTROL AND THE SENSORIMOTOR SYSTEM

When training the equine athlete, the aims are to increase stamina, speed and muscular strength as well as increase aerobic capacity, reduce the risk of musculoskeletal breakdown and improve the biomechanical skill and neuromuscular co-ordination. In order to do this successfully, the body co-ordinates have a number of different systems. For the musculoskeletal system, these include soft tissue (muscle, tendon, ligaments, nerves, fascia), bone and articular structures.

The basic functions of limb coordination, rhythm and speed through all gaits is generated and controlled in part by central pattern generators (CPG). These specialised interneuron circuits located within the spinal cord have an ability to produce rhythmic patterned locomotion independent of supraspinal (brain) input. There are separate control centres for the thoracic and pelvic limbs though they are inter-connected by long neurones to allow phasic coordination between the front and rear of the horse. Normal locomotion also depends on the ability of the central nervous system (CNS) to receive and process afferent sensory information (such as proprioceptive, visual and vestibular input) from the sensorimotor system and to initiate and control movement in an effective, coordinated, energy efficient fashion.

The relationship between neural and muscular (motor) control of movement is complex with reflexes (involuntary nervous system) as important as the voluntary activation patterns in control of spinal stability. The final motor output during locomotion is a result of the CPG's and their modulation by an intact CNS. The complex relationship between neural and muscular (motor) control of locomotion is referred to as neuromotor control.

NEUROMOTOR CONTROL IN THE SPINE AND PELVIS (AXIAL SKELETON)

As well as modulating the dynamic limb patterns of locomotion, neuromotor control is highly important in providing a stabilising 'core' of muscles their associated soft tissues to provide appropriate resistance to movement for a given joint. In the spine and pelvis, stability in man has been clearly shown to be dependent on the contribution of three elements: 1. the passive structures (including the intervertebral disks, ligaments, joint capsules and intervertebral joints), 2. the active structures (muscles) and 3. the control system (CNS) which exerts its effects on the muscles

- Spine equilibrium and stability, and resultant spinal function, are reliant on the coordination and control of muscle recruitment via neural input from the sensorimotor system.
- A coordinated pattern of when and how the muscles activate including neural feedback, compensatory mechanisms and motor adaption to changing environments are required. This includes neural feedback of changes in length and the rate of these changes in passive tissues and muscles which trigger reflex muscle activity to counter the change and feed-forward control by motor cortex whereby perturbations are predicted or anticipated and can be learned.

The importance of these mechanisms in the muscular control of the lumbar spine and pelvis have been shown in a series of experiments in people whereby the transverse abdominus, lumbar multifidus, diaphragm and pelvic floor muscles are all activated prior to and during perturbations created by rapid arm raises. This work demonstrated the predictable coordination of an array of muscles to provide a stabilising core of muscles in the spine and pelvis in a manner primarily linked to the direction reactive moments. Such neuromotor control modulates muscular recruitment to fine tune the demands of internal and external forces, so ensuring appropriate motor responses to unexpected disturbances of movement and function.

Effective neuromotor control provides maintenance of functional stability which is important in preventing excessive loading or movement that may lead to injury, degenerative changes or predispose to pain and dysfunction.

- This stabilisation is required to support the skeleton during locomotion and to ensure joints are maintained in their 'neutral zone'. The neutral zone has been defined as the area of intervertebral motion where little resistance is offered by passive structures. It is a clinically important measure of joint stability in humans and has been shown to increase with degeneration or injury.
- Unwarranted and unnecessary joint motion places the musculoskeletal system at risk of injury and is often termed 'functional instability'.

Neuromotor control principles in PT (spine and pelvis)

The principles of neuromotor control have been successfully applied to humans with back pain. Research has shown that there is a reduced and delayed muscular recruitment and stabilisation in patients with back pain, especially of the deep, core muscles of the spine and trunk. Delayed muscle response times were also correlated with poorer postural control in patients with lower back pain. This delayed onset of deep muscle activity does not reflect compromise of CNS performance caused by pain interference but has been suggested to be a result of adoption of an alternate postural strategy by the CNS, consistent with chronic adaptation to pain, and may serve to limit the amplitude and velocity of trunk excursions caused by limb movements.

However, pain adaptation may not be protective and patients with back pain are at risk of re-injury due to a failure of protection of structures from overload and unwanted movement. Similarly, in the low motion joints such as the sacroiliac joint in the pelvis (SIJ), mild articular instability or 'microinstability' may result in gradual remodelling of a joint.

Knowledge gained from this research related to the changes in neuromotor control that occur with back pain have translated to the development of rehabilitation strategies based on motor control training approaches.

It is now universally accepted that clinical benefit can be gained if motor control can be changed to optimise the load and minimise unwanted joint motion on structures of the spine and pelvis. Motor relearning strategies may focus on deep core muscles such as the transverse abdominus and multifidus and may also involve targeting specific patterns of activation of muscle groups in combined functional movements such as bracing the trunk to optimise motor control for spinal dynamic stability. There is evidence that this motor control approach can reduce low back pain intensity and functional disability which is maintained following treatment. Importantly, specific physiotherapeutic intervention in people with multifidus dysfunction following an episode of acute back pain reduced the rate of recurrence of injury to 30% in the physiotherapy intervention group compared with the controls who had a recurrence rate of 84%.

Similarly, knowledge of neuromotor control of the sacroiliac joint has contributed to the ability of clinicians to diagnose sacroiliac dysfunction in humans. Non-invasive, manual tests have a high predictive odds ratio for sacroiliac dysfunction and are currently recommended over diagnostic joint analgesia. These manual tests are described as pain provocation tests for the sacroiliac joint, and are designed to compress the sacroiliac joint articular surfaces and/or stress the extra-articular structures of the joint. Manual tests are also utilised to assess the degree of movement and the quality of motion of the sacroiliac joint during application of manual force based on the amount of hypo-/hyper-mobility. This includes analysing movement of the sacrum relative to the pelvis in weight bearing through the pelvis.

Neuromotor control principles in equine PT (spine and pelvis)

Despite obvious limitations with respect to communication of specific exercises, the principles of neuromotor control have also been successfully applied in equine PT for the spine and pelvis. Stubbs and colleagues applied the human model of researching the equine multifidus muscle to the horse and found striking similarities in structure and function. This research was used to develop and validate ultra-sonography as a tool to detect reduced multifidus cross sectional area associated with severe osseous pathology in horses.

- The use of this technique also enabled the identification of multifidus asymmetry in asymptomatic riding horses which was improved by specific physiotherapy exercises over a three month period aimed at improvement of core muscle function.

Diagnosis of equine sacroiliac disease using manual tests similar to that used in the human literature has been described and is based on biomechanical and neuromotor control principles including motion between the sacrum and ilium during the application of manual forces by a PT in vivo and in vitro.

NEUROMOTORCONTROLINTHEAPPENDICULARSKELETON

As well as controlling muscular activity in the axial skeleton, neuromotor control and the sensorimotor system are important in controlling joint position and loading of the associated soft tissues in the appendicular skeleton. Fatigue as well as injury can alter the function of active elements (muscles) as well as sensorimotor inputs and neuromotor control, principally reflected in reduced joint position sense and proprioception. Furthermore, appropriate warm-up can improve joint position sense.

Application in PT

Understanding neuromotor control and the sensorimotor system has informed treatment and rehabilitation of peripheral joint and soft tissue injuries including the ankle, knee and shoulder. Proprioceptive retraining is an important part of rehabilitation, one example of which is taping. The aim of taping techniques is to stimulate mechanoreceptive and proprioceptive activity in the skin and superficial soft tissues (fascia, ligaments and joints). Tapingaffects the sensory afferent activity from that regionvia stimulation of mechanoreceptors respondingto skin stretch and compression during joint motion, improving sensorimotor afferent input and ultimately joint position sense.

Patellar taping was shown to improve control of the knee joint in both pain free people with poor joint proprioception and in people with femoropatellar pain. Similarly the combined mechanical and proprioceptive benefits of taping for improving dynamic balance for preventing ankle sprains as well as recurrence of sprains is well documented. Taping, bracing and manual therapy are used prior to exercise based PT for an immediate effect on proprioception, while exercise based therapies are used to maintain the improvements.

Applications in equine PT

Taping has also been used clinically in horses for similar purposes. One study investigated the biomechanical effects of taping the fetlock in the forelimbs of horses which showed an effect on fetlock flexion during swing and reduced peak vertical force during stance.

Although in this model, mechanical rather than sensorimotor effects were being investigated, the results suggested that changes seen may have reflected proprioceptive adaptations.

More recent PT led research has shown clear effects of tactile stimulation of the distal hind-limb in horses, causing increased hoof flight arc, increased peak flexion angles in the hind-limb, and increased concentric activity of the tarsal musculature and will be discussed in more detail in the review in this issue on functional biomechanics.

HORSE RIDER/HORSE-TACK INTERACTION

In the past decade there has been an emergence of research and growing awareness of the interaction between the horse, its tack and the rider. Riders have a large influence of horse's gait, and can increase or decrease the expression of lameness detected by asymmetry. Furthermore, this effect varies depending on the experience of the rider with more the experienced rider more likely to increase hind limb lameness, presumably due to increasing collection and hind limb usage.

Professional riders have been shown to be more stable than novice riders, with reduced motion detected by reduced vector angles between the rider's head and the rider's back and between the rider's back to the horse's head. Experienced riders have also shown improved stability at the trot corresponding to more synchronous activation of the erector spinae and rectus abdominus muscles.

Research into the effect of the saddle, in particular in the role of increased forces and 'bridging' (where the weight of the rider is distributed on the caudal and cranial parts of the saddle but not throughout its lengths) have improved understanding of saddle induced pain.

Saddle slip has also been investigated. Despite previous assumptions about slip being due to a poorly fitting saddle or rider asymmetry, it has been shown that the saddle slip is most associated with hind limb lameness or gait abnormalities. Almost 53% of saddle slip was attributed to this and only 6% to rider asymmetry.

However, in this study rider asymmetry was present in 103 of 276 (37%) riders and even though the majority (78%) of crooked riders did not induce saddle slip, crooked riders may place additional stress in the horses' back, or indeed their own. It is already well known that elite athletes in many disciplines frequently show asymmetries, and the same is true of equestrian riders. Less elite athletes or paralympic athletes may show more marked asymmetries that require extensive PT intervention.

Asymmetry can negatively affect performance in horses in various ways from the inappropriate delivery of aides to altered biomechanics of locomotion. The important contact points of the rider and the horse are the lower limbs, pelvis and, indirectly, the hands. Rider asymmetry, injury or dysfunction can impact optimal delivery of aides and their interpretation by the horse. The relevance of the multidisciplinary team becomes significant here; the PT is well placed to identify rider asymmetry as well as assess and treat the rider as well as to ensure any suspected lameness is referred to a veterinarian and saddle problems referred to a master saddler.

Professional PTs are already highly trained in managing musculoskeletal disorders in the human athlete so the ability to assess the rider provides an important extension of the diagnostic workup. Furthermore, PT intervention can be an important part of the treatment and rehabilitation plan. Experienced riders post PT intervention to the pelvic region showed a marked improvement in symmetry compared to untreated controls.

PHYSIOTHERAPY ASSESSMENT AND TREATMENT OF THE EQUINE

Physiotherapy Assessment

Once the horse has been given a diagnosis by a veterinarian, the equine therapist needs to obtain a full history of the patient's presenting condition. This will provide important information about the horse's level of disability, the timeline and progression of the condition, and any past history that is relevant to the current presentation.

Questions to include in the subjective interview are:

- When did the horse go lame?
- How lame is the horse?
- What interventions / medications have been tried so far?
- What occurred in the lead up to the injury? (including training, shoes, boots, surfaces, supplements)
- What type of work does the horse do? What is the horse's expected level? What schooling, breeding, and training programmes does it have?
- Have there been any changes in saddles, bridles etc?
- Does pain / lameness improve when the horse has warmed up or does it get worse throughout the ride? Is it worse on small circles or with a change of direction?
- Are changes more subtle? (e.g. loss of height in piaffe / passage, dropping its foot over bigger fences, changing lead at gallop)

It can be useful to also discuss the patient's history with its grooms, and handlers - particularly when attempting to determine what other interventions the animal has received.

While obtaining the subjective history from the owner, the therapist is also able to observe the horse's demeanour, behaviour, condition, conformation, gait and posture.

Physiotherapy involves assessing the ability of the body to move and perform physical activity. It includes looking at joint mobility, muscle size and strength, coordination, balance and the ability to perform certain tasks. The physiotherapist's aims are to reduce pain and swelling and improve movement and function of the patient. They use a number of different techniques, including massage, hot and cold treatments, hydrotherapy, laser, myofascial release, joint mobilisations and acupuncture, and use exercises to increase range of motion, strengthen muscles and improve balance and coordination.

Which horses need physiotherapy?

Competition horses

These horses will be putting a lot of strain on their body due to the high intensity work that they are doing. Especially if they are at a high level of competition. Just like a human athlete, regular physiotherapy should be carried out to ensure that they are in peak physical fitness; it can help improve performance, prevent injury, and enhance mobility and suppleness, being important not only during peak training, but also during rest and recovery periods.

Routine check-ups

It's not only the elite athletes that need physiotherapy. Carrying out a routine assessment is sometimes recommended for all horses, helping to detect small problems early. Ensuring that your horse is pain free and has a good range of movement is important to allow them to live a happy and healthy life, enabling them to do the work that is required of them. In most cases a routine physiotherapy assessment is recommended every 6-12 months. However, if your horse has a history of musculoskeletal problems, they may require more frequent check-ups.

Horses that are rehabilitating after musculoskeletal injuries

Following injury or surgery, physiotherapy is important to help to reduce inflammation, improve strength and increase range of motion, with the aim of restoring the animal back to full function. Soft tissue techniques may be used to loosen up scars, swollen joints and thickened tissues after injury. A strict exercise regime will usually be created to encourage the appropriate use of the affected area.

HOW DO YOU KNOW IF YOUR HORSE NEEDS A PHYSIOTHERAPY ASSESSMENT

As well as getting a routine check-up by the physiotherapist, your horse may need to see them on other occasions. Any changes to the way your horse is performing may need assessment by a physiotherapist as these could indicate signs of musculoskeletal pain.

Signs include tension through the neck and back when putting the saddle on, reluctance to jump or canter on one rein, stiffness on one side or bucking. The signs may even be more subtle, such as facial changes, uneven shoe wear or changes in ear position when riding.

At first, it may seem like the horse is being naughty but it is important to have your horse checked over as all of these signs could be associated with nack, back or pelvic pain. Ensuring that you watch your horse closely is important in order to pick up any problems quickly.

The Injured Horse

The horse is an elite athlete, and should be given the chance to reach the optimal level of performance. Physiotherapy helps to achieve and maintain performance in the equine athlete.

Horses develop back and neck pain and other musculoskeletal injuries due to the nature of their work. Specific musculoskeletal injuries include tendon and soft tissue injuries from day-to-day work and overtraining, as well as stress fractures, fractures and nerve injuries, from falls and accidents.

Following initial veterinary diagnosis, in the acute phase of injury, physiotherapy helps to reduce pain, swelling and inflammation, and begins to restore the horse's movement. Physiotherapists can then provide full and ongoing rehabilitation to aim to restore the equine athlete's performance.

Back Pain

Back, neck and sacroiliac pain are common in the performance and recreational horse. The physiotherapists use manipulation, and other spinal mobilisation techniques to restore motion and reduce pain arising from the vertebral column and sacroiliac joint in the horse. Exercises are commonly prescribed, to help maintain the function in the spine.

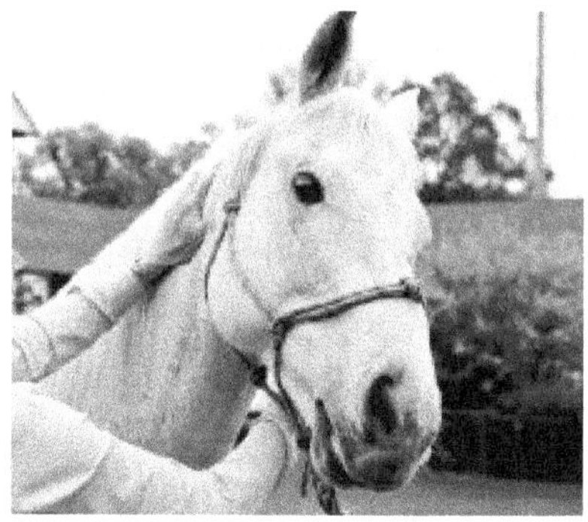

Fig. 1 Neck mobilisation

After Surgery

Physiotherapy intervention following equine arthroscopic joint surgery, surgical repair of tendons and fractures, and abdominal surgery (including colic) can enhance the horse's recovery. The correct rehabilitation ensures optimal return to function.

Prevention of Injury

Early detection of movement abnormalities, which may be indicative of orthopaedic conditions, muscle imbalances or other musculoskeletal problems, is important to help prevent development or worsening of pain and loss of performance.

The physiotherapists are well qualified to assess movement disorders, and communicate closely with veterinarians who will diagnose if there is an underlying condition.

The aged horse and arthritic joints

Physiotherapy can help to relieve aches, pain and stiffness associated with arthritis (degenerative joint disease) and the ageing process. Many horses develop degenerative joint disease early in life due to growth rates, congenital problems, previous injury and sometimes the nature of the work they perform. Performance horses can still remain competitive with arthritic changes, providing they are managed with veterinary care and with physiotherapy. Physiotherapy can help to prolong a horse's years of activity, or simply provide a better quality of life.

TREATMENT OF THE EQUINE FORELIMB

Observation

Static Observation

The therapist should observe and compare with other horses from the same breed, the patient's:

- Conformation
- Mentation
- Muscular condition and coverage (compared to horses of its age, type, level of work)
- Muscle symmetry and bony landmarks
- Weight bearing ability (compared side to side)

Dynamic Observation

Observing the horse in motion enables the therapist to establish how willing the patient is to move. Movements must be provocative enough to highlight the impairment (walking / trotting in a straight line may not adequately challenge the horse).

Movements that could be included in a dynamic assessment are:

- Horse walks away and back with the handler
-

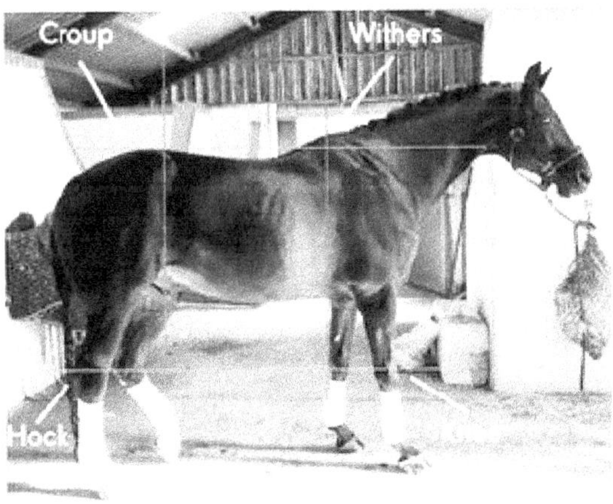

Fig. 2

- Therapist looks at the way the horse goes, if there is any reluctance to move, can the handler settle the horse?
- Repeat
- Therapist looks for symmetry of movement, flat foot placement, even strides, head nod

- Trot away and trot back
- Therapist looks for any head nod (which indicates forelimb lameness) and at stride length
- Small circles
- Therapist looks for cross over in both directions, neck bend
- Different surfaces
- Therapist looks for any apprehension, snatch back
- Lunging
- Therapist looks for symmetry, enthusiasm without the rider's weight
- Under saddle
- Looser rein, then collection

Functional Assessment

The functional assessment might include whole tasks (e.g. gait / functional activities) or components of movements. For example:

- Small circles
- Gait on a hill
- Walking on soft surfaces, over poles

Any functional test / movement can be used as both an assessment and as an intervention.

Physical Assessment

The physical examination should include:

- Active physiological movements
- Soft tissue palpation and testing
- Passive physiological joint assessment
- Passive accessory joint assessment
- Neuromechanical tissue testing

Goniometers, tape measure, and photography / video are often used as outcome measures during the physical assessment in equine physiotherapy.

Palpation

When palpating a horse, it is important to consider the following points:

- Always approach the horse with care
- Palpate for muscle type, bulk
- Remember to consider the horse's breed (i.e thin thoroughbreds vs heavier cobs)

- Allow the horse to be comfortable with you
- Check the horse's temperature, response to touch, and look for swelling, symmetry and effusion
- Compare left to right
- Look for compensatory patterns – assess the opposite musculature, and diagonal musculature

A top down approach can be useful when palpating the forelimb of a horse:

- Scapular ridge
- Spine of scapular
- Supraspinatus, infraspinatus
- Scapulohumeral joint
- Biceps bursa and biceps tendon
- Triceps and elbow, point of the olecranon
- Forearm – flexor groups. Muscles and associated tendon sheaths
- Extensors - muscles and associated tendon sheaths
- Radius – medially palpate the radial bone
- Carpus – extensors over the front of the carpus. Carpal effusion
- Accessory carpal bone, effusion in carpal sheath
- Metacarpus and splint bones
- Flexor tendons
- Suspensory ligament
- MCP joint and palmar digital flexor tendon sheath
- Pastern
- Coronary band and hoof

GENERAL MANAGEMENT PRINCIPLES

This section explores physiotherapy interventions that can be applied to the equine forelimb.

Thermal Therapy

Cold Therapy

Cold therapy is used to reduce:

- Local circulation
- Tissue swelling
- Pain sensation

It is most beneficial in the acute phase (i.e. 24-48 hours) after an injury or surgery. Cold therapy works by constricting blood vessels and reducing tissue temperature. Reduced blood flow helps to decrease oedema, haemorrhage and the extravasation (i.e. leakage) of inflammatory cells.

Heat Therapy

Heat therapy is used to:

- Increase local circulation
- Promote muscle relaxation (and thus reduce muscle spasm / pain)
- Increase tissue extensibility

Heat therapy is particularly useful for:

- Wound healing
- Promoting resorption of oedema
- Pain management
- Encouraging more effective stretching of tissues

Heat therapy should be used after the acute phase of healing.

Contrast Therapy

Contrast therapy (i.e. alternating hot / cold therapy) is often used to treat human patients, but it has not been widely researched in equine therapy. A recent study by Haussler and colleagues has looked at its potential for use in horses. They found that it is possible to achieve therapeutic tissue temperatures (i.e. <15 and >40°C) in tissues as deep as the deep digital flexor tendon with contrast therapy.

Therapeutic Ultrasound

Therapeutic ultrasound has been shown to have thermal and non-thermal benefits in both human and animal patients.

Thermal benefits include:

- Improved extensibility of collagen
- Decreased pain
- Decreased muscle spasm
- Increased blood flow

Non-thermal (i.e. biologic) effects cause changes in the cellular environment that lead to changes in cellular function. This may result in:

- Shortened inflammatory phase of healing
- Increased vascularity
- Enhanced proliferation of fibroblasts

Non-thermal ultrasound is often, therefore, used for patients with fracture or tendinopathy.

In general, ultrasound is indicated for:

- Tendons and ligaments - to minimise contraction
- Fascial planes
- Joint capsules - to improve range of motion
- Scar tissue
- Osteophytes / enthesiophytes - to decrease pain
- Muscle spasms - to slow gamma fiber transmission
- Wounds - to increase protein synthesis in fibroblasts (from 2 weeks post-injury)
- Oedema
- Nerve injuries - to encourage remyelination and regeneration of damaged axons

EXTRACORPOREAL SHOCK WAVE THERAPY

Extracorporeal shock wave therapy (ESWT) is often used to treat soft tissue and bone injuries in equine patients. Pulses are transmitted from the shockwave unit into the tissues to help stimulate healing.

It is indicated when a horse has:

- Tendinitis
- Desmitis
- Osteoarthritis
- Deep muscle pain

It is believed that ESWT:

- Reduces inflammatory mediators
- Increases angiogenic cytokines (causing vessel proliferation)
- Increases growth factors (causing tissue healing)
- Increases the number of osteoblasts
- Recruits mesenchymal stem cells
- Helps to manage pain

One recent study found that ESWT increased mechanical nociceptive threshold in horses with back pain. It can also improve the rate of healing and the prognosis of equine patients who have proximal suspensory desmitis.

JOINT MOBILISATIONS / MANIPULATIONS

Much of the information about manual techniques in equine therapy comes from human research:

- Joint mobilisation and manipulation can be used as a diagnostic tool and to guide interventions for musculoskeletal dysfunction in horses
- Soft tissue mobilisation aims to restore movement in tissues, and to enhance tissue repair, extensibility and function
- Joint mobilisation is used to restore normal, symmetric joint range of motion, end feel and to stretch connective tissues
- Manipulation is a high velocity technique that moves a joint beyond its physiologic range of motion

Manual techniques are often used to help manage musculoskeletal injuries in performance horses. It is particularly beneficial for:

- Chronic or recurring musculoskeletal conditions
- Conditions that are not easily diagnosed or not responding to conventional veterinary care

They are also indicated to help prevent negative effects of joint immobilisation and to help retrain proprioception. They have been fou to have a positive effect on pain, flexibility, muscle hypertonicity and spinal motion symmetry.

LASER THERAPY

High intensity laser therapy (HILT) is used as a non-invasive treatment option for musculoskeletal disorders in horses. Indications for low-level laser therapy include:

- Wound therapy
- Soft tissue injuries
- Osteoarthritis
- When local pain relief is required

Laser appears to:

- Have anti-inflammatory effects
- Reduce pain sensation through reduced nerve depolarisation, the release of endorphins and enhanced ATP production

A recent study found it can help to reduce pain, oedema, visual lameness and lesion percentage in horses who have tendinopathy and desmopathy. It may, therefore, help to improve the quality of life of equine patients who have chronic musculoskeletal pain.

EXERCISE

Exercise forms a key component of many rehabilitation protocols for horses. Exercise is slowly progressed depending on the horse's level of conditioning, injury status and assessment findings.

For many soft tissue injuries, hand walking is encouraged soon after injury to enhance fibre alignment and to prevent the formation of restrictive adhesions.

Hydrotherapy and Water Treadmills

Hydrotherapy is commonly used to rehabilitate equine patients, but few studies have explored its efficacy for this group of patients. Hydrotherapy has a significant effect on physiological responses in human patients and research suggest that horses may have similar responses. The benefits of hydrotherapy in people include:

- Increased joint mobility
- Promoting normal motor patterns
- Enhanced muscle activation
- Decreased incidence of secondary musculoskeletal injuries

OTHER ADJUNCTS

Massage

Massage is a popular intervention for equine athletes and horses in general. Proposed benefits include:

- Increased range of motion and stride length
- Reduced activity of nociceptive receptors
- Reduced stress response
- Enhanced exercise recovery

Many massage techniques used on horses were first developed in humans and while further research is needed, massage currently has a significant role in equine therapy.

PROPRIOCEPTIVE REHABILITATION

Proprioceptive retraining is an important part of equine rehabilitation. In human patients, taping, in particular, is often used to help stimulate mechanoreceptive and proprioceptive activity in superficial structures. Recent studies have found that tactile stimulation caused by taping can have an impact on equine gait.

Nutraceuticals (Joint Supplements)

It has been suggested that nutraceuticals (i.e. food that is said to provide medical / health benefits) may be beneficial for horses, particularly those with osteoarthritis. However, evidence for their efficacy is poor.

COMMON TYPES OF THERAPY

Treatment techniques include manual therapy such as joint mobilization and manipulations, muscle re-education through stretching and strengthening and proper movement patterning exercises. Modalities can include ultrasound, laser, electrical muscle stimulation (EMS), transcutaneous electrical nerve stimulation (TENS) and acupuncture. "Most importantly," added Scott, "a program tailored to the functional requirements of each horse is designed. The ultimate goal is to educate the horse owner in the well-being and maintenance of their equine partner."

Manual therapy (or manipulative therapy)

Manual therapy (or manipulative therapy) refers to the practice within musculoskeletal physiotherapy of therapist-applied passive or assisted active movement techniques for the management of pain and impairments in the mobility of joints, muscles and neural tissue. Joint mobilization and manipulation is performed by several professional groups including physiotherapists, chiropractors, and osteopathic physicians.

Joint mobilization consists of slow, small, passive movements applied to individual joints and surrounding soft tissue, with the purpose of increasing joint range of motion. Joint manipulation, on the other hand, involves a high-velocity, low-amplitude thrust performed at the limit of the joint's range, with the purpose of increasing joint range of motion. Both techniques are designed to reduce pain and spasm.

Other manual therapy techniques include various types of massage, myofascial release and active release therapy. These are hands-on techniques applied to muscle and surrounding connective tissue to alleviate spasm and pain and to help restore motion.

Electrotherapy

Electrotherapy is an umbrella term used to identify a range of treatments including electrostimulation of muscles and nerves, as well as the use of sound waves (ultrasound) and light (laser) to treat physical injuries.

Electrostimulation (EMS and TENS)

Electrostimulation (EMS and TENS) is the application of low or medium frequency electrical currents in order to stimulate sensory or motor nerves to produce or facilitate muscle contractions, or to provide pain relief.

Muscle stimulation can be used after injury or surgery where there has been a loss of strength of a muscle or muscle group or when the timing of the firing of the muscle has been altered due to injury. TENS is used to help reduce pain and associated spasm.

Electrodes are applied as needed over the bulk of the muscle; over motor points; over nerves; over acupuncture points, or directly over the painful area. A cool gel is placed under the electrode. This allows the current to pass through more effectively. The horse's hair should be clipped and cleaned to lower the resistance to the passage of current.

Treatment times vary from 15 minutes up to one hour. They are initially shorter to help familiarize the horse with the sensations associated with stimulation and to reduce anxiety.

Ultrasound

Ultrasound is the application of longitudinal sound waves to the body for a therapeutic effect. The sound waves directly affect the cells and stimulate healing. Sound waves are absorbed by connective tissue such as ligaments, joint capsules, tendons, fascia and muscle. The effect is either thermal or non-thermal, depending on the intensity or the pattern of absorption in the tissue.

Promotion of tissue healing is the main goal of ultrasound, and it can be used at any stage of recovery or where healing is delayed. Pain relief as well as reduction of swelling and muscle spasm are parallel effects of this type of therapy.

A cool gel is applied directly over the area of concern and the sound head is moved in a circular pattern. It is painless, and treatment time is generally between seven and 10 minutes long.

Laser (Light Amplification by Stimulated Emission of Radiation)

Laser (Light Amplification by Stimulated Emission of Radiation) is a form of light energy used to stimulate and improve healing of open wounds, ulcers and soft tissue injuries such as tendonitis. It can also be used to stimulate acupuncture points to relieve musculoskeletal pain. It is sometimes referred to as LEPT (Low Energy Photon Therapy) or LLLT (Low Level Laser Therapy).

The type (red or infrared) and frequency of the wavelength used over the area of injury and the duration of the treatment depends on several factors- and varies for individual patients. Applied by a 'cold' laser device, the process is pain-free. It has been shown, however, that the radiation of the laser beam is damaging to the retina of the eye, so it must be used with care and special protective glasses should be worn while administering laser treatment.

Acupuncture is an ancient form of Chinese Medicine involving the insertion of acupuncture needles into the skin at specific points on the body to achieve a therapeutic effect. It is used to encourage natural healing, reduce or relieve pain and improve function of affected areas of the body.

Needles are inserted and left in place for approximately 15 to 30 minutes, and may be manipulated by the therapist to strengthen or reduce the flow of energy. Most horses respond quite well to acupuncture and are not bothered by the needles.

8

BODY CONDITION SCOR-CARD OF HORSES

Body Condition Scoring (BCS) is an objective system of evaluating a horse's level of body condition (amount of stored fat) and assessing a numeric score to facilitate comparisons between horses. Many owners fail to recognize significant variations in the weight of horses or variations due to age and breed types. This often results in overfeeding or underfeeding.

If there is a negative energy balance (energy loss greater than energy intake), then weight, and subsequent body condition, will be lost. This energy balance depends on such factors as: availability of food and water, weather (e.g., ambient temperature and wind chill), reproductive activity (e.g., pregnancy, lactation) and physical activity demands for growth and health status. A positive energy balance (energy expenditure less than energy intake) will result in a horse adding fat and muscle and improving body condition.

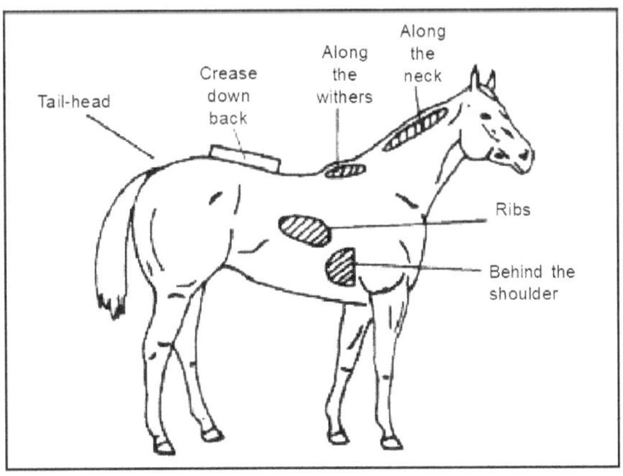

Fig 1. Diagram of Areas Emphasized in Condition Score

BODY CONDITION SCORING

Palpation and visual inspection of the ribs, tailhead area, neck and withers, and behind the shoulders, facilitates the comparison of horses with differing amounts of stored body fat, independent of body size or breed of horse.

The Body Condition Score

The body condition of horses based on the degree of fat cover is a good indicator of a horse's general health. The body condition score (BCS) allows one to access if the horse is too thin, too fat, or about right. Horses are scored on a scale from 1 (poor) to 9 (extremely fat) in six areas where they deposit fat – neck, withers, spinous processes (part of back vertebrae that project upwards) and transverse processes (portion of vertebrae that projects outward), tail head, ribs, and behind the shoulder. The subjective assessment is based on visual and physical (palpation) of the specified body regions including the hooks (tuber coxae and hip joints) and pins (tuber ischia and lower pelvic bones). Comparisons of relative adiposity can be made within or between horses. Categorization of body condition as underweight (BCS < 3, 1–9-point scale), moderate (BCS 4–6), overweight (BCS >7) or obese (BCS >8) can be used as an aid in the management of body condition for optimal health and performance

Advantages of the body condition score are

- Integration of all body areas
- Easy to perform
- Allows for classification of horses into underweight, overweight, or obese categories
- Cutoff values available to imply risk for disease

Disadvantages of the body condition score are

- The method only assesses subcutaneous fat
- Bias between evaluators may influence results
- The score can be influenced by coat length, gut fill, muscle mass, pregnancy, etc.
- The score may not be comparable between different breeds or body types.

IDEAL HORSE BODY CONDITION SCORES

Most horses, including performance horses and growing horses, should be in a body score of 5-6. For optimum reproductive efficiency, broodmares should be a 5-7, and not allowed to lose condition such that they are below a 5 during breeding season. Horses over a condition score of 7 may be at a greater risk for developing metabolic disorders such as insulin resistance.

DESCRIPTION OF INDIVIDUAL BODY CONDITION SCORES

1. Poor: Horse is extremely emaciated. Spinous processes, ribs, tail head, hooks, and pins project prominently. Bone structure of withers, shoulders, and neck easily noticeable. No fatty tissue can be felt.
2. Very thin: Animal emaciated. Slight fat covering over base of spinous processes, transverse processes of lumbar vertebrae feel rounded. Spinous processes,

ribs, tail-head and hooks and pins prominent. Withers, shoulders and neck structures faintly discernible.

3. Thin: Fat build-up about halfway on spinous processes, transverse processes cannot be felt. Slight fat cover over ribs. Spinous processes and ribs easily discernible. Tailhead prominent, but individual vertebrae cannot be visually identified. Hook bones appear rounded, but easily discernible. Pin bones not distinguishable. Withers, shoulders and neck accentuated.
4. Moderately thin: Negative crease along back. Faint outline of ribs discernible. Tailhead prominence depends on conformation, fat can be felt around it. Hook bones not discernible. Withers, shoulders and neck not obviously thin.
5. Moderate: Back level. Ribs cannot be visually distinguished but can be easily felt. Fat around tailhead beginning to feel spongy. Withers appear rounded over spinous processes. Shoulders and neck blend smoothly into body.
6. Moderate to fleshy: May have a slight crease down back. Fat over ribs feels spongy. Fat around tailhead feels soft. Fat beginning to be deposited along the sides of the withers, behind the shoulders and along the sides of the neck.
7. Fleshy: May have crease down back. Individual ribs can be felt, but noticeable filling between ribs with fat. Fat around tailhead is soft. Fat deposited along withers, behind shoulders and along the neck.
8. Fat: Crease down back. Difficult to feel ribs. Fat around tailhead very soft. Area along withers filled with fat. Area behind shoulder filled in flush. Noticeable thickening of neck. Fat deposited along inner buttocks.
9. Extremely fat: Obvious crease down back. Patch fat appearing over ribs. Bulging fat around tailhead, along withers, behind shoulders and along neck. Fat along inner buttocks may rub together. Flank filled in flush.

9

SHELTERS, STALLS AND HORSE FACILITIES

No matter what your management style or needs, the basics of a safe horse stall are the same. Many options that effect function and cost are available for horse stall features. This fact sheet provides an over- view of some basic stall features for a typical 1,000-pound horse. You should adjust the dimensions for significantly larger stall occupants.

DIMENSIONS

The size of the horse and the amount of time the horse spends in the stall help determine stall size. Larger horses require more square footage than do smaller ponies to be able to turn around, lie down, and get up comfortably. A 12-foot x 12-foot stall is the standard recommendation for a 1,000-pound horse. Many stables are successful with stalls slightly smaller than this, but walls less than 10 feet in length are not recommended. Generally, the stall wall length is 1 1/2 times the horse's length. The more time a horse spends in a stall or the more active it is, a larger stall size is justified. A divider between two standard stalls may be removed to allow more space for a mare and foal or a stall-bound horse.

An 8-foot-high stall partition is standard. Partition height needs to be at least 7½ feet to prevent horses from getting legs over the wall. Most horses can kick as high as 7 feet. An 8-foot-tall by 4-foot-wide stall doorway opening has been the recommendation for years; although this is not often seen in stables. Stall door manufacturers typically supply a doorway opening of slightly over 7 feet with a 42- to 45-inch width. These are the dimensions of the actual open area that the horse can pass through. These smaller doorway openings are adequate for horse and handler safety.

Horse barns are commonly built with a ceiling height of 10 to 12 feet with 8 feet being the minimum. A low ceiling not only inhibits air circulation, but also increases the chance that a horse may strike its head. In fact, many stables have open truss or rafter construction with no ceiling. In this case, the minimum height is the clearance to the lowest item on which a horse may strike its head, such as a light fixture or truss bottom chord.

Doors

Doors come in a wide variety of materials and configurations, although swinging and sliding doors are common (see Fig.1). Doors can cover the full length of the doorway opening, be divided into two panels (Dutch door), or partially cover half to three-quarters of the opening, which is more common with metal mesh doors.

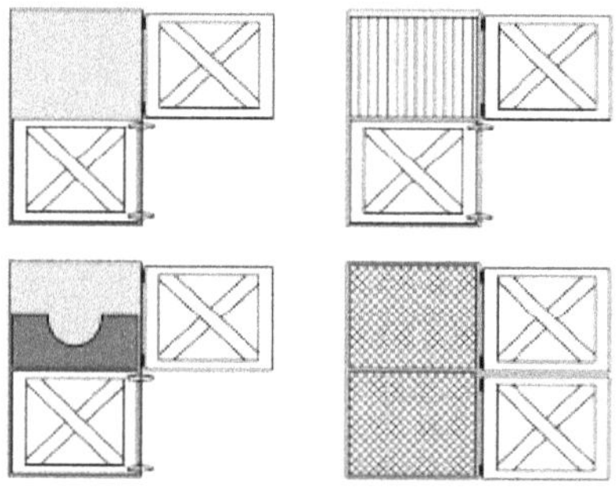

Interior Aisle Stall Doors

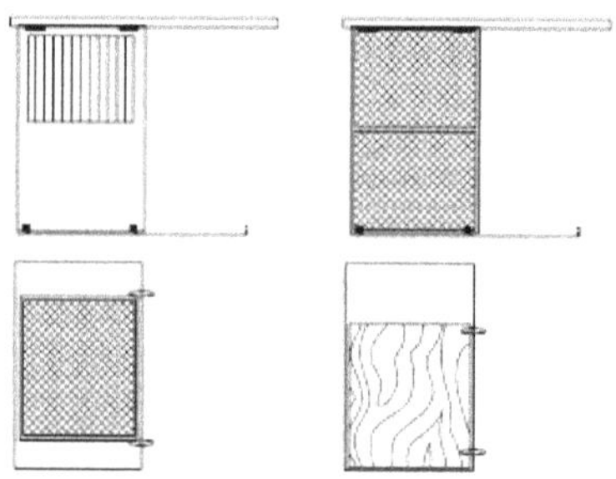

Interior Stall Doors with Safety Gate

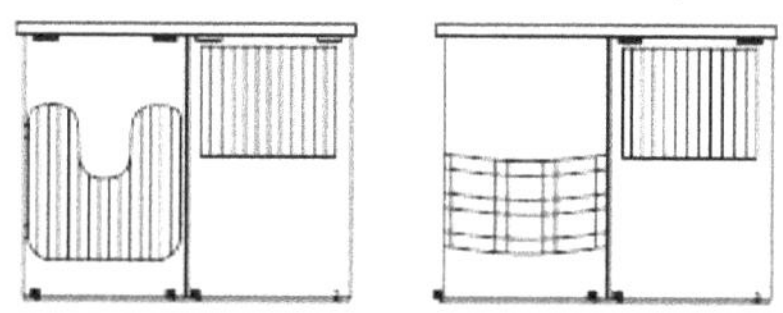

Figure 1. Examples of stall door designs

Swing doors should open into the aisle rather than into the stall. Open swing doors decrease aisle workspace but may be latched open to alleviate this problem. They also require less hardware to function properly, but heavy-duty hinges are needed to prevent sagging. Sliding doors, in addition to the overhead track, need a stop to prevent the door from opening too far and falling off the track. They also need floor-level guides to keep the lower portion in place when the horse is pawing, leaning, or kicking at the door. Full-length doors should have less than 3 inches of clearance under them to prevent the horse from getting a hoof or leg stuck.

All doors and doorjambs need to be durable, with secure latches, and free of sharp edges or protrusions. For example, door guides on sliding doors should be rounded and out of the traffic path. Door latches and other clasps that can be operated with one hand are an advantage at chore time. Position door latches out of reach of horses that may find pleasure in learning how to operate them. Horses may try to jump over doors that are half height (such as a Dutch door); however, options are available that allow a horse to hang its head out yet discourage jumping.

LIGHTING AND VENTILATION

Lighting is important for proper care and observation of stalled horses. Shadows and poorly lit areas make stall cleaning cumbersome and inhibit observation and care. For natural lighting, provide a minimum of 4 square feet of window space in each stall. Glass windows should be either out of reach (generally above 7 feet) or protected by sturdy bars or mesh. Plexiglas is a good option for window glazing.

Place electric fixtures along the front or side walls to decrease shadows in the stall. One fixture above the center creates shadows as the horse comes to the front of the stall for observation. A 100W incandescent or 20W fluorescent are suitable electric fixtures. Position fixtures at least 8-feet high to minimize contact with the horse. For further protection, provide a shatter- proof cage, which is available at most lighting supply stores.

All electrical wiring in the barn should be housed in metal or hard plastic conduit since rodents may chew unprotected wires, creating a fire hazard. Metal conduit can be used but has the tendency to rust. Position electrical wiring out of reach of horses, children, and pets.

Fresh air should be available to every horse for good respiratory health. A window, which opens for each stall, eave and ridge vents, and no ceiling (or at least a high ceiling), will enhance fresh air exchange. Storing hay and bedding over the top of the stalls is not recommended. Not only are these substances a fire hazard, but they also carry allergens and inhibit air circulation.

Open panels on the tops of stall dividers and open mesh doors help the air circulate within the stall interior. Often, the stable aisles are well ventilated while the stalls suffer from stagnant air caused by poor air circulation.

FIXTURES

Horse stall interiors, including hardware, need to be smooth, rugged, and free of projections (Fig. 3). Typical stall fixtures include a water bucket or automatic drinker, feed tub, a ring for tying the horse, and optional items such as a hay rack or ring for a hay net/bag, and environmental enrichment devices (toys). When purchasing stall fixtures, consider cost, durability, ease of replacement, and ease of cleaning, especially for feed and water buckets. Horses are fast, strong animals that have all day to work on the stall components. Choose high-quality, durable hardware for long-term, trouble-free use.

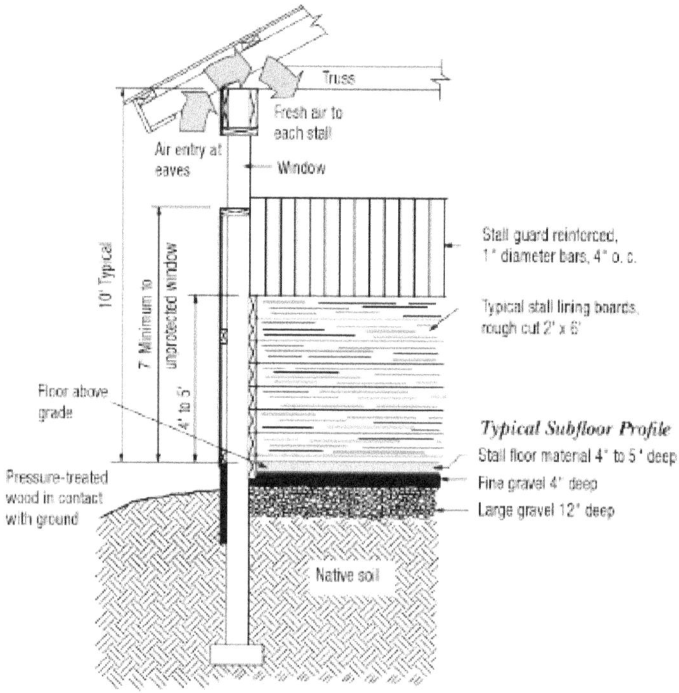

Fig. 2. Stall cross-section showing typical dimensions and components.

GRAIN AND WATER

Be sure to separate feed and water stations in the stall. A horse will drop grain into the water bucket as he chews his ration if it is within reach of the feed tub. Water and feed buckets should be fastened to the wall rather than placed on the floor where they can be tipped over. The bucket rim should be positioned just above horse chest height at nose level. This is low enough to allow the horse to reach it comfortably, yet reduce the chance of the horse stepping in it. Unfortunately, the correct placement of buckets is the ideal height for manure to be deposited in them. Fixtures to hang buckets should be smooth, free of gaps, and fastened securely to the wall. An eyehook and double-ended snap work well for buckets with a bail handle. Some manufacturers provide feed tubs and buckets with hardware for safe and secure wall attachment. The hardware should be equally safe whether the bucket is present or not. Be sure that fasteners allow easy bucket removal for frequent cleaning.

The decision to provide water in buckets or by using automatic watering devices is usually based on cost and management preferences. An automatic drinker is more expensive than a bucket to purchase and install. Drinkers reduce the time needed to complete daily activities but are not a watering "cure-all." Drinkers, like buckets, need to be checked daily to ensure that they are free of manure and contain fresh water. Any watering device needs to be cleaned of algae and debris on a regular basis. Horses will drink more water if they have a clean bucket with fresh water. Buckets allow water to be easily removed from the stall for post-exercise or treatment purposes and allow you to monitor the horse's water intake. Proper drinker placement is similar to water bucket placement in height and separation from feed tub. Some models allow two stalls to share one drinker.

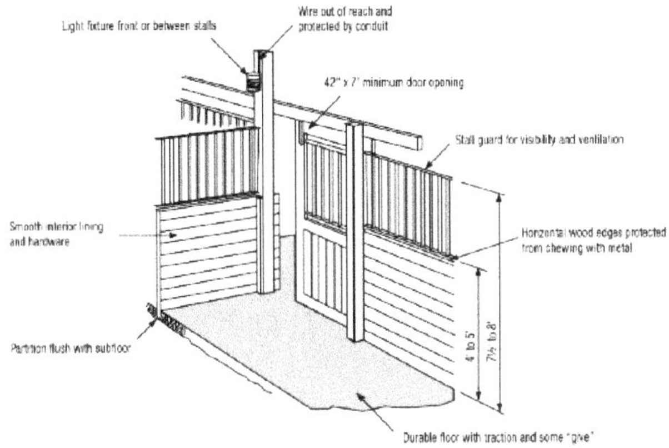

Fig. 3. Typical box stall construction.

Select an automatic drinker by considering the strength and maintenance requirements of the materials that will come in contact with the horse, the smoothness of these surfaces, water refill mechanism, and ease of cleaning. Some drinkers require the horse to lower the level of the water to refill it, whereas a refill mechanism that requires the horse nose to open a valve can be difficult or frightening for some horses to use. Valve mechanisms can also become a "toy," and some horses delight in holding the valve open and flooding the stall. In colder climates, protection is needed to prevent waterlines from freezing and breaking. Methods to consider include burying the lines, heating the barn, providing access to ground heat below the frostline, and/or using electrical heat tape on exposed waterlines.

HAY FEEDING

The ideal way to feed forage (hay) varies among owners. Hay can be fed directly off the ground, but this method allows the forage to come in contact with waste, dirt, and to be mixed with the bedding. A corner apron of concrete can minimize for- age contact with a dirty floor. A primary advantage of floor feeding is that it allows the horse to eat in a natural position.

Hay racks, hay bags, and hay nets can keep forages off the ground. Hay fixtures should be used with extreme caution since a horse's leg may become caught if the horse kicks or rears near the rack or net. Consider the horse's habits, personality, and behavior before selecting a fixture.

When a hay rack, net, or bag is used, the bottom end should be at wither height for the horse. Too high and hay dust falls into the horse's eyes and nostrils; too low and the horse may become tangled. All weld joints on racks need to be strong and smooth with rounded corners.

There is much disagreement over the proper hay feeding station. A hay rack or net is disliked by some owners due to the inhalation and irritation of hay dust and its unnatural position for a horse to eat. An alternative to a rack or net is a hay manger.

Mangers let the horse eat in a more natural position, are less prone to trap the horse, and reduce dust fall. A well-designed manger is usually made of wood, starts flush with the floor, and ends above horse chest height. Hay chaff and dust can accumulate in the bottom of the manger and must be removed regularly.

TIE RING

A ring for tying the horse is often placed at or above horse wither height. Place the ring away from the feed and water buckets and toward the back on one of the sidewalls. This keeps the horse secure when cleaning the stall or grooming and tacking. Be sure the wall is strong enough to withstand resistance from a horse, and fasteners are smooth on both sides of the wall.

FLOORING

Many stall floor options are available and should meet most of the following requirements. Horses are hard on flooring so it must be durable against pawing and use by a 1,000-pound occupant. A good floor has some "give." A floor that absorbs some of the impact and weight of a horse will reduce stress on the horse's legs and ease foot problems. The floor should be nonslip to prevent injuries, especially muscle pulls when the horse tries to stand from a lying position. Slippery floors can inhibit the horse from even trying to lie down.

Since horses have their heads close to the ground for most of the day, a non-odor (ammonia) retentive, nonabsorbent floor is beneficial. Minimize the time needed to clean and maintain the stall floor by choosing a low-maintenance material. No single flooring material seems to have all the desirable attributes. Dirt has "give" but is not durable; concrete is durable but has no "give." Some of the hardness of concrete and other unyielding materials can be overcome by using rubber mats or deep bedding. Sufficient bedding helps prevent sores or abrasions. Rubber mats and clay can be slippery when wet. For more information on flooring, see "Horse Stable Flooring Materials and Drainage."

PASTURE

The area of pasture required per horse will depend on the type of grass, ground conditions, time of year, type of horse and degree of pasture management employed. As a general rule, each horse requires about 0.5 – 1.0 hectares (or 1.25 to 2.5 acres) of grazing of a suitable quality if no extra feeding is being provided.

Each donkey requires a minimum of 0.2 – 0.4 hectares (a half to one acre). A smaller area may be adequate where a horse is principally housed and grazing areas are used only for occasional turnout.

A good pasture management programme is necessary to avoid over-grazing, to aid worm control, to maintain good drainage and to control weeds. This includes, for example, picking up droppings, rotating grazing areas and where possible, removing horses when the ground is very wet to prevent poaching (where the pasture is broken into wet muddy patches by the action of the horse's feet on the wet ground) and health problems.

In muddy conditions it is important that a horse has an adequately sized, well drained area in the pasture on which to stand and lie down, and on which to be fed and watered.

Most horse pastures have a large amount of weeds and rough grass where horses are the only grazers.

Consideration should therefore be given to grazing sheep or cattle in horse pastures to improve sward quality and assist in reducing worm burden.

DANGEROUS OBJECTS AND POISONOUS PLANTS

Fields should be kept clear of dangerous objects and poisonous plants, for example yew and laburnum, which are extremely toxic to horses and therefore horses should not have access to these (or their clippings) at any time.

Ragwort is toxic to horses and ingestion can result in fatal liver damage. Horses will eat cut ragwort as well as the living plant so the right type of disposal is essential. As cut and pulled flowering ragwort plants may still set seed, and ragwort has a 70 per cent seed germination rate, effective disposal is a key point in control. All ragwort species should be disposed of by extraction (to remove the root base) followed by incineration, controlled burning or removal to landfill.

HEDGE CLIPPINGS AND GRASS CUTTINGS

Horses should not have access to hedge clippings.

Grass cuttings are not suitable for horses to eat and care should be taken that horses do not gain access to these (that is garden waste or cut fields).

Fences should be strong enough and high enough to prevent horses from escaping (for example higher fences may be required for stallions) and designed, constructed and maintained to avoid the risk of injury with no sharp projections.

Gateways should be designed to allow for the easy and safe passage of horses, and gates should be fastened securely to prevent injury and escape. In some situations gates may need to be padlocked.

Barbed wire and sheep wire are not ideal. Where used the wire should be stretched tight in fields with horses. Where plain wire is used, measures should be taken to make sure it is sufficiently visible to the horse.

FENCE HEIGHTS FOR HORSE AND PONY PASTURES

The height of fences required will depend on the types of horses kept in the field. The British Horse Society (BHS) recommends that fences should be 1.25m (4ft) high, more specifically:

- horses: 1.08m to 1.38m (3ft 6in to 4ft 6in)
- ponies: 1m to 1.3m (3ft 3in to 4ft 3in)

Lower rail (horses and ponies): 0.5m (1ft 6in) above ground

- stallions: 1.38m to 1.8m (4ft 6in to 6ft)

Stallions may require a double fence line and possibly an electric fence line along the top of the paddock rail. This is to prevent aggression between occupants of different paddocks, as well as to contain the stallion within the allocated area.

ELECTRIC FENCES FOR HORSE AND PONY PASTURES

Electric fences should be designed, installed and maintained so that contact with them does not cause more than momentary discomfort to the horse. All power units should be correctly earthed.

Electric fencing should be clearly visible to horses to prevent injury, with extra supervision provided until they become accustomed to it. Temporary internal sub-divisions created out of electrified tape and plastic posts provide an effective internal barrier, but these should not be used as the sole boundary fence.

When grazing a number of horses, the allocation of paddocks should be considered so that horses that cause conflict are separated from the other horses. This will prevent bullying and reduce the risk of injury to subordinate horses.

COMMUNAL BARNS FOR HORSES

Groups of horses can be kept together in communal barns, but care should be taken to make sure that all horses get adequate access to hay, feed and water. Enough space should be provided to allow free movement, and to allow all the horses to lie down at the same time. Care should be taken to select groups that are compatible and aggressive horses should be segregated. Late term mares and mares with foals at foot have special requirements and it may not be suitable to house these animals in communal barns.

BEDDING FOR HORSES

Adequate and suitable bedding material is necessary in all equine accommodation to provide warmth, protection against injury and to allow the horse to lie down in comfort. Whatever bedding is used (for example straw, shavings, rubber stable mats and so on) it should be well managed and changed or cleaned regularly.

Fire is always a risk in stable areas. Advice should be sought from the local Fire Prevention Officer about statutory requirements.

Highly flammable liquid material or combustible material should not be stored in or close to stables where horses are housed. Smoking in stable areas should be prohibited.

All equipment and services (lighting units, fire extinguishers and alarm systems) should be kept clean, inspected annually by a qualified person and kept in good working order. All electrical installations should be installed, maintained and periodically inspected and tested by a fully qualified electrician.

WIRING AND FITTINGS

Wiring and fittings should be inaccessible to horses, well insulated, safeguarded from rodents and properly earthed. If using extension leads or cables care should be taken to reduce the risk of injury to the horse.

All metal pipe work and structural steelwork should be properly earthed. The risk of fire and electrocution can be reduced by having the whole installation protected by a residual current device (RCD).

Stabled horses should be capable of being released quickly if there's a fire or other emergency based on a pre-planned emergency turnout procedure.

Tethering

Tethering is not a common practice in Northern Ireland. Tethering is securing an animal by an appropriately attached chain, to a centre point or anchorage, causing it to be confined to a desired area.

Tethering is not a suitable method of long-term management of an animal, as it restricts the animal's freedom to exercise itself, to find food and water, or to escape from attacks by dogs or extreme hot and cold weather. It also risks an animal becoming entangled, or injuring itself, on tethering equipment.

Tethering may be useful as an exceptional short-term method of animal management (for example in medical cases where short-term restriction of food intake is required under veterinary advice).

Tethered horses need regular supervision. Tethered horses should be inspected no less than every six hours during normal waking hours, and clean fresh water should be available at all times. The term 'tethering' does not apply to horses that are stall-tied (a common method historically used for stabling cavalry horses).

Any horse that is stall-tied should receive regular exercise, unless this method is used under veterinary guidance, for example as part of the management of an orthopaedic condition.

RUGS

Not all horses will need a rug during inclement weather as some breeds with thick coats are capable of living outdoors throughout the year without rugs.

Some of these breeds often thrive better without rugs, as rugs can sometimes be a cause of skin irritation. However, where horses are of less hardy breeding, clipped or elderly they may require a rug to help keep them warm and dry during cold spells, during wet weather or to provide protection from flies. Turnout rugs will need to be removed when the weather (particularly temperature) improves.

Rugs and hoods should fit well, the right size to suit the horse, of the right type for the purpose intended and correctly fitted to prevent rubbing, hair loss, abrasions or restriction of movement.

The rug weight must be suited to the weather conditions and the temperature. Rugs should be regularly removed so the horse's temperature, body condition and general health can be checked. Ideally this should be done daily. Horses are very efficient at regulating their own temperature and over-rugging can impede this function.

Rugs should be cleaned and repaired as necessary and all fastenings kept in good working order. A spare rug should be available.

SUPERVISION

Horses at grass should be inspected at least once a day, preferably more often. Stabled or group-housed horses should be inspected at least twice a day. Particular attention should be paid to their gait, demeanour, feet, body condition and appetite so that early signs of disease, injury, illness or signs of parasites can be noticed and suitable treatment quickly provided.

Close examinations should be conducted at regular intervals, ideally daily, in order to identify any problems such as skin conditions that may not be seen from a distance.

A horse's hooves should be picked out on a regular basis and at the same time examined for signs of discomfort, wounds, injury, loose shoes, impacted foreign material or anything else unusual. Horses should be groomed regularly to make sure that the coat is clean, free from wounds or parasites and to detect rug, tack or harness rubbing.

The frequency required will depend on your horse's management regime and coat type. Horses living outside should not be regularly groomed as this can remove natural protective oils from their coat. They should be regularly and carefully checked over.

10

CARING FOR THE GERIATRIC HORSE

A 15-year-old horse once was considered "old," but with improved methods of management, care and conditioning, horses well past that age can continue to thrive. Such horses remain in full service, being ridden in a variety of work, leisure or competitive activities that require adequate nutrients, health care and fitness conditioning. Many older mares also are active members of broodmare bands, annually producing foals and rebreeding for the following year.

CLASSIFYING/IDENTIFYING HORSES AT LATER LIFE STAGES

The terms mature, senior and geriatric commonly are used to describe horses that have completed their growth; many owners want to know when their horse move from one classification to another. However, aging is a continuous process, so there's no discrete movement between these classes. Rather, such classifications may be used solely for purposes of illustration and discussion.

Mature Horses

Many breed associations categorize riding horses in the two-to-five year-old range as junior horses. Research has documented continued growth in four- and five-year-old horses, although such growth is comparatively small compared to earlier rates.3 Both scientific and industry consensus is that by the end of the fifth year, a horse can be considered mature. Such five-year-old horses are said to be "fullmouthed," meaning that their baby teeth are gone and all permanent incisors have erupted. By age 11, a horse is referred to as a "smooth-mouthed" horse because the cups in the teeth are no longer visible.

Senior Horses

Assignment of a horse to this classification varies, depending on whether the category refers to performance eligibility in an association or to terminology developed by horse-feed manufacturers. Most competitive horses six years old and older are considered senior horses, yet feeds developed for senior horses typically are intended for much older animals that experience changes in normal eating behavior.

Evaluation of eating behaviors in an otherwise healthy horse provides a simple way to determine the horse's status as mature or senior. In particular, as a horse reaches 15 years of age, an owner should examine its behavior when it is eating hay or grazing grass: Most older horses start "quidding," spitting out partially chewed mouthfuls of hay or grass, reflecting the changing status of their teeth. The age at which this occurs varies greatly.

GERIATRIC HORSES

Although geriatric horses cannot be defined by a particular age, 70 percent of horses 20 years old or older are found to have some condition requiring special care6 and/or management significantly different from that needed by a mature or a senior horse. (Some breed associations automatically record a 25-year-old horse as "deceased," unless notified otherwise by its owner.)

As they reach geriatric status, horses vary in their abilities to perform athletically, to eat or even to accomplish routine activities such as lying down, getting up or bending around to scratch an itch. Even so, some horses 25 years old or older still are being ridden, may remain on conventional feeding programs and have minimal-to-no special problems.

Many times, the aging process that pushes a horse into geriatric status has been hastened by an injury. Chronically foundered horses, severely arthritic horses and those with special conditions of the kidneys, liver or other organs may be classed as geriatric. Special conditions of geriatric horses may make it necessary to avoid using certain feeds.

New types of horse feeds and advanced healthcare practices have focused on older horses. "Complete senior feeds" and "equine dentistry" have become common terminology for owners of older horses.

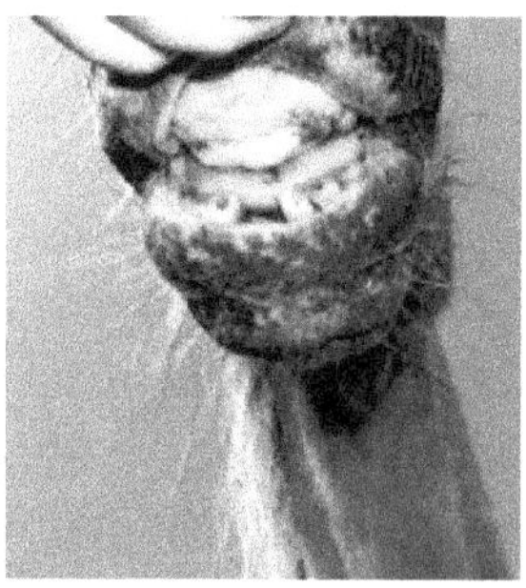

Fig. 1. The complete lack of upper incisors, missing lower incisor and worn appearance of the teeth in this geriatric horse

Equine Dentistry

At least once a year, every horse's mouth should be examined by an equine practitioner or a qualified equine dentist, who will initiate needed corrective procedures. Such dental exams should start before the horse first begins training (Fig. 1).

Nutrition and Feeding

A horse exhibiting changes in grazing or in hay consumption may be having difficulty biting and chewing such roughage; there also may be changes in overall digestion and synthesis functions in the large intestine. Dental problems that may particularly plague older horses include:

- Bit problems – During dental exams, owners routinely may be asked about older horses' responses to bit placement and bit pressure while being ridden. Such problems may be related to the "bit seat," the area where the mouthpiece actually rests, or to the presence of "wolf teeth" needing removal.
- Missing, loose or sharp-edged incisors or molars – Whatever their position, loose teeth may need to be extracted. Missing incisors (due to cribbing or to traumatic injury) may spell difficulty eating for some horses, although others get along just fine without them. Molar problems may be signaled by horses' holding their heads sideways while chewing and/or dribbling feed while eating. Because a horse's upper jaw is wider than its lower jaw, years of chewing may cause sharp enamel points to develop on the outside edges of the upper molars and on the inside edges of the lower ones. Such sharp points cause a horse to dribble feed. "Floating" with high-tech electronic devices that target only affected teeth can remove these sharp edges, but aggressive floating may risk loosening the teeth being treated. Equine dental practitioners may cautiously float teeth of older horses as needed, then encourage owners to monitor their horses' eating behavior for signs of continued difficulty.

NUTRITION AND FEEDING

The most important component of caring for geriatric horses is maintaining their body condition. Older horses often lose weight due to poor dentition, disease, parasites or due to competition with other pasture mates. It is important to take older horses' special needs into consideration to ensure they receive a well-balanced diet. An older horse may need special attention and supplemental feeding during months when there is less grass in the pasture. Geriatric horses also tend to suffer from osteoarthritis (OA), inhibiting them from grazing freely and thus reducing their intake of forage (Fig. 2).

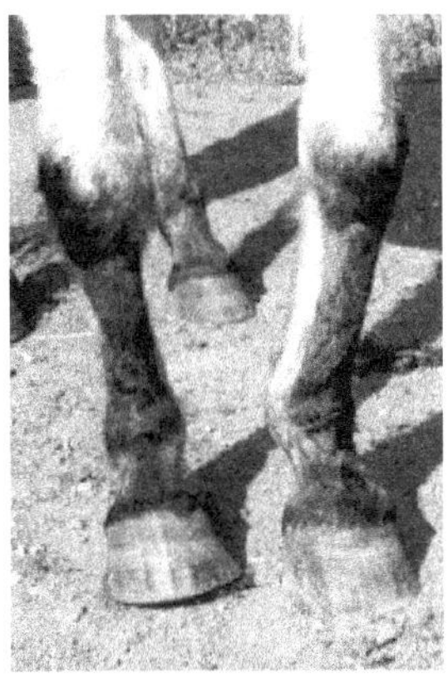

Fig. 2. A geriatric horse with severe osteoarthritis of the carpal joints . Also note the poor hoof care.

Each horse owner must decide when to change from traditional pellet or textured (sweet) feeds to those designed specifically for "old" horses. Key factors in this decision are the horses' physical ability to consume and chew roughage and its nutrient needs as influenced by likely changes in function of its large intestine.

Feeds

Although little research exists on the nutrient requirements of older horses, one study found that compared to younger horses, horses aged 20 years and older had lower apparent digestion of protein, fiber and some minerals. Consequently, manufacturers have developed "complete" feeds, many of them classified as "senior" feeds. Almost every major feed company manufactures such a feed (see Table 1).

Table 1. Typical nutrient content of some seniortype feeds for old horses.

Crude protein	12–14%
Crude fat Not less than	5%
Crude fiber Not less than	16%
Lysine	0.6–0.7%
Calcium	0.6–1.2%
Phosphorus	0.4–0.8%
Magnesium	0.15–0.30%
Sulfur	0.15–0.30%
Copper	26–55 ppm
Zinc	100–220 ppm
Vitamin A	1500–3000 IUs/lb
Vitamin E	40–80 IUs/lb
Biotin	0.4–0.5 mg/lb
Vitamin B1 (Thiamine)	2.2–2.6 mg/lb

Complete senior feeds are designed to help a horse eat, so they often are extruded or otherwise produced as soft, easy-to-chew pellets; processing sometimes involves heat treatment to gelatinize starches, making them more easily digested and absorbed in the small intestine. However, senior feeds will not effectively put additional weight on horses that have no eating problems because, compared to many other feeds, they contain too much fiber and too few calories. In one study, a specially designed feed, containing about 1300 kilocalories of digestible energy per pound, improved body-condition scores and weight gain more significantly than a traditional sweet feed, but differences were greatest in old, very thin horses.

Complete senior feeds routinely contain energy from carbohydrates and fats, with limited energy from fiber, and typically contain enough fiber so a horse does not have to eat hay or graze to maintain its digestive tract integrity. Even so, most horse owners using complete feeds also continue to offer their horses hay or grazing; such a practice helps keep a horse living as normal a life as possible for as long as possible. These feeds focus on protein quality from sources like soybean meal, known for supplying essential amino acids (lysine, threonine, methionine); on suspected needs for additional vitamins (for example, B complex) no longer synthesized in adequate amounts in the hindgut; and on carefully formulated concentrations of minerals.

MIXED FEEDS

Some horse owners mix their own feeds, using various combinations of oats; cracked, rolled or steamflaked corn; barley; soybean meal; wheat midds; and dehydrated alfalfa. If you chose to mix your horse's feed, seriously consider:

Total nutrient balance

a. Pay particular attention to mineral concentrations and to the ratio of minerals to each other and to total energy. Whether fed individually or mixed together, single grains have an inverted calcium-to-phosphorous ratio, so calcium sources such as dicalcium phosphate and calcium carbonate need to be included in appropriate amounts to achieve the proper balance.
b. Include appropriate amounts of trace minerals (sodium, potassium, chloride) to maintain dietary electrolyte balance (cation-anion balance or DCAB), important for sweating horses and for calcium deposition to minimize osteoporosis-type weakening of the skeletal system.

Vitamin A, D and E requirements of horses (not cattle)

a. Vitamin A is often added at 1500-2000 IUs/lb.
b. Vitamin D should never be added at more than 1/10th the level of Vitamin A.
c. Vitamin E's anti-oxidant role is important for hard-working horses; it usually should be added at 50 to 60 IUs/lb.

PRESENCE OF FUMONISIN

Horse owners who mix their own feed should be concerned about fumonisin, which can cause leucoencephalomalacia in horses. Recently fumonisin has been detected in corn grain at a much higher rate of incidence than in the past few years. Corn screenings or corn by-products should never be included in feeds because fumonisin can be highly concentrated in them.

EVALUATING BODY CONDITION

The eye of the horseman or the horsewoman is important in evaluating a horse's body condition, whether the owner is concerned about putting weight on a horse, getting it in shape, or enhancing a horse's thermal regulation. Significant loss in body condition is one of the worst things that can happen to an old horse, but such loss is fairly common. An old arthritic horse or a chronically foundered one does not need to carry extra weight, but with rare exceptions, thinness needs to be avoided in old horses. Older horses are notorious for having difficulty gaining weight. The owner's challenge and goal is never to let an older horse get thin in the first place.

Numerous research projects have evaluated influence of body condition on performance in broodmares and in riding horses. Maintain riding horses at body condition scores between 5 and 6. For riding horses with scores of 5, ribs cannot be seen but are easily felt; such horses' backbones or toplines basically are level. When riding horses get beyond scores of 6 and approach being considered fat, they have more difficulty with heat production. However, an older, thin riding horse will fatigue more quickly because it does not have energy needed to work. Yet, if such horses are allowed to get too fat, summer months are hard on them. Old, thin horses not being ridden will have trouble staying warm in really cold winter weather. Try also to maintain stiff, arthritic and foundered horses at body scores between 5 and 5½.

For old, thin milking mares – those that are ribby or have some backbone sticking up with the tail-head exposed – rebreeding rates will be low, often around 35 percent. Thin mares are notorious for skipping a breeding season simply because they lack the nutrient stores and nutrient supply to produce milk and support new pregnancies. In one study, milking mares with body condition scores of less than 5 were checked pregnant at 45 days, but a 12 percent pregnancy loss occurred at some time after this 45th day.

Such pregnancy losses can be avoided if old mares come into breeding season at body condition scores of 6 or 7.

Mares should not be overly fat or obese (scores of 8 or 9), but fat mares are desirable. So, if a mare set to foal in March is thin in January, take a careful, consistent approach to improving her body condition. Such improvement is easier to accomplish before foaling than after a foal hits the ground.

FEEDING TO INFLUENCE BODY WEIGHT

For too-thin older horses with no apparent chewing or eating-behavior problems, owners should use a reasonable daily amount of feed to attempt to increase body weight. Such horses should be fed two to three times per day at equal intervals, receiving feed equal to no more than ½ percent of the horse's desired body weight in grain per feeding (¾ percent of body weight per feeding is the absolute maximum that should be fed). For example, a horse that ought to weigh 1100 pounds should receive about five pounds of feed at any one feeding (but never more than eight pounds per feeding). Horses with a history of founder or colic should never receive more than ½ percent of their desired body weight in feed per feeding.

To add weight to their horses without providing a greater amount of feed, owners should select an energy-dense feed with supplemental fat (for example, corn oil) added. For instance, 10 pounds of straight oats contain about 12,500 to 13,000 kilocalories of digestible energy. If this grain were supplemented with ½ pound of corn oil, the resulting

10½ pounds of feed would contain 13,500 to 14,000 kilocalories of digestible energy. So, for riding horses and broodmares that need to gain weight, fat-supplemented feeds can be used to increase weight safely with reasonable amounts of daily feed, without increasing chances for colic or founder.

Fat-supplemented feeds also will allow owners to feed less grain to their riding horses, resulting in less total carbohydrate load and less heat production for the horse to deal with. Fat-supplemented feeds routinely are recommended for riding horses being used hard in hot weather.18 Along with daily hay intake monitored closely at no more than 1 percent of body weight, such feeds can help horses more efficiently regulate body temperature during hot summer months.

Many reputable companies manufacture horse feeds with supplemental fat sources. If you need such feeds and you feed grass hay as a roughage source, look for a 14 percent crude protein feed with a crude fat percentage in the 6 to 8 percent range. A feed with a crude fat listing of 7.5to 8 percent usually has about 5 percent supplemental fat added to it.

Heavily-stressed horses often experience exerciserelated inflammation in the ankles, knees and hocks. New research has involved feeding different sources of fat to hard-working, high-performance athletes to alter inflammatory responses. Reduced inflammation was observed when fat sources contained an optimum ratio of omega 6:omega 3 polyunsaturated fatty acids.19 Although more research is needed, owners can expect to see changes in sources of supplemental fat for horse feeds.

PASTURE ENVIRONMENT

As horses age, they often lose their place in the herd hierarchy and may be bullied by younger horses in the pasture. Therefore, it is a good idea to allow them time in the pasture alone or with another older horse. This will eliminate stress on the horse and allow them proper grazing time. Adequate pasture time is vital to minimize orthopedic issues and stiffness.

Additional considerations include placing older horses in a pasture with a flat surface and monitoring weather conditions; they often have significant OA and may have stiffness and weakness in the hind-end, predisposing them to fall in slippery conditions such as severe rain, snow, or ice.

AMBIENT TEMPERATURE AND GROOMING CARE

Geriatric horses are more sensitive to extreme weather conditions than younger horses.[2] Older horses often have hirsutism (an overlong haircoat) and are often not able to thermoregulate correctly. They may also have areas of patchy sweating. Therefore, it is important to clip them, use blankets in colder weather, and to provide a cool environment during hot months. To improve circulation, daily brushing is advisable.

PARASITE CONTROL

Deworming and pasture management are important topics that veterinary technicians can address with owners. Implementing an effective deworming program is essential for proper barn management. Rotating dewormers ensures that various species and stages of parasites are killed. While geographic locations may differ in optimal deworming programs, deworming is generally recommended every 8 weeks. False negative results from fecal exams may be misleading, and while fecal egg counts are an important part of parasite control, they do not always detect encysted larvae, which can be detrimental to older horses. Using the proper larvicidal dewormer to kill encysted parasites and help maintain a good body condition in an older horse is important to overall good health of the horse. It is also important to remove manure routinely (e.g., once a week) and maintain a low stocking density of horses in the pasture.

HOOF CARE

Costs

For mature horses, hoof care is the third most expensive horse-keeping cost, just behind nutrition and emergency/preventative healthcare. During one year, money spent on hoof care represents about 15 percent of the total cost to keep a mature performance horse.

Hoof-care expense can be expected to increase for some senior horses, and for some geriatric horses, it could represent 25 to 50 percent of annual costs. While it may cost a little money to keep a horse's feet in good shape or to manage existing hoof conditions, for a horse with a job to do, whether riding horse or broodmare, hoof care expenses represent money well spent.

Conditions and Care

Older riding horses often exhibit a variety of hoof conditions. Some are just naturally "good-footed horses," while others may have poor hoof walls or problems with the white line. Many older horses that have been in service for years show signs of navicular disease or evidence of founder.

Advances in hoof care contribute to keeping in service older horses that would otherwise be unable to move around. For horses with poor hoof-wall strength and integrity, consider supplemental biotin.

Based on research conducted in Switzerland, longterm biotin supplementation (for 9 months or longer) may improve hoof condition in about one-third of horses with hoof wall and white line problems.

However, most supplements on the market won't make nearly so much difference to hoof health as will routine hoof care, including proper and timely hoof trimming and shoeing.

HEALTHCARE ISSUES

Common Diseases of the Geriatric Horse

The following overview addresses clinical signs, diagnosis and treatment of the six most common conditions affecting geriatric horses:

Pituitary Pars Intermedia Dysfunction (Equine Cushing's disease)

With an increasing number of aged horses in the population today, there has been an increased awareness of diagnostic testing and treatment for Pituitary Pars Intermedia Dysfunction (PPID), commonly called Equine Cushing's-like disease. PPID is common in older horses and is caused by a malfunction of the pituitary gland, resulting in a tumor or enlarged gland.[3] This leads to an increased secretion of pro-opiomelanocortin (POMC)-derived peptides and ultimately to the clinical signs listed below.

A unique and consistent clinical sign of advanced PPID is the long, curly hair coat that does not shed or shed fully (hirsutism). Other clinical signs of horses with PPID include laminitis, muscle atrophy along the dorsum, fat accumulation, polydipsia, polyuria, secondary infections, lethargy, infertility, persistent lactation, hyperhidrosis, and metabolic abnormalities including hyperglycemia.[3] Diagnosis is based on clinical signs and one of three tests: Dexamethasone-suppression test to assess cortisol response; serial measurements of ACTH, insulin, and dextrose; and thyrotropin-releasing hormone stimulation. However, none of these diagnostic tests are 100% accurate and while results are usually helpful, occasionally a false negative or false positive result can occur. Therefore, if the horse is older and exhibits these clinical signs listed above, PPID should be considered. Treatment is administration of pergolide PO q 24h for the remainder of the horse's life. In addition, careful management is vital to maintaining the horse's health, including clipping the haircoat and using a blanket during the winter months, and frequent trimming of the feet (e.g., every 4 weeks)

Laminitis

Another disease that occurs in geriatric horses is laminitis, also known as founder. Laminitis is an inflammation of the laminae, causing degeneration and necrosis of the hoof. Because laminitis can be due to a plethora of diseases, the cause of this disease is not yet clear and is an active area of research by many universities. Laminitis can be an acute or chronic condition. Examples of diseases associated with acute laminitis include ingestion of large quantities of grain, strangulating intestinal lesions, or mares with placental retention. Chronic laminitis may be caused by diseases such as PPID; geriatric horses with PPID may develop laminitis as a secondary complication and it may even be the first indication that the horse has PPID. Clinical signs include lameness, depression, anorexia, and a horse's reluctance to move or lift its feet to be cleaned. Increased pulsations in the digital arteries can be palpated or sometimes visualized. Depending on the severity of the condition, the horse may stabilize with treatment; however, euthanasia is often recommended in severe cases. Treatment is directed at the primary disease causing laminitis (e.g., administration of pergolide to horses with PPID), supportive care and pain management. It is important to keep the horse comfortable and supportive treatment includes shoeing changes, deep bedding in the stall, and nonsteroidal antiinflammatory drugs (NSAIDs). Also, these horses seem to have a higher rate of foot abscesses, which must be treated aggressively. It is important in these cases not to mistake laminitis for abscess formation and vice versa. Laminitis in non-PPID horses is often associated with a degree of third phalanx (P3) rotation, while horses with PPID often do not have rotation or only minimal rotation of P3.

Heaves

This disease is more appropriately known as Recurrent Airway Obstruction (RAO). A similar disease can occur in young horses and is known as Recurrent Airway Inflammation. It is a condition that can be acute or chronic and can affect a horse year-round or seasonally. Another form of the disease is actually worsened by outside exposure in the summer and on hot, humid days. Treatment includes keeping the horse inside in the heat of the day. This is commonly seen in the southeast United States, but is not limited to that region.

Because a horse with RAO is reacting to an allergen in its environment (e.g., dust), care should be taken to minimize exposure to dust and known offending allergens. Providing adequate pasture time, minimizing dusty bedding and stalls, and soaking hay before feeding are important steps to alleviate RAO in the geriatric equine patient. Clinical signs include: cough, tachypnea, dyspnea, flared nostrils, wheezing, and a heave line, which is caused by increased exhalation and subsequent overdevelopment of external abdominal oblique muscles. Diagnosis is based on history, clinical signs, physical examination and diagnostic tests including transtracheal and bronchioalveolar lavage using an endoscope, radiographs, and blood tests. The most important part to controlling RAO is minimizing allergens and dust in the horse's environment.

Uveitis

Equine recurrent uveitis, also referred to as moon blindness, is one of the most common ocular diseases of the horse and the most common cause of blindness in equine patients. It is an immune-mediated disease characterized by periods of inflammation and inactive periods where inflammation may be difficult to discern. Clinical signs include photophobia, swelling and reddening of the conjunctiva, excessive tear production or discharge from the eye, corneal edema, and constriction of the pupil (miosis). Uveitis can be the result of trauma to the eye or caused by systemic disease including leptospirosis, brucellosis, onchocerciasis, strangles, equine influenza, or tooth abscessation. The diagnosis of uveitis includes a thorough ophthalmic exam and additional diagnostic tests, such as a CBC and serum chemistry panel. Treatment is based on the underlying clinical disease and use of topical and systemic antiinflammatory and antimicrobial medications to reduce intraocular inflammation and further damage to the eye. If the condition is chronic, sometimes surgical intervention may involve vitrectomy (removal of the vitreous) or a suprachoroidal cyclosporine implantation in which a cyclosporine disk is implanted under the scleral flap. It is important to treat uveitis quickly because recurrent episodes can lead to other chronic conditions such as adhesions between the iris and the lens, cataracts, retinal degeneration and, most importantly, blindness.

Euthanasia

As always, the subject of euthanasia can be difficult to discuss with an owner. Many times these horses have been members of the family for several decades. As veterinary technicians, we need to recognize the bond between owners and their horses and understand the loss they are feeling. We can help provide compassion and support at a time when they are needed the most.[7]

When the owner decides to euthanize his/her horse, some medical issues need to be taken into consideration. Whether the veterinarian chooses to use a needle or insert a catheter, it is helpful to clip the area over the jugular vein. As with any aged animal, these horses can be thin and it can be difficult to locate the jugular vein. Due to the large size of these animals, disposal also can be a concern. The owner may choose to bury or cremate the horse. If burial is elected, the owner should contact local authorities because of possible restrictions in their township.

ESSENTIAL VACCINATIONS

Unfortunately, annual immunizations are easily forgotten. Nature, however, reminds horse owners of the need to vaccinate their animals, by means of emerging (new) infectious diseases like West Nile virus. Failure to keep horses on regular, annual immunization programs can result in a lost horse.

Consult a veterinarian who knows horses to find out what immunizations are absolutely necessary in your area. Most equine practitioners will recommend a basic vaccination program (including rabies vaccine), along with other immunizations based on the needs of individual horses.

DE-WORMING

There are several ways to de-worm your horse; you need to match your chosen method to your particular situation. For example, a few horses grazing a large pasture should be evaluated differently from a few horses in semi-confinement on a few acres in close contact with each other. Select an appropriate de-worming strategy, then stay on schedule.

Broad-spectrum tube worming is effective, although this method is not utilized so much as in the past because of the advent of paste wormers and dailyfeed wormers. Remember that just because you put a paste de-wormer in your horse's mouth, that does mean the horse swallowed it. It's especially important to watch the old, smart horses carefully, because they are notorious for holding paste in their mouths until you leave, then spitting it out onto the ground. Even if you choose a daily-feed de-wormer, start your program with one dose of a paste de-wormer.

GLOSSARY

Abdomen - the middle section of the body, between the chest and the pelvis.

Abdominal cavity - the body cavity between the chest and the pelvis.

Abdominocentesis - surgical procedure in which a needle is inserted into the abdomen to withdraw fluid.

Abortion - the end of a pregnancy before the expelled fetus can survive independently, either by spontaneous abortion (miscarriage) or by a medical termination of pregnancy.

Abscess - a pocket of pus, usually caused by a bacterial infection.

Acariasis - disease caused by a mite of the order acarina.

Acaricide - a chemical agent used to kill mites.

Ace inhibitor - any of a class of drugs intended to lower blood pressure by widening blood vessels. Ace stands for angiotensin-converting enzyme.

Acidic - a liquid that has a ph lower than 7.

Acquired - conditions that are not inborn and that develop during the animal's life.

Acromegaly - a disorder of excessive growth hormone secretion by the pituitary gland, resulting in excessive growth of bones in the legs.

Actinobacillosis - disease caused by bacteria of the genus *actinobacillus.*

Actinomycosis - a bacterial infection in humans, swine, and cattle that causes hard masses to form in the mouth and jaw.

Acupuncture - a procedure adapted from chinese medical practice in which specific body areas are pierced with fine needles for therapeutic purposes.

Acute - a condition that has a brief or short course; signs often develop suddenly and may be severe.

Acute pain - the short-term sharp, throbbing, aching, or burning sensation in response to a stimulus (twisting, crushing, or burning) or tissue injury (bruises, wounds, and surgical incisions).

Addison's disease - a deficiency of adrenal gland hormones.

Adenocarcinoma - a malignant tumor formed in the epithelium, or covering tissue, of an organ.

Adenoma - a benign tumor formed in glandular tissue.

Adenovirus - a virus of the family adenoviridae.

Adrenal gland - a small, paired gland located near the kidneys that produces cortisol, epinephrine, and other hormones.

Aerosol - a suspension of particles dissolved in liquid and dispersed in a fine mist.

Aflatoxicosis - poisoning caused by consumption of foods contaminated with a toxin produced by the fungus *aspergillus flavus.*

African horse sickness - an equine viral disease that is widespread in africa. It is characterized by signs of lung and blood system impairment, and is most frequently transmitted by midges or mosquitoes.

Agalactia - partial or complete lack of milk flow from the mammary gland.

Agent - anything that produces an effect. For example, viruses and bacteria are agents that cause disease.

Aggression - behavior that is related to conflict between individuals; includes both threats and attacks.

Agonist - a drug or other chemical that can bind to a receptor or cell to trigger a response typical of a naturally occurring substance.

Agouti - a mottled coat color in rodents, characterized by fur with bands of different colors.

Airway - passage for air from the nose or mouth to the lungs.

Algal poisoning - a toxic and often deadly condition caused by heavy growths of blue-green algae in drinking water.

Alkaline - a substance with a ph higher than 7; also referred to as basic.

Alkaloidosis - poisoning by alkaloids, plant toxins that damage the liver.

Allergy - an abnormally high sensitivity to certain substances, such as pollens, foods, or microorganisms.

Alloimmune reaction - a type of immune reaction that occurs when the body produces antibodies against the tissues of another animal. This may occur, for example, when one animal receives a blood transfusion from another animal of the same species but with a different blood type.

Alopecia - a partial or complete loss of hair in areas where it is usually found.

Alternative therapy - therapy used instead of conventional treatments (for example, homeopathic treatment).

Alveoli - plural form of the word alveolus.

Alveolus - tiny air-holding sac formed at the end of air passageways in the lungs, where the barrier between the air and the blood is a thin membrane.

Amino acid - a chemical compound that forms the basic building block of proteins.

Amoeba - a type of protozoa, or single-celled organism. Some are parasitic and can cause infection in animals.

Amphetamine - a class of drugs that stimulates the central nervous system and the cardiovascular system.

Amphibian - a class of cold-blooded animals that spends at least part of their life cycle living in water.

Amputation - the removal of a limb or other part of the body.

Amyloid - a type of abnormally folded protein that may collect in various body tissues and interfere with their function.

Amyloidosis - disease characterized by accumulation of abnormal protein deposits.

Anabolic - pertaining to a metabolic process in which complex molecules are created from simpler ones.

Analgesia - treatment given to control pain; a deadening or absence of the sense of pain without loss of consciousness.

Analgesic - a class of drugs that relieve pain.

Anaphylactic shock - a rare, life-threatening, immediate allergic reaction to something that has entered the body, such as food, an injection, or an insect sting. Also called anaphylaxis.

Anemia - an abnormally low red blood cell count caused by insufficient intake of iron in the diet, blood loss, or other medical conditions.

Anesthesia - a lack of all sensation, particularly sensitivity to pain. It can be induced medically or result from trauma, and it can be limited to a small area (local anesthesia) or affect the entire body (general anesthesia).

Anesthetic - an agent used to induce anesthesia, including injectable drugs and inhaled gases.

Anestrus - an interval of sexual inactivity between 2 periods of estrus in female mammals that breed cyclically.

Aneurysm - a dilation or bulging of a blood vessel caused by a weakening of its walls.

Animal-assisted therapy - using animals as therapy for the sick or elderly in nursing or other rehabilitation centers because of the positive effect such visits have on residents and patients.

Animal welfare - human efforts to reduce and prevent pain and suffering and promote well-being in animals.

Anorexia - a lack or loss of appetite.

Anoxia - lack of oxygen in the blood or body tissues.

Antacid - a medication that neutralizes acidity, especially in the stomach.

Antagonist - a drug or substance that nullifies the effect of another substance.

Anterior - located toward the head or the front end of the body.

Anterior uvea - part of the front portion of the eye, including the iris and ciliary body.

Anthelmintic - a class of drugs used to treat infection with parasitic worms.

Anthrax - an often-fatal infectious disease caused by *bacillus anthracis* bacteria that may infect all warm-blooded animals, including humans.

Antibacterial - destroying or inhibiting the growth of bacteria.

Antibiotic - a class of drugs used to destroy bacteria while remaining safe for the human or animal being treated.

Antibiotic resistance - ability of a microorganism (such as bacteria) to resist the effects of an antibiotic drug.

Antibody - a molecule produced by the immune system that attacks a particular foreign substance (antigen) in the body.

Anticholinergic - a class of drugs that block acetylcholine receptors in nerves.

Anticoagulant - a substance that stops blood from clotting.

Anticonvulsant - a class of drugs used to prevent or relieve convulsions.

Antidepressant - a class of drugs designed to relieve depression in humans; may also be used to help control behavior problems in pets.

Antidote - a substance that counteracts the effect of a poison or toxin.

Antiemetic - one of a group of drugs used to retard or stop vomiting.

Antifungal - a class of drugs that destroy or prevent the growth of fungi.

Antigen - any substance that can stimulate an immune response.

Antihistamine - a class of drugs used to relieve allergy signs by blocking the inflammatory action of histamines.

Anti-inflammatory - medication that prevents or reduces inflammation.

Antimicrobial - a large group of drugs used to fight infections caused by bacteria, fungi, and viruses.

Antineoplastic - a group of chemical agents or drugs used to combat cancer.

Antioxidant - a substance that inhibits oxidation of other compounds.

Antiparasitic - any of a group of drugs used to combat infestation with parasites.

Antiseptic solution - a solution of a substance that kills or inhibits the growth of microbes.

Antitoxin - a compound that neutralizes a specific toxin.

Antivenin - an antidote to a particular venom; a serum that counteracts venom.

Antiviral - compound that kills or inhibits the growth of viruses.

Anus - the opening at the end of the intestinal tract where solid wastes are pushed out of a body.

Aorta - the largest artery in the body. It carries blood away from the heart on its way to distribute oxygen to all body tissues except the lungs.

Aortic arch - the curved portion between the ascending and descending portions of the aorta.

Aortic valve - a heart valve comprising 3 flaps that controls the flow of blood from the left ventricle into the aorta.

Aplasia - incomplete or incorrect development of a body part.

Aquatic - describes organisms that live in water.

Arboreal - describes species that spend most or all of their lives in trees.

Arrhythmia - an abnormal pattern of contraction of the heart, caused by a disturbance in conduction of the normal electrical impulses within the heart.

Arsenical - a substance (a drug or insecticide) containing arsenic.

Arterial dilator - a drug that dilates the small arteries, making it easier for the heart to pump blood away from itself.

Artery - blood vessel that carries oxygen-rich blood away from the heart and toward the body's tissues.

Arthritis - inflammation of a joint; often characterized by swelling, pain, and redness.

Arthroscopy - examination of the interior of a joint, such as the knee, using a type of endoscope that is inserted into the joint through a small incision.

Artificial insemination - introduction (with a syringe or other device) of semen into the uterus without sexual contact.

Ascarid - a class of roundworms whose larvae can cause disease.

Ascites - a condition in which fluid collects in the abdomen.

As-needed dosing - administering pain medication only when the animal shows recognizable signs of pain.

Aspergillosis - a fungal infection caused by several species of *aspergillus* fungi.

Asphyxiation - a severe lack of oxygen resulting from inability to breathe.

Aspiration - the use of a suction device to withdraw fluid from the body.

Aspiration pneumonia - inflammation caused by inhalation of food particles or fluids into the lungs.

Asthma - a respiratory condition marked by recurring episodes of labored breathing, wheezing, and coughing, triggered by oversensitivity to environmental conditions.

Astringent - a substance that causes tissues, such as mucous membranes, to shrink or dry out.

Atherosclerosis - a hardening of an artery caused by deposits made of cholesterol, other fatty substances, or cellular debris that accumulates inside the artery.

Atopy - allergy characterized by itching and redness of the skin; may also include discharges from the eyes or nose.

Atria - plural form of the word atrium.

Atrial fibrillation - irregular contraction of the atria (upper heart chambers) caused by abnormal electrical activity in the heart.

Atrial standstill - a failure of the electrical impulses in the upper chambers of the heart, which results in a lack of contraction of those chambers.

Atrial thrombosis - a heart condition caused by a blood clot in the atrium of the heart.

Atrioventricular valve - the valve between the upper (atrial) and lower (ventricular) chambers of the heart.

Atrium - the upper chamber of the heart that receives blood from the veins and pushes it into the ventricle.

Aural plaque - in horses, a white growth caused by a virus that develops in and around the ears.

Autoimmune - an immune response that is developed against the animal's own tissues.

Autonomic nervous system - specialized set of neurons controlling and regulating basic, unconscious bodily functions such as breathing and heart beat.

Avian tuberculosis - a slowly spreading, chronic infection of birds caused by the bacteria *mycobacterium avium* and characterized by gradual weight loss.

Awn - a slender, bristle-like appendage found on the spikelets of many grasses.

Axon - extensions of neurons that transmit electrical charges away from the cell body.

B cell - a type of white blood cell that produces antibodies.

Bacteremia - the presence of bacteria in the bloodstream.

Bacteria - the plural form of the word bacterium.

Bacterial disease - disease caused by invading bacteria or an overgrowth of usually harmless bacteria.

Bacterium - a microscopic, single-celled organism that may cause disease or may be a harmless, or even helpful, part of an animal's normal internal or external environment.

Barbering - excessive chewing of hair or feathers that leads to bald patches of skin.

Baroreceptors - nerve endings in blood vessels that are sensitive to blood pressure changes.

Basal cells - cells at the base of the top layer of the skin.

Basking - the behavior of a cold-blooded animal lying in the sun to increase its body temperature.

Basophil - a type of white blood cell that releases histamine as part of the body's allergic response.

Benign - something that is nonharmful or noncancerous.

Besnoitiosis - infectious disease caused by protozoa of the genus *besnoitia*, transmitted by certain biting flies and ticks, found in africa, france, and mexico.

Beta cells - cells in the pancreas that produce insulin.

Biceps brachii tendon - tendon of the biceps brachii, a major muscle of the upper front leg that acts to bend the elbow joint.

Biopsy - the removal of a small sample of tissue or fluid for examination. A sample is obtained in a way suited to the type of tissue and its location; it might be drawn out with a hollow needle and syringe, scraped with a curette, or cut away with a scalpel.

Bladder - a stretchable, membranous sac-like structure in the body that holds fluids; the term is used most often to refer to the urinary bladder.

Blastoma - a tumor composed of previously healthy young cells that never mature normally, but mutate into a cancer.

Blastomycosis - a disease caused by *blastomyces* fungi that can affect several species of animals or humans; infection may occur in the skin, lungs, or other body organs.

Blepharitis - inflammation of the eyelids.

Blind spot - the small circular area, insensitive to light, where the optic nerve enters the eye. *See also* optic disk.

Blister - a fluid-filled bump on the skin.

Blood cell count - the number of red blood cells, white blood cells, and platelets in a sample of blood. Also called a complete blood count (cbc).

Blood cells - any of the cells contained in blood. *See also* erythrocyte, leukoctye, platelet.

Blood clot - a mass of blood cells, protein, and platelets, also known as a thrombus, that forms whenever there is a break or tear in a blood vessel.

Blood poisoning - a disorder, also known as septicemia, in which bacteria or their toxins circulate in the bloodstream.

Blood pressure - the force exerted by the blood against the walls of the blood vessels, especially the arteries.

Blood transfusion - a procedure in which another animal's blood is introduced into the body to counteract blood loss, anemia, or other conditions.

Blood typing - the identification of blood groups in order to match donor blood with the recipient's blood for a blood transfusion.

Bloodborne - carried by or transmitted through blood.

Bloodstream - the flow of blood through the circulatory system of an organism.

Body cavity - an enclosed space in the body that contains organs, such as the cranial, spinal, thoracic, and abdominal cavities.

Boid snakes - snakes related to boa constrictors. The group includes pythons.

Bone marrow - a soft tissue filling the spaces of the spongy tissue found at the ends of long bones. It produces red blood cells, most types of white blood cells, and platelets.

Borreliosis - disease caused by bacteria of the genus *borrelia*. *See* lyme disease.

Botulism - infection caused by ingesting food or dead flesh containing toxins produced by the bacterium *clostridium botulinum*, or by absorbing toxins in the gastrointestinal tract. It results in rapid paralysis and death.

Brachycephalic - short-headed or broad-headed.

Brachygnathia - abnormal shortness or recession of the lower jaw.

Brachytherapy - a cancer treatment that involves internal radiation therapy.

Brackish - water that is a mixture of fresh and salt water.

Bradycardia - a slower than normal heart rate.

Brain - the controlling center of the nervous system in vertebrates, connected to the spinal cord and enclosed in the cranium.

Brain stem - one of the 3 main sections of the brain; it controls many basic life functions.

Brain stem auditory evoked response (baer) - records electrical activity in the pathway from the sound receptors in the ear to the brain stem and cerebrum.

Breed - a group of animals or organisms having common ancestors and certain distinguishable characteristics.

Breeding - sexual reproduction of animals, either spontaneously or planned and supervised by human beings.

Broad-spectrum antibiotics - antibiotics that are effective against a wide range of bacteria.

Bronchial - relating to the bronchi, the bronchial tubes, or the bronchioles, the body's airways.

Bronchitis - inflammation of the bronchial airways.

Bronchoscopy - interior examination of the airways with an endoscope.

Buck - the male of certain mammal species, such as rabbits, antelope, and deer.

Budgerigar - a small australian parrot commonly kept as a pet; also called a budgie or parakeet.

Bumblefoot - a foot abscess in sheep, guinea pigs, or birds caused by a localized bacterial infection.

Bursa - a fluid-filled body sac located between a tendon and a bone or at points of friction.

Calcification - the abnormal hardening or stiffening of a body part caused by deposits of calcium.

Calcinosis - the abnormal depositing of calcium salts contributing to hardening of a part or tissue of the body.

Calcinosis cutis - a condition in which calcium deposits form in the skin; they can appear as small, thickened, "dots" on the abdomen.

Calcitonin - hormone secreted by the parathyroid glands that regulates levels of calcium in the bloodstream.

Calcium deficiency - a lack of calcium in the body that can result from insufficient calcium or vitamin d in the diet and can cause bone deformities.

Caloric - relating to heat or calories.

Cancer - a malignant tumor or growth that destroys healthy tissue.

Cancer pain - pain resulting from primary tumor growth, a spreading cancerous disease, or the toxic effects of chemotherapy or radiation.

Candidiasis - a fungal disease caused by *candida albicans* that affects the mucous membranes and the skin.

Canidae - scientific name for dogs, foxes, and wolves.

Canine - relating to animals of the canidae family, primarily dogs.

Canine distemper (hardpad disease) - a highly contagious, usually fatal viral disease of dogs, ferrets, mink, raccoons, and other mammals.

Canine herpesviral infection - a severe, often fatal, viral disease of puppies, sometimes referred to as fading or sudden-death syndrome. In adult dogs, it may be associated with upper respiratory infection or an inflammation of the vagina marked by pain and a pus-filled discharge (in females) or inflammation of the foreskin of the penis (in males).

Canine thrombopathia - a hereditary disorder of blood platelets that causes bleeding from the nose and gums, and tiny purple or red bruises as a result of bleeding under the skin.

Canine tooth - long, pointed tooth used primarily for holding food in place in order to tear it.

Cannibalism - the act of eating a member of an animal's own species.

Capillary - the smallest type of blood vessel, which connects small blood vessels that branch off from arteries and veins.

Capsule - a medication consisting of an active ingredient and fillers, enclosed in a cylindrical coating usually made of gelatin; designed to be taken by mouth.

Carcass - the dead body of an animal.

Carcinogen - a cancer-causing substance or agent.

Carcinoma - an invasive, malignant tumor derived from epithelial tissues (tissues that make up the skin, glands, mucous membranes, and organ linings).

Cardiac - of or relating to the heart.

Cardiac output - the amount of blood pumped from the heart during a specified period of time.

Cardiac shunts - abnormal openings between chambers of the left and right sides of the heart.

Cardiac tamponade - a buildup of fluid in the sac around the heart, which increases pressure on the heart and gradually interferes with its ability to pump blood.

Cardiomyopathy - a disease in which the heart muscle is weakened.

Cardiopulmonary resuscitation (cpr) - an emergency procedure, often employed after cardiac arrest, in which massage of the heart, artificial respiration, and drugs are used to maintain the circulation of oxygenated blood to the body. Also called cardiopulmonary-cerebral resuscitation (cpcr).

Cardiovascular system - the body system that consists of the heart and the blood vessels (veins and arteries).

Carnivore - a flesh-eating animal.

Carpal - relating to bones in the wrist; a wrist bone.

Carpal joint - any of the joints between the carpal bones.

Carrier - an animal that, without becoming ill, harbors or spreads disease-causing microorganisms.

Cartilage - a somewhat elastic connective tissue that is found at the ends of bones and helps reduce friction as joints move.

Castration - most often refers to surgical removal of the testicles; less commonly may refer to removal of the ovaries.

Cataract - condition in which the lens of the eye progressively loses transparency, which often results in loss of vision.

Cathartic - a drug given to increase the passage of gastrointestinal contents, to cleanse the bowel before radiography or endoscopy, to eliminate toxins from the gastrointestinal tract, and to soften feces after intestinal or anal surgery.

Catheter - a thin flexible tube that is inserted into a body cavity, duct, or vessel to allow passage of fluids.

Cationic - a substance or class of detergents that are locally corrosive, causing skin, eye, and mucous membrane injury similar to that of alkaline corrosive agents.

Ceiling effect - situation in which an increased dose of a pain-relieving drug provides incrementally smaller gains in pain relief.

Cell - the smallest functioning unit in the structure of an organism.

Cell body - the center portion of a neuron.

Cellular infiltrates - gas, fluid, or dissolved matter that enters cells or tissue.

Centesis - procedure in which a needle is inserted into a structure (for example, the chest or urinary bladder) of an animal to remove fluid or air.

Central nervous system - the part of the nervous system that includes the brain and spinal cord.

Cercariae - parasitic larvae of trematode worms.

Cerebellar hypoplasia - lack of development of the cerebellum, the section of the brain that controls motor function.

Cerebellum - the cauliflower-shaped brain structure located just behind the cerebrum and above the brain stem.

Cerebrospinal fluid - the fluid surrounding the brain and spinal cord.

Cerebrum - one of 3 main sections of the brain; area where sensory and motor nerve activity is coordinated.

Cesarean section - a surgical procedure in which the abdomen and uterus are cut open and the young are delivered through the abdomen.

Cestode - intestinal parasitic worm of the class cestoda, with a flat, segmented body; tapeworms.

Chelonians - tortoises and turtles.

Chemotherapy - the use of chemical agents to treat diseases, especially cancer.

Cherry eye - swelling and inflammation of the third eyelid, especially in dogs.

Chlamydiosis - infection with a bacteria of the genus *chlamydia.*

Chlamydophila - bacteria that cause serious respiratory infections in birds.

Cholesteatomas - cysts on the eardrum that may extend into the middle ear.

Chondrosarcoma - a malignant tumor of cartilage.

Chordae tendineae - strands of connective tissue in the heart that connect the valves to the papillary muscles of the heart's ventricles.

Choroid - a membrane between the retina and sclera of the eye.

Chromosome - dense strands of material in the cell nucleus that carry the individual's genetic material (dna).

Chronic - a condition that persists over a long period of time, often months or longer.

Chronic pain - pain that persists for longer than the expected time frame for healing, or pain associated with progressive, noncancerous disease, such as osteoarthritis.

Cilia - tiny, hairlike projections that line the outer part of cells in some tissues, including the lower respiratory tract.

Cilia-associated respiratory bacillus - bacteria that can cause chronic respiratory disease in rats and mice; transmitted by direct contact.

Ciliary muscles - the muscles in the eye that change the shape of the lens in order to keep vision in focus.

Cleft palate - a congenital abnormality that creates a gap along the center of the roof of the mouth.

Cloaca - in amphibians, fish, birds, and reptiles, an opening through which the digestive, urinary, and reproductive tracts exit the body.

Cloacal prolapse - a condition in which the cloaca protrudes outside the body.

Cloacitis - inflammation of an animal's cloaca. *See* cloaca.

Clostridia - bacteria that can cause severe intestinal disease or spread toxins through the bloodstream.

Clot - a collection of red blood cells, white cells, and platelets, bound together by protein fibers, that plugs holes in blood vessels.

Coagulation - the process by which liquid blood is transformed into a clot.

Cobalt therapy - a type of radiation therapy that uses radioactive cobalt to treat cancer.

Coccidia - a group of protozoan parasites (small, single-celled organisms) that infect the intestinal tract of animals.

Coccidioidomycosis - a dustborne, noncontagious infection caused by inhalation of fungal spores.

Coccidiosis - a serious disease in cattle, sheep, goats, hogs, poultry, and rabbits, and less serious in dogs, cats, and horses. It is caused by protozoans (coccidia) that invade and may destroy the lining of the intestines.

Cochlea - a snail-shaped cavity in the inner ear, containing the organs of hearing.

Coelomitis - inflammation of the coelom, or abdomen, in retiles.

Cognitive dysfunction - senility; similar to alzheimer's disease in people.

Cold-blooded - animals that do not maintain a constant internal body temperature; instead, their temperature is greatly influenced by their environment.

Colibacillosis - a form of diarrhea caused by *escherichia coli* bacteria.

Colic - severe abdominal pain caused by spasm, obstruction, or distention of the intestines; there are many possible causes.

Colitis - inflammation of the colon.

Collagen - a fibrous protein that forms tendons, ligaments, and connective tissue; also found in skin, bone, and cartilage.

Colon - the large intestine.

Colonoscopy - examination of the inside surface of the colon using a tube inserted through the rectum.

Colony - a group of organisms of one species that live and interact closely with each other in an organized fashion.

Colostrum - the watery fluid rich in antibodies and nutrients that is produced by a mother after giving birth and before producing true milk.

Colt - a young male horse.

Colubrid - a snake of the colubridae family, including adders, vipers, cobras, rattlesnakes, and coral snakes.

Combination chemotherapy - using a combination of drugs that target different sites or that employ different mechanisms to maximize destruction of cancer cells.

Companion animal - any animal kept by humans for companionship or pleasure rather than for utility; a pet.

Compensatory mechanism - any one of several specific responses the body uses in combating heart disease to maintain normal circulation.

Complementary therapy - therapy used in addition to conventional treatments.

Compulsive behavior - otherwise normal behaviors that occur out of context or so often that they interfere with normal activity.

Computed tomography (ct) - a computer-enhanced x-ray procedure used to detect abnormalities in various body organs.

Conduction - passage of the electrical impulses that govern the pumping of the heart.

Conformation - the structure or outline of an item or entity, determined by the arrangement of its parts.

Congenital defect - an abnormality that is present at birth, as a result of either heredity or environmental influence such as a toxin or infection.

Congestion - an abnormal buildup of fluid in an organ or area of the body.

Congestive heart failure - a condition marked by weakness, shortness of breath, or an excessive buildup of fluid in the tissues or body cavities when the heart fails to maintain adequate blood circulation.

Conjunctiva - the mucous membrane lining the inside of the eyelids.

Conjunctivitis - inflammation of the mucous membrane lining the inside of the eyelid. Also called pink eye.

Constipation - difficulty in passing bowel movements; incomplete or infrequent passing of hard stools.

Constricted toe syndrome - a condition in newly hatched birds in which a tough ring of tissue forms around a toe joint, partially cutting off circulation.

Contagious - describes a condition that can spread from one organism to another.

Contaminated - unclean or polluted because of contact with harmful substances.

Contraction - pumping action of the heart muscle or other muscles.

Contrast procedure - specialized x-ray technique in which the animal is given a dye that shows up on the x-ray film to help provide more detailed images of body organs.

Convulsion - *see* seizure.

Coprophagia - eating feces.

Cornea - the transparent outer part of the eye that covers the iris and pupil and admits light into the eyeball.

Coronavirus - a family of viruses that chiefly cause respiratory infections.

Corticosteroid - any of the steroid hormones made by the adrenal gland or their synthetic equivalents; commonly used to reduce inflammation.

Cortisol - a steroid hormone produced by the adrenal gland that regulates carbohydrate metabolism and maintains blood pressure.

Counterconditioning - a method for reducing unwanted behavior by teaching a pet to replace it with a more favorable behavior.

Counterirritant - a substance that, when applied, irritates the skin and thereby reduces the inflammation of underlying tissue.

Counterpressure - pressure applied to reduce bleeding.

Cranial - relating to the skull, or cranium; toward the head end of the body.

Cranium - the portion of the skull enclosing the brain.

Cream - a semisolid mixture made for application to the skin or mucous membranes.

Crop - in many birds, a pouch in the gullet where food is stored and sometimes partially digested before passing to the stomach.

Cross matching - blood typing test done to ensure that a blood donor and recipient have compatible blood types.

Crotalids - snakes of the genus *crotalidae*, including pit vipers (rattlesnakes, for example).

Cryptococcosis - a fungal disease that may affect the respiratory tract (especially the nasal cavity), central nervous system, eyes, and skin (particularly of the face and neck of cats).

Cryptorchidism - a developmental defect marked by the failure of one or both testes to descend into the scrotum.

Cryptosporidiosis - intestinal infection with *cryptosporidium* parasites, the primary sign of which is diarrhea.

Cryptosporidium - a genus of single-celled protozoal parasites that causes intestinal infection in several species, including humans.

Ct scan - *see* computed tomography.

Culture - a method of encouraging a microorganism to grow in a laboratory in order to identify specific bacteria or viruses that may be present.

Cushing's disease - a hormonal disease characterized by overproduction of cortisol from the adrenal gland; most often caused by a tumor of the pituitary gland in the brain.

Cutaneous - of or relating to the skin.

Cyst - a closed, fluid-filled growth in otherwise normal tissue.

Cystitis - inflammation of the bladder.

Cystocentesis - extraction of a sample of urine directly from the bladder using a needle and syringe.

Cytokine - a protein secreted by cells of the immune system that helps regulate inflammatory responses.

Cytology - the study of the structure and function of individual cells.

Cytotoxic - substance that is poisonous to cells.

Debilitated - having greatly decreased energy and strength.

Debulking - a surgery done to remove part of a cancer or tumor.

Decongestant - a medication that reduces mucosal congestion.

Defecate - to expel feces from the intestinal tract.

Defibrillation - a process of shocking the heart in a specific way to restore a coordinated heart beat and a pulse.

Deficiency - a lack of something that is required for normal body function.

Degeneration - a condition that causes a gradual deterioration in the structure or function of a body part.

Degenerative joint disease - a form of arthritis characterized by gradual loss of cartilage of the joints. Also called osteoarthritis.

Dehydration - a lack of sufficient water within the body.

Dendrite - extension of a neuron that receives signals from other neurons and transmits electrical charges to the cell body.

Dental abscess - an infected cavity in a tooth, soft tissue surrounding the teeth, or bone of the jaw.

Dental malocclusion - a misalignment of the teeth in which the upper and lower surfaces fail to come together properly.

Depression - in animals, this usually refers to lowered activity and lack of interest in surroundings.

Dermatitis - inflammation of the skin.

Dermatologist - a specialist in the treatment of skin disorders.

Dermatophytosis - a fungal infection of the skin. Also known as ringworm.

Dermis - the middle layer of the 3 layers of the skin.

Descending aorta - the part of the aorta that passes through the chest and into the abdomen, supplying blood to the trunk and rear legs.

Desensitization - a way to gradually teach a pet to tolerate a situation by carefully exposing it to that situation in small steps.

Detergent - a cleansing substance, especially a liquid soap.

Dewlap - loose skin on the underside of an animal's neck; this is normal in many species.

Diabetes insipidus - a metabolic disorder caused by a lack of antidiuretic hormone, which leads to production of large amounts of dilute urine and excessive thirst.

Diabetes mellitus - a metabolic disorder characterized by a deficiency in the hormone insulin and an accompanying inability to properly digest sugars; signs include excessive urination, too much sugar in the blood, thirst, hunger, and weight loss.

Diagnosis - the identification of a disease based on its signs, physical examination, and appropriate tests.

Diaphragm - a thin muscle that separates the abdominal and thoracic cavities and expands the chest during respiration.

Diarrhea - the abnormally frequent discharge of soft or liquid feces.

Diastole - the first half of a heartbeat, during which the upper chambers of the heart (atria) contract and send blood into the lower chambers (ventricles).

Diestrus - a short period of sexual inactivity between 2 estrus periods, during which the uterus is prepared for a fertilized egg.

Dietary indiscretion - unhealthy eating, as of trash, large amounts of table scraps, or other inappropriate food.

Digestion - the process by which an animal processes food and absorbs nutrients.

Digestive tract - the system of organs responsible for digestion.

Dilate - to widen or enlarge.

Dilated cardiomyopathy - a heart disease in which the heart is enlarged and the heart muscle is weakened.

Direct life cycle - a pattern in which a parasite needs only 1 host in which to grow, breed, and reproduce itself.

Discharge - any fluid that emerges from a sore or infection.

Disinfectant - a chemical used to kill germs.

Dislocation - displacement of a body part, especially of a bone, from its usual fitting in a joint.

Displacement activity - the resolution of a behavior conflict by performing a seemingly unrelated activity such as grooming or sleeping.

Disseminated intravascular coagulation - a condition in which small blood clots develop throughout the bloodstream, blocking small blood vessels and destroying the platelets and clotting factors needed to control bleeding.

Dissemination - the spread of a disease-causing organism throughout the body, causing signs in multiple parts of the body.

Distemper - an airborne viral disease of dogs and some related animals such as raccoons; signs include fever, vomiting, diarrhea, loss of appetite, dehydration, tremors, weakness, and incoordination.

Distended - swollen or expanded, as by pressure from within; dilated.

Distillation - the evaporation and subsequent collection of a liquid by condensation as a means of purification.

Diuretic - a medicine usually prescribed to reduce fluid overload; increases urine production.

Dna - deoxyribonucleic acid; the molecule that encodes genetic information in the nucleus of cells and is capable of self-replication.

Doe - a female of any of several species, including rabbits and deer.

Dormant - existing in a temporarily inactive form or state, or biological rest.

Duodenum - the first and smallest portion of the small intestine, beginning at the stomach.

Dustborne - carried by exterior or interior dusts, often used to describe bacteria transmitted in this way.

Dysecdysis - improper or incomplete shedding of the skin in reptiles.

Dysplasia - abnormal growth, development, or placement of body parts.

Dystocia - abnormal or difficult birth.

Dystrophy - a degenerative condition caused by a nutritional defect or disorder.

Ear canal - the tube connecting the external ear with the eardrum.

Ear mites - tiny organisms resembling ticks that can infect the ear canal of animals, especially dogs and cats.

Eardrum - the membrane at the end of the ear canal that transmits sound waves to the middle ear.

Ecdysis - the act of molting, or shedding, an outer skin layer.

Echocardiography - a type of ultrasonography used to examine the heart.

Eclampsia - a condition marked by a sudden drop in blood calcium levels, caused by the production of milk after giving birth; often leads to convulsions and coma.

Ecosystem - a community of interdependent living organisms and the environment they inhabit.

Ectoparasite - a parasite that lives on its host's skin, hair, or feathers, such as fleas and ticks.

Ectotherm - an animal that cannot regulate its own body temperature and is instead dependent on the temperature of its surroundings (for example, reptiles and amphibians); commonly referred to as cold blooded.

Ectropion - a slack eyelid edge that is turned outward.

Edema - the abnormal accumulation of fluid in a tissue.

Egg binding - a condition in birds and reptiles in which the female is unable to lay a developed or partially developed egg.

Ehrlichiosis - a tickborne bacterial infection that affects white blood cells.

Elapid - a member of a family of venomous snakes with hollow fangs, such as cobras.

Electrocardiogram (ekg) - a recording of the heart's electrical activity made by attaching a set of electrodes to the skin.

Electrocardiography - recording of the electrical activity of the heart.

Electrolytes - ions, or salts, such as sodium and potassium, that are present in blood and other bodily fluids and help regulate various metabolic processes.

Electromyography - an electrical recording of muscle activity that aids in the diagnosis of diseases affecting muscles and peripheral nerves.

Elisa - an abbreviation for enzyme-linked immunosorbent assay, a test used to detect a disease-causing agent such as a virus.

Elokomin fluke fever - an infectious disease of dogs acquired by eating raw fish infected with flukes that carry the disease-causing bacteria.

Emaciation - a condition in which the animal is abnormally thin, generally as the result of malnutrition or disease.

Embolism - obstruction of a blood vessel by a blood clot that breaks off from its point of origin and lodges elsewhere.

Embolus - portion of a blood clot that breaks free and travels through the cardiovascular system.

Embryo - the earliest stage of development of an animal in the womb, before any of the major body organs have formed.

Emphysema - abnormal accumulation of air in tissues; often affects the lungs and causes breathing difficulties.

Emulsifier - a chemical agent used to bind together substances that normally do not bind.

Emulsion - a suspension of one liquid in another with which the first will not mix (for example, oil and water).

Encephalitis - inflammation of the brain; often caused by an infection.

Encephalitozoonosis - a protozoal infection of rabbits and occasionally of mice, guinea pigs, rats, and dogs that affects multiple organs; also called nosematosis.

Encysted - enclosed in a cyst, sac, bladder, or vesicle (for example, an *encysted* tumor).

Endocarditis - inflammation of the membranes lining the heart cavity.

Endocrine - related to glands that deliver hormones into the bloodstream.

Endoparasite - a parasite that lives inside its host, such as a heartworm.

Endoscope - an instrument for examining visually the interior of a bodily canal or a hollow organ such as the colon, bladder, or stomach.

Endoscopic gastric biopsy - a sample of stomach tissue taken with an endoscope, a long, flexible tube equipped with a camera and other instruments that is inserted through the mouth into the stomach.

Endoscopy - a procedure in which a tube called an endoscope is inserted into a hollow organ. The tube generally has a camera for maneuvering and frequently has tools such as forceps or scissors attached.

Endotoxin - a substance found in the cell walls of some bacteria that causes toxic shock, fever, and inflammation in mammals.

Endotracheal tube - tube inserted into the trachea to deliver oxygen or anesthetic gas.

Engorge - to fill with blood.

Enterolith - a hard mass composed of magnesium ammonium phosphate crystals that forms around a foreign object (such as a stone or nail) in the large intestine, most commonly in horses.

Enterotoxemia - the presence of bacterial toxins in the bloodstream.

Entropion - a turned-in edge of the eyelid, which leads to irritation of the eyeball from the eyelashes.

Enzootic - a disease that is continually present in a particular location.

Enzyme - a protein that speeds up a biological process such as digestion.

Eosinopenia - a decrease in the number of eosinophils (a type of white blood cell) in the bloodstream.

Eosinophil - a type of white blood cell that plays a role in the immune response by ingesting bacteria and other foreign cells, immobilizing and killing parasites, and participating in allergic reactions.

Eosinophilia - an increase in the number of eosinophils (a type of white blood cell) in the bloodstream.

Epidemic - an outbreak of a contagious disease that spreads rapidly and widely.

Epidermis - the outer layer of the 3 layers of the skin.

Epidural anesthesia - injection of pain-relieving or numbing drugs into the space surrounding the spinal cord to decrease sensation in parts of the body below that portion of the spinal cord; often used to provide anesthesia for surgery.

Epilepsy - an inherited disease that causes seizures; generally requires treatment with anticonvulsants.

Epithelial - having to do with the skin (epithelium).

Epizootic lymphangitis - a fungal disease that affects the skin, lymph vessels, and lymph nodes of the limbs and neck of horses.

Equine - related to or having to do with horses.

Equine granulocytic ehrlichiosis - an infectious disease of horses caused by a bacterium found in the bloodstream and transmitted by ticks.

Equine infectious anemia - an incurable, viral bloodborne infection of horses transmitted by blood-sucking insects.

Equine morbillivirus pneumonia - a short-term, often fatal, viral respiratory infection of horses caused by the hendra virus.

Equine protozoal myeloencephalitis - protozoal infection of the nervous system of horses.

Equine sarcoid - *see* sarcoid.

Equine viral arteritis - a short-term, contagious, viral disease of the horse family that affects multiple body systems.

Erosion - a shallow or superficial ulcer or sore, typically on the skin.

Erythrocyte - a red blood cell.

Erythropoiesis - the formation and production of red blood cells.

Erythropoietin - a hormone secreted by the kidneys that triggers the production of red blood cells in bone marrow.

Esophagus - the muscular tube that connects the throat to the stomach.

Estrous - of, relating to, or being in heat (estrus).

Estrous cycle - the recurring physiological and behavioral changes that take place from one period of estrus (heat) to another.

Estrus - a recurring period of increased sexual desire during which a female mammal will allow sexual activity and is capable of conceiving.

Euthanasia - the deliberate, painless killing of an incurably ill or injured animal; also called putting to sleep or putting down.

Excretion - the process for removing waste matter from the blood, tissues, or organs.

Exertional rhabdomyolysis - a metabolic disorder caused by intense exercise in which toxins from muscle injury can damage other tissues, especially the kidneys.

Exoskeleton - a skeletal structure outside the body, as in insects.

Exotic pets - nontraditional pets; animals that are not domesticated.

Expectorant - a medicine that thins airway secretions, making them easier for the animal to cough up.

Exposure - contact with or proximity to some environmental condition, toxin, or infectious agent.

Eyelid atresia - a congenital condition in which the eye opening is reduced or closed entirely over otherwise normal eyes.

Failing heart - any heart with a reduced ability to contract.

Farcy - a contagious, incurable bacterial infection of horses that may affect the skin or lungs. Also called glanders.

Farrier - a person who makes and fits horseshoes.

Fasting - withholding food from an animal for a certain length of time.

Fatal - causing or capable of causing death.

Fatty acid - one of the major components of fat, used by the body to supply energy and build tissues.

Fecal - relating to or consisting of feces.

Feces - the solid waste from an animal.

Feed hopper - a simple device that uses gravity to keep a trough or bowl filled with food as animals eat.

Feline - of or having to do with cats.

Feline distemper - *see* feline panleukopenia.

Feline infectious enteritis - *see* feline panleukopenia.

Feline infectious peritonitis - a progressive viral infection of cats that affects multiple body systems and causes a variety of signs.

Feline leukemia virus - a cancer-causing virus of cats that infects cells of the immune system and frequently results in death.

Feline lymphoma - a tumor of the immune system that is the most frequently diagnosed cancer of cats.

Feline panleukopenia - a viral infection of cats that affects multiple body systems; most infections cause no signs, but if signs are present the infection is serious and usually fatal.

Femur - the large bone of the upper hind limb; also known as the thigh bone.

Fertility - the ability to produce offspring.

Fertilization - the combination of a sperm cell and an egg cell into a developing organism.

Fetal - having to do with a fetus or its development.

Fetal membranes - the thin layers of tissue that surround the embryo during its development. Also called amniotic sac.

Fetus - a developing animal from the stage at which the major organs form until birth. *See also* embryo.

Fever - abnormally high body temperature.

Fibrocartilage - a type of strong, relatively inelastic connective tissue.

Fibroma - a benign tumor formed in fibrous or connective tissue.

Fibromatosis - a thickening and invasive growth in tendon sheaths.

Fibropapillomatosis - a condition characterized by the presence of abnormal growths of tissue (fibrous papillomas) in both the epidermal and dermal skin layers.

Fibrosarcoma - a malignant tumor that arises from cells that produce connective tissue, predominantly found in the area around bones or in soft tissue.

Fibrosis - the formation of excessive, dense, tough connective tissue.

Fibrous osteodystrophy - generalized loss of mineral salts throughout the skeleton due to an increased rate of bone destruction resulting from hyperparathyroidism (excess parathyroid hormone secretion). Also known as osteitis fibrosa cystica.

Fibrous tissue - tissue consisting primarily of high-strength fibers, such as ligaments and tendons.

Filly - a young female horse.

Filtration - the process of removing waste and particulate matter from water.

First aid - emergency medical treatment given until more thorough, professional veterinary treatment can be obtained.

Fistulous withers - a condition in which connective tissue in a horse's withers region becomes infected and inflamed.

Flagellate - a single-celled organism with one or more flagella, whip-like appendages used for locomotion.

Flashing - scratching (as pertains to fish).

Flea - a small, wingless insect that lives on the skin of mammals or birds and feeds on their blood.

Flexor tendons - any of several tendons that act to bend a joint.

Flora - bacteria that normally live in a part of the body, such as the intestines.

Fluke - any of almost 6,000 species of parasitic flatworms.

Fluorescein staining - a test that uses orange dye (fluorescein) and a specialized light to detect foreign bodies or scratches in the eye.

Fly strike - a condition in which flies lay their eggs on wounds, dead skin, or skin covered with feces. The maggots that hatch can destroy large areas of skin. Also called cutaneous myiasis.

Foal - the offspring of a horse or other equid, up to the age of 1 year.

Forceps - a surgical instrument used to grasp and hold tissue.

Forebrain - the front segment of the brain that includes the cerebrum, thalamus, and hypothalamus.

Foreskin - the loose fold of skin that covers the glans of the penis. Also called prepuce.

Fossorial species - an animal that is specially adapted for digging.

Fracture - the partial or complete break of a bone.

Frostbite - tissue damage caused by freezing temperatures, which can result in tissue death if exposure is extensive.

Fry - newly hatched fish.

Fungal - caused by, or related to, a fungus.

Fungus - a classification of living things that are immobile but cannot gain energy from sunlight, as plants can; some cause infections in animals and people.

Fur mite - external parasites that live on the skin and fur and cause itching.

Fur slip - a condition in chinchillas in which patches of fur are lost due to rough handling or fighting.

Gait - the manner of walking or moving.

Gastrin - a hormone that prompts the release of gastric acid in the stomach, usually secreted by the stomach and small intestine.

Gastrinoma - a tumor of the pancreatic islet cells.

Gastroenteritis - inflammation of the stomach and intestine, often resulting in diarrhea, vomiting, and cramps.

Gastrointestinal - having to do with the stomach and intestines.

Gastrointestinal system - the internal organs responsible for digestion, including the stomach and the intestines.

Gastrostomy - insertion of a tube directly into the stomach for the purpose of providing nutrition.

Genetic - having to do with genes or heredity.

Genitalia - external sex organs.

Geotrichosis - a rare fungal infection caused by *geotrichum candidum*, a fungus found in soil, decaying organic matter, and contaminated food.

Gestation - the period of development of an animal inside its mother's womb.

Giardia - a water-dwelling, single-celled microorganism that causes diarrhea in many species, including humans.

Giardiasis - a gastrointestinal disorder caused by infection with *giardia* microorganisms, characterized by diarrhea, stomach cramps, nausea, and vomiting.

Gingivitis - inflammation of the gums.

Glanders - a contagious, incurable, slowly progressive bacterial infection of horses that may affect the skin or lungs. Also called farcy.

Glaucoma - an eye disorder marked by increased pressure within the eye, which can damage the interior of the eye and lead to blindness.

Gliding membrane - a flap of skin which allows an animal to glide but not fly, as is found in sugar gliders and flying squirrels. Also called a patagium.

Globin - a globular protein that combines with heme to form hemoglobin. *See* hemoglobin.

Glomerulonephritis - inflammation of the glomeruli of the kidney.

Glomerulonephrosis - a common disease of older rats involving inflammation of the blood vessels in the kidney.

Glomerulus - structure in the kidney made up of special blood vessels that help filter blood; each kidney contains thousands of these.

Glossitis - inflammation of the tongue.

Glucagon - a hormone that helps convert stored carbohydrates into glucose (sugar) so they can be used as energy.

Glucocorticoid - a type of corticosteroid (*see* corticosteroid) that is involved with metabolism of carbohydrates, protein, and fat. They are frequently used in medicine for their anti-inflammatory and immuno-suppressive properties.

Glucose - a simple sugar that is one of the body's main sources of energy.

Glucosuria - the presence of glucose, a sugar, in the urine.

Gnat - a small, 2-winged biting fly.

Goiter - an enlarged thyroid, often caused by iodine deficiency.

Goitrogen - a goiter-producing substance.

Gonads - the sex organs that produce reproductive cells (sperm and eggs). In the male, these are the testes; in the female, the ovaries.

Gout - a painful inflammation of joints, often in the foot, that is most often caused by a buildup of uric acid and salts.

Granule - a small grain or particle; or a compound of powder particles that have been formed into larger pieces.

Granulocyte - a specialized type of white blood cell, produced in the bone marrow, that plays a role in immune responses to invading microorganisms.

Gray patch disease - a herpesviral infection of the skin that affects turtles, characterized by sores that spread across the turtle's body.

Growth plate - zone of cartilage near the ends of long bones where new bone is formed.

Gut loading - the process of feeding prey animals highly nutritious food in order to pass the nutrients on to animals that eat them.

Guttural pouch - areas of the eustachian tubes that form a bag or pouch, located under the base of the skull in horses.

Habituation - a simple form of learning that involves the ending of, or decrease in, a reaction to a situation as a result of repeated or prolonged exposure to that situation.

Halogenated - combined or treated with a halogen (fluorine, chlorine, bromine, iodine).

Hardpad disease - *see* canine distemper.

Head tilt - a condition in which the head is kept tipped to one side; can be caused by many different diseases, including inner ear infection and neurological problems.

Heart disease - any structural or functional abnormality of the heart that impairs its normal functioning.

Heart failure - any heart abnormality that results in failure of the heart to pump enough blood to meet the body's needs.

Heat exhaustion - a condition caused by overexertion in high temperatures or overexposure to the sun.

Heat stroke - a collapse brought on by prolonged periods of heat stress or heat exhaustion. Signs include cessation of sweating or panting, extremely high body temperature, and unconsciousness.

Helminth - a general term for a group of parasitic worms.

Hemangiosarcoma - a rare, rapidly growing, highly invasive cancer that originates from cells that line blood vessels (endothelial cells).

Hematology - the study of blood, its chemistry and components.

Hematoma - a mass of blood, generally clotted, that forms in an organ or body cavity due to a ruptured blood vessel.

Hematopoiesis - the formation and development of the various blood cells.

Heme - a complex molecule containing iron that combines with globin to form hemoglobin.

Hemoglobin - the iron-rich compound in blood that carries oxygen throughout the body.

Hemolysis - a condition in which red blood cells are ruptured.

Hemorrhage - bleeding; escape of blood from a broken blood vessel.

Hemostasis - a process that stops blood flow, particularly clot formation.

Hemostatic - a compound that inhibits bleeding.

Hepatic - related to or affecting the liver.

Hepatic encephalopathy - a syndrome that occurs as a result of liver disease; signs include circling, head pressing, aimless wandering, weakness, poor coordination, blindness, excessive drooling, aggression, dementia, seizures, and coma.

Hepatitis - inflammation of the liver.

Hepatopathy - general scientific term for liver disease.

Herbicide - one of a group of chemicals used to destroy weeds.

Herbivores - animals, such as rabbits or horses, that eat only plants.

Hereditary - transmitted genetically from parent to offspring.

Hernia - the protrusion of a body part through the lining that normally encloses it.

Herpesvirus - any of a group of viruses that cause disease in humans and animals. Herpesviruses often cause sores or rashes and generally remain in the body even when not causing signs.

Hibernation - a state of inactivity and unconsciousness, generally during the winter months.

Histiocytoma - a soft tissue giant cell tumor.

Histology - the anatomical study of the microscopic structure of tissue.

Histoplasmosis - a noncontagious infection caused by a soil fungus, occurring when airborne spores are inhaled.

Hives - the least severe type of anaphylactic (allergic) reaction. Small bumps occur on the skin. The hair may stand up over these swellings and sometimes they itch.

Hock - the ankle joint of rabbits, horses, and other 4-legged animals that walk on the same bones that form the toes in humans.

Hormone - a compound produced by a gland in the body that stimulates other parts of the body and controls their activity.

Host - a living animal or plant on or in which a parasite lives. *See* parasite.

Hot packing - a supportive treatment that involves application of moist heat to reduce inflammation.

Human-animal bond - the emotional relationship existing between humans and companion animals.

Husbandry - the care provided to maintain domestic animals.

Hutch - a pen or coop for a small animal, such as a rabbit.

Hutch burn - a disease caused by wet and dirty hutch floors in which the area surrounding the anus and genital region becomes inflamed and chapped, and then infected with disease-causing bacteria.

Hydration - the process of providing an adequate amount of fluids to body tissues.

Hydrocephalus - a condition in which excess fluid accumulates within the skull because of a blockage in the normal channels that allow it to flow out of the skull.

Hygiene - actions taken to maintain cleanliness and health.

Hygroma - a cyst or sac filled with fluid.

Hyper- - prefix meaning over, above, too much, too high, excessive.

Hyperadrenocorticism - a disease caused by production of too much cortisol. Also called cushing's disease.

Hypercalcemia - abnormally high levels of calcium in the blood, characterized by weakness, nausea, confusion, and lethargy.

Hyperextension - extension of a joint beyond its normal range of motion.

Hyperlipemia - excessive levels of fat in the blood.

Hyperparathyroidism - an excess of parathyroid hormone in the blood.

Hyperplasia - an abnormal increase in the number of cells in an organ or tissue with consequent enlargement.

Hypertension - an increase in the body's blood pressure.

Hyperthermia - abnormally high body temperature.

Hyperthyroidism - a disorder caused by an excess of the thyroid hormones.

Hypertrichosis - a common endocrine disorder resulting from chronic excess of the hormone cortisol (cushing's disease). Signs include development of an abnormally long or heavy hair coat, excessive thirst and urination, increased appetite and weight, an enlarged abdomen, and bulging eyes.

Hypertrophy - enlargement of an organ or tissue.

Hyperuricemia - abnormally high levels of uric acid in the blood, caused by excessive production or insufficient excretion of the compound.

Hypo- - prefix meaning below, less than normal, deficient, too little, too low.

Hypoadrenocorticism - a deficiency of adrenal gland hormones. Also called addison's disease.

Hypocalcemia - abnormally low levels of calcium in the blood.

Hypoglycemia - abnormally low levels of glucose in the blood, often caused by a deficiency of insulin, characterized by trembling, weakness, hunger, confusion, unconsciousness, and in severe cases, death.

Hypoparathyroidism - disorder characterized by low calcium levels, high phosphate levels, and either temporary or permanent insufficiency of parathyroid hormone.

Hypoplasia - a condition of abnormal development in which a body part remains small, immature, or underdeveloped.

Hypoproteinemia - abnormally low levels of protein in the blood.

Hypothalamus - the part of the brain below the thalamus that functions to regulate bodily temperature and certain metabolic processes.

Hypothermia - abnormally low body temperature.

Hypothyroidism - a deficiency of thyroid hormone, which can cause weight gain, constipation, and cold sensitivity.

Hypoxia - condition in which the level of oxygen in the blood is too low; anoxia.

Idiopathic - used to describe a disorder or disease that has no apparent cause.

Immersion - a method of administering medication to or treating fish by placing them in a tank containing the medication.

Immune - resistant to infection or disease.

Immune response - the body's reaction to an infectious agent or other foreign "invader." This includes recognition of the invader and development of a protective defense.

Immune system - the system within an animal that recognizes an infectious agent or other foreign "invader" and mounts an immune response. The immune system includes various organs, such as the thymus gland, spleen, and lymph nodes, as well as specialized cells found throughout the body.

Immune-mediated - describes a process initiated or controlled by the immune system.

Immunization - the process of making an individual immune to a given disease, generally through vaccination.

Immunized - rendered resistant to toxins or infectious agents, especially by injection or vaccination.

Immunodeficiency - an inability of the immune system to produce a normal immune response.

Immunoglobulin - protein antibodies produced by the body to fight a disease.

Immunomodulator - a drug that helps regulate the immune system's activity.

Immunostimulant - a drug or agent that increases an immune response.

Immunosuppressed - a state in which the immune system is inhibited by medications during the treatment of other disorders, or by stress or infection.

Immunosuppression - interference with the normal function of the immune system.

Immunotherapy - any of several treatments of disease that involve inducing, enhancing, or suppressing an immune response.

Impedance - obstruction of normal flow or passage, such as an obstruction of blood flow.

Implant - a drug, such as a long-lasting tablet, inserted under the skin.

Incisor - front teeth that are used to grasp or cut food.

Inclusion body disease - any disease characterized by inclusion bodies, small foreign bodies within cells.

Incontinence - the inability to control urination or defecation.

Incubation period - the time after an infection has been contracted but before any signs are apparent.

Infection - a disorder that occurs when microorganisms invade the body and multiply. Infectious microorganisms include bacteria, viruses, fungi, and parasites.

Infectious - a condition that is passed from animal to animal by a virus, bacterium, or other agent.

Infectious canine hepatitis - a contagious viral disease of dogs with signs that vary from a slight fever and congestion of the mucous membranes to severe depression, severe reduction in white blood cells, and deficiency of blood clotting.

Infertility - the inability to produce offspring.

Infest - to live as a parasite in or on.

Infestation - the act of infesting or state of being infested.

Infiltrate - material deposited within the space between cells in a tissue.

Inflammation - a localized protective response to injury or other tissue damage. The response includes increased blood flow in the surrounding capillaries (causing redness), swelling, increased temperature in the area, and pain.

Inflammatory - characterized or caused by inflammation.

Influenza - a respiratory infection caused by an influenza (flu) virus.

Ingest - to take food or liquid into the body by swallowing or absorption; eat.

Inhalation - the act of breathing in.

Inherited - passed genetically from parents to offspring.

Inhibitor - a substance that restrains or retards physiological, chemical, or enzyme action.

Initiation - the first step in the transformation of healthy cells into cancerous cells.

Inoculation - introduction of a substance into the tissues or fluids of the body; this is often done for the purpose of preventing or curing certain diseases.

Inorganic - composed of minerals rather than living material; without carbon.

Insect growth regulator - a class of drugs that helps control pests such as fleas by disrupting their development and maturation.

Insecticidal - of or related to a chemical substance used to kill insects.

Insulin - a hormone secreted by the pancreas that is essential for digestion, especially that of carbohydrates. *See also* diabetes mellitus.

Insulinoma - a common pancreatic islet tumor that affects the insulin-secreting beta cells.

Interdigital furunculosis - abscesses on the webbing between the toes.

Interferon - protein produced by immune cells that helps fight viral infection. *See also* cytokines.

Intermediate host - an animal in which juvenile parasites reside before passing to the final host animal to develop into adults and breed.

Intestinal protozoan - any of a number of single-celled microorganisms that infect or dwell within the intestines. Many cause disease, but others are harmless or even beneficial.

Intestine - the part of the digestive tract between the stomach and the anus, divided into the small intestine and the large intestine.

Intoxication - another term for poisoning or toxicosis.

Intramuscular - directly in or into the muscle.

Intraocular - having to do with, entering, or residing within the interior of the eye.

Intravascular - inside the blood vessels.

Intravenous - a method of administering fluids or medications directly into a vein. Also known by the abbreviation iv.

Intubation - insertion of a breathing tube into the trachea.

Intussusception - the doubling up of a section of intestine on itself in accordion-like folds, causing obstruction.

Invasive - a tumor that tends to spread locally into adjacent tissues.

Invertebrate - an animal without a backbone, such as an insect or spider.

Involuntary - spontaneous or automatic; not controllable by the conscious mind.

Iodine deficiency - insufficient iodine in the diet that can lead to goiter.

Iodine toxicity - harmful effects, which may include goiter, of an excess of iodine in the diet.

Iris - the muscular diaphragm in the eye that controls the size of (and therefore the amount of light passing through) the pupil.

Irradiation - bombardment with radiation, generally as a treatment for tumors.

Islet cell tumor - a cancer of the islet cells of the pancreas.

Islet of langerhans - cluster of 3 kinds of endocrine cells scattered throughout the pancreas that secrete several hormones, including insulin.

Isolation - the process of keeping diseased or potentially diseased animals separate from other susceptible animals.

Jaundice - a condition characterized by yellowing of the skin, eyes, and mucous membranes caused by an excess of bile products in the blood.

Joint - the site where 2 or more bones meet. Joints may be movable or immovable.

Joint mice - fragments of cartilage in joints.

Jugular - of, relating to, or located in the region of the neck or throat.

Keratin - the hard protein that makes up hair, fingernails, claws, horns, scales, and the shafts of feathers.

Keratinization - creation of new skin cells near the base of the epidermis that migrate upwards, producing a compact layer of dead cells on the skin surface.

Keratoacanthoma - a benign skin tumor of dogs that includes a cyst filled with keratin.

Ketosis - a condition resulting from excess buildup of ketones, a waste product, in the blood.

Kidney - either of a pair of abdominal organs that filter waste from the blood and help maintain proper water and salt balance.

Kidney failure - loss of normal function of the kidneys, which can be either a short- or longterm condition.

Kit - the young of any of a number of mammals, such as foxes and rabbits.

Laceration - a cut or tear in the skin.

Lacrimal gland - the gland near the eye that produces tears.

Lactation - the production of milk by a female mammal.

Lactobacillus species - a group of bacteria that create lactic acid and play a normal, often beneficial, role in many animals' bodies.

Lagenidiosis - a fungal infection of dogs that affects the skin and blood vessels.

Lagophthalmos - an inability to completely close the eyelids due to malformation.

Lameness - an inability to walk or move normally, often, but not always, caused by pain in the limb.

Larva - an immature form or life stage of an insect or parasite.

Larvae - plural form of the word larva.

Larval - of or pertaining to larvae.

Larynx - the part of the throat often called the "voice box" in humans.

Latent - in an inactive or hidden stage.

Laxative - a drug used to promote bowel movements.

Leg banding - the process of putting coded bands onto the legs of captive birds, generally while they are young, for purposes of identification.

Legg-calvé-perthes disease - deterioration of the top of the femur (the femoral head) seen in young miniature and small breeds of dogs, characterized by a lack of blood supply and destruction of blood vessels of the bone.

Lens - the transparent, oval-shaped part of the eye that focuses light on the retina.

Leptospirosis - an infection characterized by fever and jaundice caused by bacteria of the genus *leptospira.*

Lesion - any abnormal change in the structure or function of a part of the body.

Lethargy - lack of energy; apathy.

Leukemia - a cancer of the blood and bone marrow, characterized by increased numbers of white blood cells.

Leukocyte - blood cell type involved in immune responses; commonly called white blood cells.

Leukocytic - having to do with leukocytes.

Leukocytosis - an increase in the number of white blood cells in the bloodstream.

Leukogram - a diagnostic blood test that counts the number of different white blood cells circulating in the bloodstream.

Leukopenia - a decrease in the number of white blood cells in the bloodstream.

Libido - sexual drive; desire to mate.

Lice - a group of small, wingless insects that live on the skin of birds and mammals and suck their blood.

Life cycle - a description of all the stages in the life of an organism.

Ligament - a band of tough, fibrous tissue connecting bones or cartilage at a joint, or supporting an organ.

Liposarcoma - a benign tumor of fatty tissue.

Listeriosis - an infection by the bacteria *listeria monocytogenes* which can affect the nervous system, or lead to abortion or blood poisoning.

Liver - a large abdominal organ with many functions, such as filtering and removing toxins from the blood, storing glycogen, and producing and secreting bile.

Localized - restricted or limited to a specific body part or region.

Lockjaw - a spasm of the jaw muscles that keeps them tightly closed, most frequently caused by tetanus. *See also* tetanus.

Long bones - any of several elongated bones of the legs (for example, the femur and humerus) that have a roughly cylindrical shaft.

Lordosis - an abnormal inward curving of the spine in the lower area of the back.

Lumpectomy - surgical excision of a tumor with minimal removal of surrounding tissue.

Lumpy jaw - the most common and least severe form of actinomycosis, a bacterial infection that causes hard masses to form in the mouth and jaw.

Lung - either of 2 spongy, saclike respiratory organs that occupy the chest cavity and provide the blood with oxygen while removing carbon dioxide during respiration.

Luxation - dislocation.

Lyme disease - tickborne infection of animals and humans caused by *borrelia burgdorferi* bacteria that can cause rash and arthritis. Also known as lyme borreliosis.

Lymph node - small organ of the immune system that contains cells that fight infections, neutralize toxins, and produce antibodies.

Lymph - a clear, watery fluid derived from body tissues that collects through the lymphatic system and is then returned to the bloodstream.

Lymphadenitis - inflammation of the lymph nodes.

Lymphangitis - inflammation of lymphatic vessels.

Lymphatic system - the network of small vessels that collects the fluid surrounding the cells and returns it to the bloodstream.

Lymphocyte - white blood cells that produce antibodies, neutralize toxins, and fight infections and cancer.

Lymphocytic choriomeningitis - a viral infection of mice characterized by fever, vomiting, neck stiffness, and slow pulse.

Lymphocytosis - an increase in the number of lymphocytes in the bloodstream.

Lymphoid - of or relating to the lymph or lymphatic tissue.

Lymphoma - a cancer of certain white blood cells that begins in a lymph node or other lymphoid tissue.

Lymphopenia - a decrease in the number of lymphocytes in the bloodstream.

Macrophage - a type of white blood cell, larger than most, that consumes infectious agents and other foreign cells and destroys them.

Maggot - the legless, soft-bodied, wormlike larva of any of various flies, often found in decaying matter.

Magnetic resonance imaging (mri) - an advanced, noninvasive diagnostic imaging technique that uses powerful magnets to examine tissues and organs.

Malabsorption - faulty or abnormal absorption of nutrients from the digestive tract.

Malaise - a feeling of illness or depression.

Maldigestion - abnormal breakdown and absorption of foods from the digestive tract.

Malignant - cancerous; a tumor that invades other nearby tissues or spreads throughout the body.

Malnourished - affected by an improper or insufficient diet; undernourished.

Malocclusion - *see* dental malocclusion.

Mammals - animals that produce milk to feed their young and have 4 limbs and at least some hair.

Mammary - of or relating to the mammary glands of a female mammal.

Mammary glands - the organs that produce milk.

Mange - any of several skin disorders caused by an infestation of mange mites.

Marking - depositing urine or feces to send a social signal, such as claiming territory.

Marsupials - mammals, chiefly but not exclusively from australia, that carry their young in an external pouch.

Masking behavior - behavior to hide injury or weakness, especially by prey animals.

Mass - another word for a tumor or growth.

Mast cell - a cell that secretes histamine found in connective tissue.

Mastitis - inflammation of the mammary glands, often caused by bacterial infection.

Maternal immunity - the resistance to disease provided by antibodies passed through the mother's first milk (colostrum) to newborn mammals, usually lasting for several weeks.

Mechanism - a process by which something is accomplished.

Megakaryocyte - a large cell found in bone marrow that produces platelets.

Melanoma - a type of skin tumor, often malignant, that contains dark pigment.

Melioidosis - an uncommon bacterial infection, usually of rodents, that can be passed to humans.

Membrane - a thin layer of tissue that lines an organ or body cavity.

Meninges - thin layers of tissue that line the brain and spinal cord.

Meningitis - inflammation of the meninges.

Meningoencephalitis - inflammation of the brain and of the membrane lining the brain and spinal cord.

Metabolic activity - the chemical processes occurring within a living cell or organism that are essential to maintenance of life.

Metabolic bone disease - any of several diseases of the bones caused by an imbalance of calcium and other minerals in response to abnormal metabolism.

Metabolic disorder - any disorder in which normal body processes are disturbed, leading to an increase or decrease in the end products of those processes.

Metabolic rate - metabolism over time; the speed at which metabolism occurs.

Metabolism - the physical and chemical processes that take place in the body to maintain life.

Metacarpal bones - bones in a vertebrate animal's forefoot similar to the bones in the human hand between the wrist and the fingers.

Metastasis - the spread of a malignant tumor to distant parts of the body.

Metastatic calcification - abnormal, hardened deposits of calcium in soft tissues.

Metastatic tumor - a tumor formed from cells that have traveled from the original tumor to another site in the body.

Metatarsal bones - bones in a vertebrate animal's hind foot similar to bones in the human foot between the toes and the ankle.

Metritis - inflammation of the uterus.

Microbiology - the study of small organisms such as bacteria, viruses, fungi, and other single-celled life forms.

Microchipping - a method of identifying pets that involves the insertion of a small glass-encased electronic chip under the skin.

Microfilaria - immature life stage of heartworms that is found in the bloodstream.

Microhabitat - the small, specialized environment in which an organism lives.

Microorganism - a bacterium, virus, or other organism that is too small to see without a microscope.

Midges - gnatlike flies that are often found near water; some species bite and feed on blood.

Miliary dermatitis - skin irritation with small, solid, bumps typically spread over the back, neck, and face.

Mineralocorticoids - hormones produced by the adrenal cortex that help control the body's balance of sodium and potassium salts.

Mineral - a solid crystalline substance arising from inorganic processes. Many minerals are nutrients that are needed for normal body functions.

Mite - any of a number of very small arachnids, related to spiders and scorpions, many of which live as parasites on various species of animals.

Mitral valve - the valve between the left chambers of the heart, through which the blood flows from the atrium to the ventricle.

Molar - a large grinding tooth in the back of the mouth.

Mold - any of various fungi that often cause disintegration of organic matter.

Molt - in birds, the normal loss of feathers in preparation for the growth of new feathers. In reptiles, the normal shedding of skin; also called ecdysis.

Mongolian desert mice - another term for gerbils, related to their origin.

Monkeypox - a viral disease, similar to but milder than smallpox, originally detected in monkeys.

Monocyte - a type of white blood cell that plays a role in immune defense by moving from the bloodstream into the tissues, enlarging, and becoming a macrophage. *See also* macrophage.

Monocytopenia - a decrease in the number of monocytes in the bloodstream.

Monocytosis - an increase in the number of monocytes in the bloodstream.

Mortality - the rate of death in a population.

Mosquito - a winged insect that feeds on blood and can transmit disease.

Motor - relating to motion, or body movement.

Motor function - the ability to produce body movement by complex interaction of the brain, nerves, and muscles.

Motor neurons - nerve cells that carry signals from the brain that control muscle activity.

Mri - *see* magnetic resonance imaging.

Mucosa - *see* mucous membrane.

Mucous membrane - the layer of cells that lines the tubular organs of the body, such as the digestive and respiratory tracts.

Mucus - a slippery secretion produced by glands of the mucous membranes.

Multifocal - relating to or arising from many locations.

Murmur - a vibration heard coming from the heart or major blood vessels.

Muscle - a tissue composed of fibers capable of contracting (and thus producing motion).

Muscular wasting - the steady loss of muscle mass and strength.

Musculoskeletal - having to do with the muscles, bones, and joints.

Mustelidae - latin term for the scientific family that includes ferrets, mink, and skunks.

Mutation - a spontaneous, permanent change in genetic material that is passed to the organism's offspring.

Muzzle - an animal's nose and jaws.

Mycetoma - infection of the skin and underlying tissues that has the appearance of a nodule or tumor.

Mycobacterial infections - *see* mycobacteriosis.

Mycobacteriosis - infection by mycobacteria, a group that includes the bacteria responsible for leprosy and tuberculosis.

Mycoplasma - the smallest known type of bacteria, which lack cell walls.

Mycosis - fungal infection.

Mycotoxicosis - disease caused by toxins produced by fungi.

Myelography - a specialized x-ray procedure in which a dye is injected into the cerebrospinal canal to outline the spinal cord.

Myiasis - maggot infestation. Also known as strike.

Myocardial disease - a disorder of the heart muscle.

Myocarditis - a local or widespread inflammation of the heart muscle with degeneration or death of the heart muscle cells.

Myocardium - the muscular tissue of the heart.

Myopathy - general term referring to any skeletal muscle disease.

Myositides - diseases that produce a mainly inflammatory reaction in muscle.

Myositis - inflammation of a muscle, characterized by pain, tenderness, and sometimes spasm in the affected area.

Myxomatosis - a severe viral disease in rabbits, characterized by the formation of myxoma, or soft, gelatinous tumors, and subsequent swelling around the head, face, and genitals.

Nagana - an often fatal disease of vertebrates transmitted by the bite of the tsetse fly; may affect multiple body systems and often causes anemia.

Nares - the openings of the nose.

Nasal - having to do with the nose, often its interior.

Nasal cavity - the air-filled space above and behind the nose, on either side of the septum.

Nasal discharge - material, typically mucus, emerging from the nose.

Nasogastric tube - a feeding tube that is inserted through the nose into the stomach.

Nasolacrimal duct - a duct that moves tears from the eye to the nose.

Nebulization - conversion of a substance, such as a medication, from a liquid or solid state into a fine mist or vapor.

Necropsy - an animal autopsy.

Necrotic dermatitis - inflammation of the skin characterized by localized death of tissue.

Necrotic meningoencephalitis - a disease caused by infection of the brain with microorganisms, with signs that may include depression, lethargy, labored breathing, loss of appetite, bluish skin, and a pus-like discharge from the nose.

Nematode - a parasitic worm; also called a roundworm.

Neonatal - having to do with newborn offspring.

Neoplasia - the formation of a tumor.

Neoplasm - a tumor.

Neosporosis - an infectious disease of dogs and other animals caused by the protozoan parasite *neospora caninum*.

Nephritis - inflammation of the kidney.

Nephrotic - of or relating to the kidneys.

Nephrotic syndrome - signs of disease in the kidney that may include protein in the urine, low levels of protein in the blood, a buildup of fluid in the abdomen, shortness of breath, and swelling in the legs.

Nerve - specialized tissues that transmit electrical impulses serving to relay sensory or motor information between the nervous system and body organs.

Nest box - a man-made box provided for animals to nest in.

Neuroendocrine tissue tumors - tumors that can develop from neuroendocrine cells (found in tissues that have both nervous system and hormone-producing functions) in the adrenal or thyroid glands.

Neurologic - of or pertaining to the nervous system.

Neurologic signs - impairments of perception or behavior caused by damage to the central nervous system.

Neuromuscular - having to do with the terminations of nerves in muscle tissue.

Neuron - the specialized cells of the nervous system responsible for transmitting electrical signals.

Neuropathic pain - pain resulting from damage to a nerve or some other part of the central nervous system.

Neurotransmitter - a chemical released by a nerve cell that passes signals to other nerve cells, or to muscles or glands.

Neuter - to remove the internal reproductive organs (that is, the ovaries and uterus or testes) of an animal in order to prevent reproduction.

Neutropenia - a decrease in the number of neutrophils in the bloodstream.

Neutrophil - a common type of white blood cell that engulfs and destroys bacteria and other foreign cells.

Neutrophilia - an increase in the number of neutrophils in the bloodstream.

Nevus - a congenital pigmented area on the skin; sometimes called a birthmark.

Newcastle disease - a contagious viral disease in birds, whose signs include coughing, sneezing, diarrhea, tremors, and twitching.

Nictitating membrane - a thin membrane in many animals that can extend across the eye to protect it; also called the third eyelid.

Nit - the small egg of a louse, typically found glued to hair.

Nitrates - chemical compounds that can be used by plants and algae as food, or removed by water filtration.

Nocardiosis - a chronic, noncontagious disease caused by *nocardia* bacteria found in soil, decaying vegetation, and other environmental sources.

Nocturnal - an animal that is active only or primarily at night.

Nodule - a small, irregular, rounded mass.

Noncontagious - not contagious; not communicable by contact.

Nonregenerative anemia - a decrease in the number of red blood cells, which the bone marrow is not able to fully compensate for by creating new red blood cells.

Nonsteroidal anti-inflammatory drug (nsaid) - a group of medications other than corticosteroids that relieve pain, fever, and inflammation.

Nonviremic - animals that, despite being infected by a virus, show no evidence of it in the bloodstream.

Nuclear scintigraphy - a diagnostic procedure involving dosing the animal with a radioactive element. This element is then detected within the body by means of a special camera attached to a computer, which generates the image.

Nutrient - a substance that nourishes a living thing.

Nutrition - a source of nourishment; food.

Nutritional deficiency - a lack in the type or amount of nutrients an organism receives.

Nutritional osteodystrophy - defective bone formation, as in rickets, caused by an imbalance of calcium and phosphorus in the diet.

Nymph - the larval form of certain insects.

Nymphomania - prolonged estrus or sexually receptive behavior in a female animal.

Nystagmus - abnormal, involuntary, usually rapid movement of the eyeballs as a result of dizziness, head injury, or disease.

Obstruction - blockage of a passage in the body, as of the intestines.

Ocular - of or relating to the eye.

Ocular fundus - the back layer of the eye opposite the pupil where light is detected by specialized nerve cells.

Ointment - a healing salve intended for external application.

Oncologist - a cancer specialist.

Oncology - the field of medicine dedicated to the study, diagnosis, and treatment of cancer.

Oocyst - a fertilized egg in the process of development; a zygote.

Oomycosis - infection with oomycetes fungi, most common among fish.

Opaque - something through which light cannot pass.

Ophthalmoscope - an instrument for viewing the interior of the eye.

Opiate - a class of narcotic drugs derived from opium that can reduce pain, induce sleep, and suppress coughing.

Opioid - any of a class of synthetic drugs that are not derived from opium but have similar properties. *See* opiate.

Opportunistic agent - an infectious substance or microorganism, not normally dangerous, that can cause disease when the body's immune system is impaired or weakened.

Opportunistic infection - an infection by a microorganism that normally does not cause disease but becomes capable of doing so when the body's immune system is impaired or weakened.

Optic disk - the point on the retina where the optic nerve enters the eye. Also called the blind spot.

Optic nerve - the nerve that connects the eye to the brain and transmits visual information; also called the second cranial nerve.

Optimal temperature zone - the preferred temperature range for a species.

Oral - having to do with the mouth.

Oral cavity - the interior of the mouth.

Orbit - the part of the skull that encloses and protects the eye and related structures.

Organ - a structure composed of various types of tissues that has a specific function; most organs function as part of an organ system.

Organic - relating to a substance derived from a living organism; containing carbon.

Organism - an individual form of life, such as a plant, an animal, a bacterium, or a fungus.

Osmoregulation - maintenance of an optimal balance in the concentration of salts in the body's fluids.

Osteoarthritis - *see* degenerative joint disease.

Osteochondritis dissecans - a condition usually seen in young animals in which the immature joint cartilage separates from the underlying bone.

Osteochondrosis - a condition in which immature joint cartilage separates from the bone and floats loosely in the joint cavity, where it can cause inflammation and interfere with proper bone formation.

Osteomalacia - a condition in adult animals in which the bones soften because of an imbalance in calcium and phosphorus metabolism.

Osteomyelitis - inflammation of the bones caused by a bacterial infection.

Osteoporosis - a condition marked by loss of bone mass due to poor nutrition, age, or nursing.

Osteosarcoma - a malignant bone tumor.

Otitis - inflammation of the ear.

Otitis externa - inflammation of the external ear canal.

Otitis interna - inflammation of the inner ear.

Otitis media - inflammation of the middle ear.

Otoscope - an instrument with a light and a magnifying lens to aid visual examination of the ear canal.

Outbreak - a sudden occurrence or appearance, as of a disease.

Ovary - the female reproductive organ that produces eggs, as well as the hormones estrogen and progesterone.

Ovariohysterectomy - the surgical removal of the ovaries and uterus.

Over-the-counter - sold directly to the public without a doctor's prescription.

Ovulation - the release of an egg (ovum) from the ovary for possible fertilization.

Oxygenate - to treat, combine, or infuse with oxygen.

Oxytocin - a hormone that stimulates milk flow, causes the uterus to contract during and after birth, and increases maternal behavior.

Paecilomycosis - an infection caused by fungi of the genus *paecilomyces* that affects the lungs and other organs.

Palliative - a drug or medicine used to relieve or soothe the signs of disease.

Palpation - examination by finger pressure to detect growths, changes in underlying organs, and unusual tissue reactions to pressure.

Pancreas - a large gland that secretes digestive enzymes and hormones, such as insulin, that regulate blood sugar levels.

Panhypopituitarism - a disorder in which the pituitary gland and nearby tissues, including the hypothalamus, are compressed or damaged, leading to a lack of several different hormones.

Papilloma - a wart or other benign growth on the skin or other vascular tissues.

Papillomatosis - any condition marked by the presence of many papillomas. *See* papilloma.

Papule - a small, hard, round bump or protuberance on the skin.

Paralysis - partial or total loss of motor function or sensation in part of the body.

Paramyxovirus - any of a group of viruses including those that cause measles, mumps, rubella, and newcastle disease.

Paranasal - adjacent to the nasal cavity.

Parasite - any living organism that lives inside, with, or close to another living creature (called a host) and uses the host as a source of food, shelter, or other requirements.

Parasitic - of, related to, or caused by a parasite.

Parasitism - a close relationship in which one species, the parasite, benefits at the expense of the other, the host.

Parathyroid glands - glands that secrete parathyroid hormone and calcitonin.

Parathyroid hormone - a hormone that acts with vitamin d and another hormone, calcitonin, to regulate the levels of calcium in the body.

Parvovirus - a family of viruses including a type that causes a highly contagious intestinal disease of dogs.

Passerine - describes the group of perching birds and songbirds such as jays, blackbirds, finches, warblers, and sparrows.

Paste - a semisolid drug dosage form for treating animals.

Pasteurellosis - infection with *pasteurella* bacteria, which most frequently infect the respiratory tract.

Patagium - *see* gliding membrane.

Patella - kneecap; a flat triangular bone located at the front of the knee joint.

Patellar luxation - displacement of the kneecap.

Patent ductus arteriosus - a heart defect in which the ductus arteriosus (the temporary fetal blood vessel connecting the aorta and the pulmonary artery) does not close at birth.

Pathogenic - producing disease, or having the capability to cause disease.

Pathologic - relating to or caused by disease.

Pathologist - a veterinarian or physician who specializes in examining tissue samples to identify the cause of disease or death.

Pectoral muscle - any of the muscles that connect to the chest at one end and to the bones of the front limbs at the other end.

Pelvic canal - the passage from the abdomen through the bones of the pelvis to the outside of the body.

Penicillosis - infection by mold of the genus *penicillium*, which usually affects the nose and sinuses.

Penis - the external male organ of copulation, used to transfer semen to the female and to expel urine.

Pentastomes - worms that infest the respiratory system of birds, reptiles, and mammals. Also called tongue worms due to their appearance.

Perianal - situated or occurring around the anus.

Pericardial disease - disease of the pericardium, the sac surrounding the heart.

Pericardiocentesis - insertion of a needle through the pericardium (the sac surrounding the heart) to withdraw fluid.

Pericarditis - inflammation of the sac or lining around the heart.

Pericardium - the sac-like membrane surrounding the heart.

Periodontal - of or relating to the gums.

Perioperative - the period immediately before and after a surgical procedure.

Peripheral nervous system - the parts of the nervous system outside of the brain and spinal cord.

Peritoneal cavity - the space between the membranes lining the abdominal cavity and the abdominal organs.

Peritoneal lavage - rinsing of the peritoneal cavity with saline or other fluids as a part of a diagnostic test to look for signs of infection or inflammation.

Peritoneum - the membrane lining the abdominal cavity and the organs found within it.

Peritonitis - inflammation of the peritoneum, often caused by infection or injury to the gastrointestinal tract.

Permeability - the rate at which a liquid or gas passes through a membrane or other porous material.

Persistent - tenaciously or obstinately continuing, often for a long time.

Pesticide - a chemical that kill pests, especially insects.

Ph - a measure of the acidity or alkalinity of a fluid or damp substance.

Phaeohyphomycosis - a fungal infection that usually occurs because of contamination of tissue at the site of an injury.

Phagocyte - a cell that ingests and kills other substances, especially microorganisms.

Phagocytosis - the process by which cells engulf and digest microorganisms and cellular debris; an important defense against infection.

Phalanx - any of the bones that form the digits, corresponding to fingers and toes in humans.

Pharmacology - the science that deals with the chemistry, development, uses, and metabolism of drugs.

Pharynx - the throat.

Pheochromocytoma - a tumor of the adrenal gland that is able to secrete adrenaline (epinephrine) and other hormones.

Pheromone - a chemical secreted by an animal that influences the behavior or development of others of the same species; often serving to attract the opposite sex.

Phobia - an intense and excessive fear of something.

Photoperiod - the amount of time per day that an organism is exposed to sunlight or artificial light.

Photoreceptor - any structure that senses the presence of light.

Photosensitization - a condition in which skin is overly sensitive to sunlight; distinct from sunburn.

Pica - the eating of non-food items, such as gravel or dirt.

Pigmentation - the deposition of coloring matter (pigment) in a cell or tissue.

Pink eye - *see* conjunctivitis.

Pinna - the large visible portion of the external ear.

Pinworm - any of a group of small, parasitic nematodes that live in the intestines of vertebrates.

Piping - refers to the activity of fish swimming near the surface of the water trying to gulp air.

Pituitary - related to the pituitary gland of the brain that produces hormones critical for control of many bodily functions.

Pituitary dwarfism - disorder of the pituitary gland in which a shortage of growth hormone leads to smaller than normal size.

Pituitary gland - a small, oval, endocrine gland attached to the base of the brain which secretes hormones that control many other endocrine glands.

Placenta - the organ that connects the fetus to the mother in most mammals and regulates the exchange of nutrients between them.

Placental - of or relating to the placenta.

Plague - an acute and sometimes fatal bacterial disease, transmitted primarily by the fleas of rats and other rodents.

Plasma - the clear, yellowish fluid portion of blood or lymph in which cells are suspended.

Plasmodial organisms - single-celled protozoal parasites that live within the bloodstream and cause malaria.

Platelet - a type of small blood cell responsible for clotting. Also called a thrombocyte.

Pleura - the membranes lining the outside of the lungs and the chest cavity.

Pleural cavity - the space between the membranes lining the chest wall and the lungs.

Pleurisy - inflammation of the lining around the lungs (the pleura), causing pain, cough, chest tenderness, and shortness of breath.

Pneumonia - inflammation of the lung tissue, often accompanied by inflammation of the trachea and other large airways; also known as pneumonitis.

Pneumonitis - *see* pneumonia.

Pneumothorax - air in the space between the lungs and the chest wall.

Pododermatitis - inflammation of the skin near the foot or hoof.

Poison - a substance that causes illness, injury, or death if ingested.

Polioencephalomalacia - a neurologic disease that leads to softening and degeneration in the outer layer of the brain.

Poll evil - bacterial infection and inflammation of a sac surrounding a tendon near the base of the skull in horses.

Polyarteritis nodosa - inflammation of the walls of arteries that affects multiple organs.

Polycythemia - an increase in the number of red blood cells circulating in the bloodstream.

Polydactyly - the presence of extra toes, which is a common inherited condition in cats.

Polyp - a growth or mass projecting from the tissue of a membrane, sometimes tumorous.

Polyphagia - excessive appetite or overeating.

Polysaccharide - a complex carbohydrate such as starch or cellulose, made up of sugar molecules in a chain structure.

Porphyrin - a protein molecule that is one of the building blocks of hemoglobin, the molecule that carries oxygen in the bloodstream.

Portosystemic shunt - a congenital defect in the blood vessels of the liver that reduces the ability of the liver to process waste products.

Positive inotrope - any of a class of drugs used to help the heart muscle contract.

Postpartum hypocalcemia - *see* puerperal hypocalcemia.

Powder - a formulation in which a drug powder is mixed with other powdered fillers to produce a final product.

Predation - the hunting and eating of other animals.

Predilection - a particular liking or preference.

Predisposing factor - a condition or situation that increases the susceptibility to a particular disease or injury.

Pregnancy toxemia - an often-fatal metabolic condition of pregnant guinea pigs, cows, and sheep, more common in those that are overweight, in which a buildup of toxins occurs in the bloodstream.

Prenatal - of or relating to the period before birth.

Prepuce - a retractable fold of skin covering the penis in many mammals.

Prevalent - widely or commonly occurring.

Priapism - an abnormal, persistent erection of the penis, often caused by spinal cord injury or injury to the penis.

Primary factor - the main cause, or one of the main causes, of a disease or injury.

Prognathia - abnormal protrusion of the jaw, commonly the lower jaw.

Prognosis - the prospect of survival or recovery following a disease or injury.

Progressive - tending to become more severe or wider in scope.

Prokinetic - a drug that in creases the movement of food through the gastrointestinal tract.

Prolapse - the displacement of a body part from its usual position.

Proliferative enteropathy - a disease of the intestinal tract in young pigs characterized by severe diarrhea and anemia; possibly caused by bacteria.

Promoter - an agent that facilitates the development of cancer in cells.

Promotion - the second step in the development of cancer.

Prophylaxis - administering antibiotics as a preventive measure to keep an infection from developing.

Prostate gland - an organ of the male reproductive system that creates part of the fluid portion of semen.

Prostration - total exhaustion or weakness; collapse.

Protein - complex molecules made of amino acids that include many substances (such as enzymes, hormones, and antibodies) necessary for the proper functioning of an organism.

Protocol - a method or regimen of treatment.

Protozoa - plural of protozoan.

Protozoal - of, related to, or caused by protozoa.

Protozoan - any of a large group of single-celled, usually microscopic organisms, that may be parasites.

Protrusion - something that sticks out.

Pruritus - severe itching; usually signalled by scratching.

Pseudomyiasis - false strike (maggot infestation); the presence of fly maggots in the gastrointestinal tract (from ingestion) but without tissue infestation.

Psittacine - of or belonging to the family psittacidae, which includes parrots, macaws, and parakeets.

Psychotropic drug - any of a group of drugs that are used to modify an animal's behavior, including antidepressants, anti-anxiety drugs, and sedatives.

Puberty - the phase during which an animal becomes sexually mature.

Puerperal hypocalcemia - a life-threatening decrease in calcium usually seen in dogs 2 to 3 weeks after giving birth, caused by the loss of calcium from producing milk.

Puerperal tetany - *see* puerperal hypocalcemia.

Pulmonary - of, relating to, or affecting the lungs.

Pulmonary artery - the artery that carries venous blood from the right ventricle of the heart to the lungs.

Pulmonary edema - fluid in the lungs.

Pulmonary hypertension - high blood pressure in the blood vessels of the lungs.

Pulmonary valve - the valve that releases blood out of the right ventricle of the heart into the pulmonary artery.

Pulse - the rhythmic throbbing of arteries produced by the regular contractions of the heart.

Pupa - the nonfeeding, transformative stage between the larva and adult in insects.

Pupil - the black circle in the center of the iris in the eye; the hole through which light enters the eye.

Pus - a thick, yellowish-white fluid seen in wounds and sores and containing white blood cells, microorganisms, and tissue debris.

Pustules - small, inflamed, elevations of the skin filled with pus.

Pyloric stenosis - a muscular constriction between the stomach and intestines.

Pyoderma - any skin disorder that includes formation of pustules or pimples.

Pyometra - a disorder characterized by the accumulation of a large amount of pus in the uterus.

Pythiosis - a disease caused by *pythium insidiosum*, an organism similar to a fungus, which can affect the skin or gastrointestinal tract in dogs or cause skin disorders in horses or cats.

Q fever - a bacterial infection that mainly affects the respiratory or reproductive tracts of ruminants such as cattle and sheep, although other domestic animals, including dogs and cats may be infected. Also known as query fever.

Quadriceps - large muscle at the front of the thigh that acts to extend the knee.

Qualitative - of or related to a categorical observation of an object, for example breed or sex.

Quantitative - of or related to a numerical observation of an object, such as 5 pounds or 3 meters.

Quarantine - to keep an animal separate from other animals to avoid spreading a disease or infection.

Queen - a mature female cat, especially one kept for breeding purposes.

Rabbit calicivirus disease - a highly infectious, contagious, and mostly fatal disease of domestic rabbits that affects the digestive system and causes internal bleeding. Also called viral hemorrhagic disease.

Rabbitpox - an often fatal, generalized, viral disease of rabbits that causes pox marks on the skin as well as discharges from the nose and eyes.

Rabbitry - a place where rabbits are kept or bred.

Radiation - high-intensity energy waves emitted by radioactive elements, for example, x-rays.

Radiation therapy - the use of radiation or radioactive substances to treat disease.

Radiography - an imaging technique that produces an image on film or other sensitive surface by radiation, such as x-rays passing through an object.

Radioisotope irradiation - a type of radiation therapy. *See* radiation therapy.

Radiotherapy - *see* radiation therapy.

Radius - the shorter and thicker bone in the lower forelimb of animals.

Radon - a colorless, radioactive gaseous element used in radiotherapy.

Range (as in range plants) - extensive open land area where livestock wander and graze.

Rash - a temporary outbreak on the skin's surface that is often reddish and itchy.

Receptor - a sensory nerve ending that responds to one of several stimuli, such as touch, temperature, light, taste, or pain.

Recurrence - a repeated occurrence; reappearance or repetition.

Recurrent - happening again and again.

Reflex - an unconscious, automatic movement that occurs in response to sensory stimulation, for example the extension of the knee when the tendon below the knee is tapped.

Regenerative anemia - a form of anemia in which the bone marrow responds to the decreased number of red blood cells by increasing red blood cell production.

Regurgitate - to flow in the opposite direction than normal, as in backward flow of blood within the heart; to bring undigested food up from the esophagus (rather than the stomach) to the mouth.

Reinfestation - a reoccurrence of an infestation, as by fleas.

Reinforcement - reward; any event that increases the chances that a certain behavior will be repeated.

Relapse - the return of an illness, especially after a period of apparent health or improvement.

Remission - a decrease in or a temporary disappearance of the signs of disease.

Renal - of, relating to, or in the region of the kidneys.

Replicate - reproduce.

Reproduction - the process that gives rise to offspring.

Reproductive system - the organs involved in reproduction.

Reptile - any of a class of air-breathing, usually ectothermic (cold-blooded), vertebrate animals, generally covered in scales or plates; examples include lizards, snakes, and turtles.

Resistance - an organism's ability to keep from being affected by an infection; ability of a microorganism to withstand the effects of a previously effective drug or dosage.

Resistant - having the capacity to withstand; relating to or conferring immunity.

Resorption - the process of reclaiming an established organ or structure in order to use its nutrients.

Respiratory - of, relating to, used in, or affecting respiration (breathing).

Respiratory failure - inadequate gas exchange or airflow in the respiratory system.

Respiratory sinus arrhythmia - the small variations in heart rate in healthy, quiet animals that are caused by pressure changes in the chest associated with breathing.

Respiratory system - the organs responsible for breathing, including the lungs, trachea, mouth, nose, and throat.

Respiratory tract - the passages through which air enters and leaves the body.

Reticulocyte - an immature red blood cell.

Retina - the rear inner surface of the eye, responsible for picking up light and transmitting it to the brain as visual signals via the optic nerve.

Retrovirus - any of a family of viruses that store their genetic material as single-stranded rna rather than 2-stranded dna.

Reverse osmosis - purification process by which water is forced through an extremely fine membrane and a carbon filter to remove even more compounds than are removed during normal filtration.

Rhabdomyolysis (sporadic exertional) - severe cramping and stiffness of muscles following heavy exercise, leading to disintegration of muscle fibers; also called tying up.

Rhinitis - inflammation of the nose.

Rhinosporidiosis - a chronic, nonfatal, fungal infection, primarily of the lining of the nasal passages and, occasionally, of the skin.

Rickets - a nutritional disorder of young animals caused by a lack of phosphorus or vitamin d, leading to malformation of bones and lameness.

Rickettsiae - a group of small bacteria that can live only within cells and that cause several diseases, including rocky mountain spotted fever, in animals and people.

Ringtail - a ring-like constriction of the tail, affecting mice, rats, or hamsters, caused by low humidity and high temperatures, and eventually causing gangrene and loss or partial loss of the tail.

Ringworm - a fungal skin infection affecting many animals and humans; dermatophytosis.

Rna - ribonucleic acid; a nucleic acid found in all living cells essential for the manufacture of proteins and carrying genetic information.

Rocky mountain spotted fever - an infection of humans, dogs, and other animals that is caused by *rickettsia rickettsii* bacteria, transmitted by ticks.

Rodenticide - a compound used to poison rodents.

Root canal - the central cavity of a tooth that extends down into the roots of the tooth.

Rotavirus - a genus of viruses that cause intestinal infection in young animals of several species, including birds and pigs.

Roughage - another term for fiber, which aids digestion.

Roundworm - *see* nematode.

Ruminant - any of various hoofed, even-toed, mammals such as cattle, sheep, goats, and deer, characteristically having a 4 compartment stomach and chewing a cud consisting of partially digested food.

Saline - a solution of salt (sodium chloride) and purified water that has the same concentration of salts as the bloodstream.

Saliva - the clear liquid containing digestive enzymes and immune cells that is secreted into the mouth by the salivary glands.

Salmon poisoning disease - an infectious disease in which the infective agent is transmitted through the various life cycle stages of a flatworm known as a fluke. *See* elokomin fluke fever.

Salmonellosis - infection with *salmonella* bacteria, most often characterized by gastrointestinal signs such as diarrhea.

Sanitation - measures and actions to maintain health through good hygiene.

Sarcocystosis - disease in which the muscles and other soft tissues are invaded by intermediate life stages of single-celled organisms of the genus *sarcocystis.*

Sarcoid (equine) - fibrous tumor masses that resemble large warts. They commonly occur on the lower legs of horses.

Sarcoma - a malignant tumor formed in connective tissue, bone, cartilage, or certain types of muscle.

Scabies - infestation by mites of the genus -*sarcoptes*, which affect dogs, cats, horses, pigs, and other species; sarcoptic mange.

Scar tissue - the pale, inflexible connective tissue that forms at the site of an injury.

Scintigraphy - *see* nuclear scintigraphy.

Sclera - the white outer coating that covers the eyeball, except for the central round area covered by the transparent cornea.

Scoliosis - a congenital sideways curvature or deformation of the spine.

Scraping - cellular material obtained for examination by scratching a specific tissue with a clinical instrument.

Screwworm - the larval stage of certain disease-spreading flies.

Scrotum - the external pouch of skin and muscle containing the testes in male mammals.

Scurvy - a nutritional disorder caused by a lack of vitamin c and characterized by bleeding of the skin and mucous membranes, tooth loss, weakness, and spongy gums.

Scute - an external bony or horny plate or scale covering the skin of some reptiles, such as the shell of a turtle.

Sebaceous gland - a skin gland that secretes the oil known as sebum into the hair follicles and onto the skin.

Seborrhea - a disease of the sebaceous glands characterized by excessive secretion of sebum or an alteration in its quality, resulting in an oily coating, crusts, or scales on the skin.

Sebum - oily secretion from the sebaceous gland that helps lubricate the skin.

Secondary hyperparathyroidism - the excessive secretion of parathyroid hormone by the parathyroid glands in response to hypocalcemia (low blood calcium levels).

Secretion - the process of secreting (generating) a substance from cells, or bodily fluids such as saliva, mucus, or tears.

Sedate - to administer sedatives, bringing about a relaxed state.

Sedative - a drug or other agent that induces sedation, a state of calm, restfulness, or drowsiness.

Sedentary - an adjective used to describe an animal or human that exercises little.

Seizure - any of several types of interruption in normal bodily control or thought processes, often characterized by uncontrollable stiffness or jerking of the body, face, or limbs.

Semen - the viscous, whitish fluid containing sperm and seminal fluid that a male ejaculates during breeding.

Semiaquatic - an animal that frequents water but does not completely live in it.

Semilunar valves - valves between the heart and the aorta, and between the heart and the pulmonary artery.

Sensory - of or relating to sensations of pain, position, touch, temperature, taste, hearing, vision, and smell.

Sepsis - illness resulting from the persistent presence of microorganisms or their toxins in the bloodstream. Also called septicemia or blood poisoning.

Septal defect - a hole in the membrane, or muscle wall, dividing the chambers of the heart.

Septic shock - a life-threatening condition caused by an infection in the bloodstream in which blood pressure falls dangerously low and many organs malfunction because of inadequate blood flow. *See* sepsis.

Septicemia - *see* sepsis.

Septicemic cutaneous ulcerative disease (scud) - a bacterial disease in turtles in which the scales are pitted.

Serotype - a group of related microorganisms that are neutralized by the same antibodies.

Service animal - companion animal that is trained to help a person with disabilities, aid law enforcement personnel, help search for lost people, or other tasks.

Sheath - an enveloping tubular structure, such as the tissue that encloses a muscle or nerve fiber.

Shock - a condition of sudden failure of the circulatory system, brought on by excessive blood loss, severe infection, or nervous system dysfunction, among other causes.

Sign - indication or evidence of disease, for example weakness, coughing, or diarrhea.

Silage - animal feed made by storing green plant material, as in a silo.

Sinoatrial node - the heart's natural pacemaker, which generates rhythmic impulses that cause contractions of the muscle fibers of the heart.

Sinus (cardiology) - a dilated channel or receptacle containing chiefly venous blood.

Sinus (respiratory system) - any of several bony cavities in the head connected to the nasal cavity.

Sinus arrest - a pause or cessation of cardiac sinus pacemaker activity.

Sinusitis - inflammation of the lining of the sinuses in the head.

Skeletal disorder - disease affecting the development or structure of the bones.

Skin appendage - a small or secondary attachment to the skin, such as hair follicles, oil and sweat glands, and claws.

Skin tenting - condition that occurs when a small section of skin is pinched away from the body does not snap back to its original position. It can be used to indicate the degree of dehydration of an animal.

Small intestine - the long, narrow part of the digestive tract that lies between the stomach and the colon.

Smear - a medical screening or diagnostic procedure in which a sample of cells (blood, for example) is collected and spread on a microscope slide for examination.

Soft tissue - any of the body tissues other than bone and cartilage.

Solution - a drug dosage form that is dissolved in liquid, usually water.

Solvent - a substance in which other substances are dissolved to create a solution.

Somatostatin - a hormone produced chiefly by the hypothalamus that inhibits the secretion of growth hormone and various other hormones.

Soundness - freedom from injury, disease, or illness; without damage.

Spasm - a sudden, involuntary contraction of a muscle or group of muscles.

Spawning - the process by which some animals, such as certain fish, reproduce.

Spay - to remove the internal reproductive organs (ovaries, uterus) of a female animal in order to prevent reproduction.

Species - a subdivision of a basic biological group, the genus, containing individuals that resemble one another and that may interbreed.

Spina bifida - a congenital defect in which the spinal column is imperfectly closed.

Spinal - of, relating to, or situated near the spine or spinal cord.

Spinal cord - the long bundle of nerve tissue that runs from the brain to the end of the spinal column and connects to the majority of the peripheral nerves.

Spine - the backbone of a vertebrate.

Spirurid - a worm, transmitted by mosquitoes or ticks, that may cause skin sores or infect the stomach lining, body cavity, or blood vessels.

Splay leg - a leg or pelvic socket deformity causing the legs to spread out (splay).

Spleen - a glandlike, lymphoid organ that is part of the immune system and that stores blood cells and produces some types of white blood cells.

Splint - a rigid device used to prevent motion of a joint or of the ends of a fractured bone.

Sporadic - happening or appearing at irregular intervals.

Spore - a reproductive cell, produced by bacteria or fungi, capable of developing into a new individual without fusing with another reproductive cell.

Sporocyst - the first sac-like reproductive stage in many parasitic flatworms that buds off cells.

Sporotrichosis - an infectious disease caused by a yeast-like organism that affects many species, including humans, and that often takes the form of localized, ulcerated skin sores.

Spot-on - a solution of active ingredients for application to the skin which typically contains a cosolvent and a spreading agent to ensure that the product is distributed to the entire body.

Squamous - referring to the portion of the epithelium (skin) composed of flat, plate-like cells.

Squamous cell carcinoma - a form of skin cancer that usually originates in sun-damaged areas.

Stamina - endurance.

Star-gazing - a sign of neurologic disease in which the neck is twisted backward and the animal appears to be looking up into the sky.

Stenosis - a constriction or narrowing of a duct or passage; an obstruction.

Stereotypic behavior - repetitious, relatively unvaried actions that have no obvious purpose or function.

Stethoscope - an instrument used to magnify sounds produced within the body in order to determine health or diagnose disease.

Stifle joint - knee joint; the tendons, ligaments, and other tissues that connect the upper and lower long bones of the rear leg.

Stillbirth - unintentional death of the fetus in the uterus.

Stimulant - a drug or other agent that produces an increase in function of an organ or body part.

Stimulation - to cause physical reaction in something such as a nerve or organ.

Stimulus - an agent or condition that elicits a reaction or response from an organism.

Stomatitis - inflammation of the mouth.

Strain - a group of organisms of the same species, having distinctive characteristics but not usually considered a separate breed or variety.

Strike - maggot infestation, or myiasis.

Stunting - a reduction in overall growth or progress.

Stye - an infection of one or more of the glands at the edge of the eyelid or under it.

Subcutaneous - located just beneath the skin.

Subcutis - the innermost of the 3 layers of the skin.

Subspectacle abscessation - a common bacterial eye infection in snakes.

Substrate - ground covering such as newsprint, sand, peat moss, potting soil, wood shavings, or cypress mulch that are used to cover the bottom of cages for animals such as rodents or reptiles.

Subvalvular - located below one of the heart valves.

Superficial - located at the surface, or only affecting the surface.

Superficial flexor tendon - a tendon that flexes the joints of the lower leg.

Supplement - something added to complete a thing, make up for a deficiency, or extend or strengthen the whole.

Supportive care - a wide range of nonspecific treatments for sick or injured animals designed to relieve the signs of illness and that may include injectable fluids, supplemental feeding, heat, or removal of stress.

Suppression - the reduction or stoppage of a normal bodily function.

Supravalvular - located above one of the heart valves.

Surgery - medical procedure to treat injury or disease involving an operation, such as removal or replacement of a diseased organ or tissue.

Susceptibility - the likelihood of being affected or infected; vulnerability.

Suspension - a dispersion of insoluble or poorly soluble drug particles in a liquid.

Suspensory ligament - a ligament that provides support for the fetlock joint in horses.

Suture - any of the fine threads of specialized material used surgically to close a wound or join tissues; also the act of surgically closing a wound or joining tissues using a stitch or stitches.

Syndrome - a group of signs that occur together and signal a particular abnormal condition.

Synostosis - an abnormality in which 2 adjacent bones, such as vertebrae, fuse together.

Synovial fluid - fluid contained within a joint cavity that helps lubricate the joint.

Synovial membrane - membrane surrounding a joint between bones.

Systemic - a disease or condition that affects or spreads throughout the entire body rather than being confined to a single location. Also called generalized.

Systole - the second half of the heartbeat, characterized by the sound of the aortic and pulmonary valves closing, when the ventricles contract.

T3, t4 - two iodine-containing hormones produced by the thyroid gland that act on many cellular processes to regulate metabolic rate.

Tablet - a solid pellet made up of one or more compressed powdered drugs and perhaps fillers to be taken by mouth.

Tachycardia - a rapid heartbeat.

Tarsal joint - the hock, or ankle joint of the lower rear leg.

Tarsal - of, relating to, or situated near the bones of the ankle.

Tartar - a hard deposit of organic material that forms on teeth.

Temperate - mild or restrained in behavior or attitude. As refers to climate, neither very hot nor very cold.

Tendinitis - inflammation of a tendon.

Tendon - an inelastic band of tough fibrous connective tissue attaching a muscle to a bone or other part.

Tension pneumothorax - a buildup of air in the space between the lungs and the chest wall; can lead to collapse of a lung.

Tentative diagnosis - early, most likely diagnosis based on the history, physical examination, and signs of a disorder.

Teratogen - agents or factors that cause or increase the incidence of a congenital defect.

Terrestrial - living on the ground or underneath its surface.

Testes - the reproductive organs in a male vertebrate, which produce sperm and the hormone testosterone.

Tetanus - an often-fatal disease characterized by spastic contraction of muscles and caused by a toxin produced by *clostridium tetani* bacteria. Also called lockjaw.

Tetany - continuous, spastic contraction of muscles, causing rigidity of limbs.

Tetralogy of fallot - a complex congenital heart defect that produces a bluish tinge to skin and membranes caused by insufficient oxygen in the blood.

Therapy - treatment for an illness.

Thermography - an imaging technique that records the heat emitted by bodies as infrared radiation; used to diagnose musculoskeletal disorders.

Third eyelid - *see* nictitating membrane.

Third phalanx - the outermost bone of a finger or toe.

Thoracentesis - procedure in which a needle is inserted into the chest cavity to withdraw excess fluid.

Thoracic - of, relating to, or situated in or near the chest (thorax).

Thorax - the chest cavity, encased by the ribs and containing the heart, lungs, and other organs.

Thrombocyte - *see* platelet.

Thrombopoietin - a hormone that regulates the production of blood platelets.

Thrombosis - obstruction of an artery by a blood clot.

Thrombus - a blood clot formed in an artery or vein, frequently causing blockage of the blood vessel.

Thymus - a gland in the upper chest or the base of the neck that is the site of maturation of some types of lymphocytes, a class of white blood cell.

Thyroid gland - an endocrine organ in the base of the neck that regulates metabolism.

Thyroid hyperplasia - enlargement of the thyroid gland. Also known as goiter.

Tick - parasitic invertebrates with 8 legs that suck blood and can transmit several diseases.

Tick fever - *see* rocky mountain spotted fever.

Tissue - interconnected cells that perform a similar function within an organism.

Tonometer - a device for measuring pressure, particularly pressure inside the eye.

Tonsillitis - inflammation of the tonsils.

Tonsil - a small mass of lymphoid tissue in the throat.

Topical - involving local application to a part of the body, especially on the skin; for instance, a topical ointment.

Torpor - a state of deep unconsciousness, usually brought on as a result of environmental conditions such as low temperature.

Torticollis - a twisting of the neck to one side, resulting in the head being tilted; can be caused by an ear infection or neurologic disease. Also called wry neck.

Toxemia - a condition brought on by toxins in the blood, especially those produced by bacteria or a metabolic disturbance.

Toxic - containing or being a toxin; poisonous.

Toxicant - a toxic substance.

Toxicity - the degree to which something is poisonous.

Toxicology - the branch of science that studies how poisons affect animals and people and how they respond to poisons.

Toxicosis - disease or condition resulting from poisoning.

Toxin - a poisonous material; most often used to describe poisons produced by plants, animals (such as venomous snakes), and some bacteria.

Toxoid - a substance that has been treated to destroy its toxic properties but retains the capacity to stimulate production of antibodies that can neutralize the original toxin.

Toxoplasmosis - infection by *toxoplasma* microorganisms, which can cause serious damage to the central nervous system, especially in young animals.

Trachea - the thin-walled, cartilaginous tube that connects the throat to the lungs. Also called the windpipe.

Tracheal intubation - insertion of a tube into the trachea to help an animal breathe or to administer anesthesia.

Tracheobronchitis - inflammation of the trachea and large airways (bronchi).

Tracheostomy - an emergency procedure for inserting a tube through the neck into the trachea to allow breathing.

Tranquilizer - any of a class of drugs used to produce a calming or soothing effect.

Transdermal - describes a medication delivery form that is absorbed through the skin into the bloodstream, such as a patch or an ointment.

Transformation - the 2-step process of development of cancerous cells from healthy cells, consisting of initiation and promotion.

Transfusion - the transfer of whole blood or blood products, such as packed red blood cells, from one individual to another.

Transmission - the passing of an infection from one individual to another.

Trauma - damage to living tissue caused by an outside source; a wound.

Trematodes - parasitic flatworms.

Treponematosis - infection by bacteria of the genus *treponema*, which includes syphilis.

Trichinellosis - a parasitic disease caused by a type of roundworm, transmittable to humans and often associated with eating undercooked pork. Also called trichinosis.

Tricuspid valve - the valve between the right chambers of the heart, through which blood flows from the right atrium to the right ventricle.

Trocarization - a technique used to relieve the pressure in the abdomen when it becomes distended with gas due to an intestinal blockage.

Tube feeding - delivery of nutrients, either a special liquid formula or pureed food, through a tube advanced through the nose or mouth into the stomach.

Tuberculosis - disease of many animal species and humans caused by infection with bacteria of the genus *mycobacterium*, which typically affects the respiratory system.

Tularemia - a highly contagious bacterial infection found especially in wild rabbits and rodents that may also affect humans, and which may be transmitted by ticks or direct contact with an infected animal.

Tumor - an abnormal, usually well defined, mass of tissue within an animal; can be either malignant (cancerous) or benign.

Tympanic bullae - the round bones behind the ears.

Tyzzer's disease - a common infection of rabbits and rodents, caused by *clostridium piliforme* bacteria, that typically affects the digestive system. Other species are occasionally affected.

Ubiquitous - existing everywhere.

Udder - another term for the mammary glands of farm animals, including cows, pigs, and horses.

Ulcer - a sore of the skin or of a mucous membrane (for instance, the mouth or stomach lining) characterized by erosion and loss of surface tissue.

Ulcerate - to develop an ulcer.

Ulcerative dermatitis - a skin disorder characterized by formation of ulcers in multiple locations; can be a result of itching and scratching caused by another condition.

Ulna - one of the 2 long bones of the lower part of the front leg.

Ultrasonography - a diagnostic test that uses a machine which emits ultrasonic sound waves, or sounds above the range that humans can hear, to produce a 2-dimensional image of the inside of a body cavity.

Ultraviolet (uv) radiation - light energy radiating from the sun that is not visible to the human eye and that can cause sunburn and increase the risk of skin cancer.

Umbilical - related to or situated in the umbilical cord, the navel, or the area surrounding the navel.

Umbilical cord - the flexible tube connecting the fetus to the placenta, through which nutrients are delivered and waste is expelled.

Unconscious - lacking awareness and the capacity for sensory perception; not conscious.

Unthriftiness - failure of a young animal to grow or gain weight at a normal rate in spite of an adequate diet and absence of obvious illness.

Upper airways - the portion of the respiratory tract that extends from the nostrils or mouth through the throat (pharynx).

Urate - a salt formed from uric acid. *See* uric acid.

Uremia - a buildup of toxic chemicals in the blood that occurs when the kidneys are not functioning properly.

Ureter - the narrow tube that connects the kidney to the bladder.

Urethra - the tube from the urinary bladder through which urine exits the body.

Uric acid - a weak acid present in the urine, which can lead to gout or other disorders in birds if it builds up to high levels.

Urinalysis - laboratory analysis of urine, used to aid in the diagnosis of disease.

Urinate - to expel liquid waste from the body by contracting the urinary bladder.

Urine scalding - skin inflammation caused by prolonged contact with urine.

Urogenital tract - relating to or involving the organs of the urinary tract and the reproductive system.

Urolith - a buildup of mineral salts in any part of the urinary tract; also called a urinary calculus or stone.

Urolithiasis - a condition brought on by the formation of stones (calculi) in the urinary system of an animal.

Urticaria - *see* hives.

Uterus - the organ of the female reproductive system in which the fetus develops.

Uvea - the middle layer of the eye, which includes the iris and the muscles that control it.

Uveitis - inflammation of the uvea.

Vaccination - the administration of a substance to produce immunity against a specific disease; immunization.

Vaccine - a product, including dead or weakened forms of an infectious agent or molecules that are part of the agent, that prompts the immune system to develop defenses against that specific organism.

Vagina - the lubricated muscular tube of female mammals that connects the cervix to the vulva, forming the external opening of the genitals.

Valve - a membranous structure that closes to prevent the backward flow of material through a canal or passage.

Valvular disease - disease resulting in failure of the heart valves to open or close properly.

Vascular - of, characterized by, or containing vessels that carry fluids, such as blood or lymph, through the body of an animal.

Vascular network - the collection of vessels that carry or circulate bodily fluids.

Vasculitis - inflammation of the blood vessels.

Vasodilator - any of a class of drugs intended to lower blood pressure by widening blood vessels, thus increasing blood flow.

Vector - an organism, such as a tick or mosquito, that carries an infectious agent between susceptible animals. A vector may also be mechanical (nonliving), such as clothing or equipment.

Vein - any of the system of blood vessels that carry blood toward the heart.

Venae cavae - the 2 largest veins, which return blood from the body to the right atrium.

Venereal disease - a contagious disease typically spread through sexual activity.

Venom - a poisonous fluid injected by the bite or sting of an animal.

Venous dilator - a drug that dilates the veins coming to the heart and increases the amount of blood that enters the heart.

Ventricle - either of the 2 lower chambers of the heart.

Ventricular fibrillation - a common arrhythmia of the heart characterized by chaotic, ineffective contraction of the heart muscle.

Vertebra - any of the bones forming the spinal column.

Vertebrate - an animal with a backbone, such as fish, reptiles, mammals, and birds.

Vesicle - a small, raised area of skin, containing fluid; blister.

Vesicular stomatitis - an acute viral disease of horses and pigs, transmitted by mosquitoes and other insects and signaled by excessive drooling, loss of appetite due to mouth blisters, and lameness due to foot ulcers.

Vestibular system - the organs in the inner ear that control balance.

Veterinarian - an individual trained and licensed to treat the medical conditions of animals; a doctor of veterinary medicine.

Veterinary dermatologist - a veterinarian specializing in the treatment of skin disorders.

Veterinary family practice - also known as "bond-centered practice," in which the veterinarian establishes a lifelong relationship with families and their animals and cares not only for the medical welfare of the animal, but also for the social health of its family.

Vipers - a group of highly poisonous snakes whose long fangs fold back when not in use.

Viral - of, relating to, or caused by a virus.

Virus - a tiny infectious agent consisting of a genetic material (rna or dna) in a protein coat, which relies on host cells to reproduce.

Visceral - relating to or affecting one or more of the soft internal organs of the body, especially those within the abdominal cavity.

Visceral gout - an inflammatory buildup of uric acid metabolites in the internal organs of reptiles or birds, leading to pain and discomfort.

Visceral leishmaniasis - a chronic, severe disease of humans, dogs, and certain rodents caused by protozoa, characterized by skin lesions, lymph node enlargement, weight loss, anemia, lameness, and kidney failure.

Vitamin - any of a group of compounds that are essential for proper body function and growth.

Vitamin d - a fat-soluble vitamin required for normal metabolism of calcium and phosphorus.

Volume overload - a form of heart failure that results in an increase in the size of the one or both ventricles, the lower chambers of the heart.

Vulva - the external female reproductive organs.

Warm-blooded - an animal that maintains a relatively constant and warm body temperature independent of environmental temperature. Also called homeothermic.

Wart - a hard, rough lump growing on the skin.

Water mold - an aquatic fungus living chiefly in fresh water or moist soil.

Water salinity - a measure of the amount of salt in water.

Weaning - the process of getting an infant mammal adjusted to eating food rather than drinking its mother's milk.

Wheal - a localized area of fluid buildup in the skin that may be pale or reddened and may itch; a hive.

White blood cell - any of a group of infection-fighting blood cells. *See* leukocyte.

Withers - the ridge between the shoulder blades of a horse.

Womb - another word for uterus. *See* uterus.

Worms - soft-bodied organisms, many of which are parasitic and infect animals and/or humans.

X-ray - a high-energy form of electromagnetic radiation that can be used to produce images that allow a veterinarian to see inside the body; also used to describe the pictures produced by the rays, which are also called radiographs.

Yeast - a small, single-celled fungus that ferments carbohydrates; some types can infect humans and animals.

Yellow fat disease - a condition in cats involving inflammation of the fatty tissue, thought to be due to an excess of unsaturated fatty acids in food combined with a deficiency of vitamin e.

Zinc toxicity - a typically chronic form of poisoning caused by consumption of items containing the metal zinc and characterized by lameness and stiffness.

Zoonosis - a disease that can be passed from animals to people.

Zoonotic risk - the likelihood that a disease will be passed from an animal to people.

Zygomycosis - a fungal infection of the lining of the mouth, nasal passages, and tissue beneath the skin, or the sides of the head, neck, and body.

BIBLIOGRAPHY

A.Q.H.A. 2003. Official handbook of rules and regulations. 51st edition. American Quarter Horse Association. Amarillo, Texas. 253 pgs.

Bentz AI: The Geriatric Horse, in McCurnin DM, Bassert JM, (ed): *Clinical Textbook for Veterinary Technicians,* ed 7, Philadelphia, PA, Elsevier, 2009.

Boersema, JH, Eysker, M, Nas JW. Apparent resistance of Parascaris equorum to macrocylclic lactones. *Vet Rec* 81-150:279 .2002

Cooper, S.R. et al. 1995. "Effects of dietary cationanion balance on blood ph, acid-base parameters, serum and urine mineral levels and parathyroid hormone." In Proceedings: 14th Equine Nutrition and Physiology Symposium. Ontario, California. p. 42.

Corning, Susan, Equine Cyathostomins: a review of biology, clinical significance and therapy. *Parasites and Vectors.* 2009 2(Suppl2):SI

Couto et al., Environmental Influence in cyathostominae ecology. 2008. *Veterinari Medicina* 53(5): 243-249

Equine Uveitis, in Aiello SE, (ed): *The Merck Veterinary Manual,* ed 8, Whitehouse Station, NJ, Merck & Co., Inc., 1998, pp 360-362.

Gibbs, P.G. et al. 1998. Report on the Texas horse industry. Texas Cooperative Extension. Equine Science Section. Department of Animal Science. Texas A&M University. 28 pgs.

Jones, L.L. et al. 1993. Population estimates for the Texas horse industry. Departmental Information Report No. 94-2. Texas A&M University. 25 pages.

Linford, RL: Laminitis (Founder), in Smith, BP (ed): *Large Animal Internal Medicine,* ed 4, St. Louis, MO, Mosby Elsevier, 2009, pp1224-1227.

McFarlane D: Pituitary and Hypothalamus, in Smith, BP (ed): *Large Animal Internal Medicine*, ed 4, St. Louis, MO, Mosby Elsevier, 2009, pp 1340-1344.

N.R.C. 1989. Nutrient requirements of horses. 5th revised edition. National Research Council. Washington, D.C.

Part I: Baseline Reference of 1998 Equine Health & Management. Washington, DC: USDA:aphis, 1998; 7, 9, 12, 21, 44-46. 2. Ralston SL. *Management of Geriatric Horses.* Available at www.ker.com, October 2008.

Proudman, C, Edwards G. Are tapeworms associated with equine colic? A case control study. *Equine Vet J* 6-224:(3)25;1993

Ralston, S.L. 1993. Management of old horses. Rutgers Cooperative Extension. New Jersey Agricultural Experiment Station. #FS715. 4 pgs.

Reinemeyer and Nielsen. Parasitism and Colic. Vet Clin. *Equine* 245-233 :(2009)25

Scrutchfield, W.L., J. Schumacher and M.T. Martin. 1996. "Correction of abnormalities of the cheek teeth." Proceedings: American Association of Equine Practitioners 42:11.

Slater JD: Medical Nursing, in Coumbe, K (ed): *Equine Veterinary Nursing Manual Oxford*, UK, Blackwell Science Ltd, 2001, pp 249-283.

INDEX

www.ingramcontent.com/pod-product-compliance
Lightning Source LLC
LaVergne TN
LVHW062117200926
848484LV00007B/1693